'The topic of behavioural addictions in women has been significantly under researched at a global level for far too long. This book greatly addresses the research gap in this field and makes essential reading for all in the clinical realm and in research.'

Henrietta Bowden-Jones, *OBE, Professor, National Clinical Advisor on Gambling Harms, Vice President of the Royal Society of Medicine*

'This is a much-needed book for anyone working in the behavioural addictions field written and collated by some of the leading female researchers and practitioners. If you want an insightful and engaging female perspective on behavioural addictions, then this is the book read.'

Mark Griffiths, *PhD, Distinguished Professor of Behavioural Addiction and Director, International Gaming Research Unit, Psychology Department, Nottingham Trent University*

'This book focuses on global female perspectives on a range of behavioural addictions. There is an important need to understand better girls and women and how they may experience and be impacted by behavioural addictions involving gambling, gaming, internet use, love, sex, pornography viewing, eating and other behaviors. This impressive book includes over 30 chapters detailing aspects of often difficult-to-identify clinical concerns and how they may be impacting the health of women and girls, all communicated from womens' perspectives. This book sheds new light on many important topics, and provides a lens through which to view these from international vantage points. As such, this is an essential book that contributes to promoting female health and well-being.'

Marc N. Potenza, *MD, PhD, Director of Division on Addictions Research at Yale, Director of Yale Center of Excellence in Gambling Research and Director of Women and Addictions Core of Women's Health Research at Yale*

'Taking into consideration the most important yet most understudied areas of behavioural addictions research, one would certainly point to gender issues first. The current book is a huge step to address this gap. The book edited by Fulvia Prever, Gretchen Blycker, and Laura Brandt provides an excellent collection of papers studying women-specific aspects of behavioural addictions, covering a wide range of perspectives, and with a special focus on aetiology, needs, and treatment issues. Moreover, the global perspective of the book, with contributions from all over the world, makes it especially unique and important.'

Zsolt Demetrovics, *Chair of the Centre of Excellence in Responsible Gaming, University of Gibraltar; Head of the Addiction Research Group at ELTE Eötvös Loránd University and President of the International Society for the Study of Behavioural Addictions*

Behavioural Addiction in Women

Behavioural Addiction in Women gives insight into ongoing research efforts and clinical developments across the globe, focusing specifically on women with behavioural addictions.

The book brings together an international network of clinicians and researchers to offer a unique transcultural female perspective on female-specific aspects of addiction, which is underrepresented in the available literature. By compiling both research and clinical spotlights focusing on women with behavioural addictions across the six continents, the book is an important first step toward building a shared knowledge base on the subject, starting from the importance of female-specific diagnostic criteria, to new therapeutic strategies, prevention programs, and harm reduction approaches. This book will help us gain a better understanding of ongoing work and where to allocate our attention and efforts for helping a vulnerable, and – in many areas of the world – still underserved, and economically disadvantaged, population.

The book will be of great interest to researchers and clinicians in the field of addiction.

Fulvia Prever is a psychotherapist with a particular focus on women, gambling, and behavioural addictions. She has been an executive psychologist for 38 years in the Addiction Clinic of the Italian NHS in Milan, and she is the Scientific Director of the Women & Gambling Project, SUN(N)COOP, international referee for Women, Gambling & Behavioural Addiction for EASG and ISSBA, and president of the Varenna Foundation.

Gretchen Blycker, LMHC, LMT, RYT, PhD candidate, is a board-certified sex therapist in private practice and an adjunct faculty member at the University of Rhode Island. For the last 25 years she has been integrating a holistic framework for promoting sexual wellbeing, healthy relationships, healing from sexual trauma and treating compulsive sexual behaviours as well as addressing their relational impact.

Laura Brandt, PhD, is currently an Assistant Professor in Psychology at The City College of New York. To address the complexity of substance use disorders in her research, she draws from psychological, applied medical and data science, and takes an implementation perspective on interventions that target addictive behaviours.

Behavioural Addiction in Women

An International Female Perspective on
Treatment and Research

**Edited by Fulvia Prever,
Gretchen Blycker, and Laura Brandt**

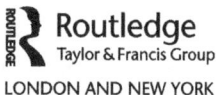
Routledge
Taylor & Francis Group

LONDON AND NEW YORK

Designed cover image: © Giuseppe Pagani, a free interpretation of Amedeo Modigliani's "naked lying woman"

First published 2023
by Routledge
4 Park Square, Milton Park, Abingdon, Oxon OX14 4RN

and by Routledge
605 Third Avenue, New York, NY 10158

Routledge is an imprint of the Taylor & Francis Group, an informa business

British Library Cataloguing-in-Publication Data
A catalogue record for this book is available from the British Library

Library of Congress Cataloging-in-Publication Data
Names: Prever, Fulvia, editor. | Blycker, Gretchen, 1974- editor. | Brandt, Laura, 1985- editor.
Title: Behavioural addiction in women : an international female perspective on treatment and research / edited by Fulvia Prever, Gretchen Blycker and Laura Brandt.
Description: Abingdon, Oxon ; New York, NY : Routledge, 2023. | Includes bibliographical references. |
Identifiers: LCCN 2022060602 (print) | LCCN 2022060603 (ebook) | ISBN 9781032067032 (hardback) | ISBN 9781032067025 (paperback) | ISBN 9781003203476 (ebook)
Subjects: LCSH: Compulsive behavior--Diagnosis. | Compulsive behavior--Treatment. | Women--Mental health. | Women--Counseling of.
Classification: LCC RC533 .B4466 2023 (print) | LCC RC533 (ebook) | DDC 616.85/840082--dc23/eng/20230414
LC record available at https://lccn.loc.gov/2022060602
LC ebook record available at https://lccn.loc.gov/2022060603

ISBN: 978-1-032-06703-2 (hbk)
ISBN: 978-1-032-06702-5 (pbk)
ISBN: 978-1-003-20347-6 (ebk)

DOI: 10.4324/9781003203476

Typeset in Times New Roman
by MPS Limited, Dehradun

This book is dedicated to Nancy Petry and Kimberly Young, two great ladies who shed light on our path of understanding behavioural addiction and who left us too soon with an important heritage to help women achieve a better quality of life.

Contents

Preface

Behavioural Addiction in Women: An International Female Perspective on Treatment and Research brings together an international network of clinicians and researchers with expertise in behavioural addiction and related issues, with chapters reflecting ongoing work with women across the world in both group and individual settings. Our primary aim is to raise awareness about and interest in ongoing research efforts and clinical developments across the globe, focusing specifically on female-specific aspects of behavioural addictions from a unique female perspective. This book resembles an important first step toward building a shared knowledge base on behavioural addictions in women from diverse cultural backgrounds, their specific needs, and effective and promising intervention approaches.

Acknowledgment

The editors have opted to donate their royalties to the SUN(N)COOP Women's Group for Gambling Problems in Milan, Italy, to support free social and clinical activities as well as research.

Contributors

Abdul Aziz, Dr. Melisa Abdul Aziz is a psychiatrist in a government hospital in Malaysia. She is a co-founding member of MYSIA. Dr. Abdul Aziz has been featured in several local TV programs in an attempt to promote cyber-wellness in Malaysia.

Achab, Sophia Achab is a psychiatrist-psychotherapist with expertise in research and care response to behavioural addictions since 2006 and 12 years of leadership of the pioneering facility ReConnecte with a fit-for-purpose care for patients and relatives suffering from behavioural addictions. She is a public health advisor since 2013 in Switzerland and for the WHO regarding Internet use and misuse.

Andronicos, Mélina Andronicos, PhD is a psychologist. She has been working as a research project manager in the Service of Addiction Medicine at the Lausanne University Hospital in Switzerland. Her interests are focused on improving the accessibility of mental health care and suicide prevention.

Bahar, Dr. Norharlina Bahar is a consultant child and adolescent psychiatrist and founder of MYSIA and an international board member of the International Society of Internet Addiction (ISIA). She has served as a working group member in a series of annual WHO expert meetings on implications of addictive behaviour and gaming disorder.

Baharudin, Dr. Azlin Baharudin is an associate professor of psychiatry and a consultant psychiatrist at National University of Malaysia. She is now the head of the Department of Psychiatry and Mental Health from the same university.

Bhang, Soo-young Bhang, MD, MPH, PhD, is a child and adolescent and addiction psychiatrist, majored in Public Health in her Master's degree, and received a doctorate in comparing brain imaging findings from the East and the West. She is the director of the Nowon-gu Addiction Management Center in Seoul, Korea, the director of the Eulji Student Mental Health Research Center, and Associate Professor in the

Department of Psychiatry, Nowon Eulji University Hospital, Seoul. As a clinician and researcher, she is very interested in trauma and internet addiction among children and adolescents, especially in creating policies or systems, and is also paying attention to women being underestimated in the diagnosis of ADHD, which is closely related to the development of addiction.

Blanca, Debora Blanca is a psychologist and psychoanalyst specialized in pathological gambling. She is the director of Lazos en Juego as well as a lecturer in Argentina, Spain, Italy, and Poland. She published four books in Argentina.

Blycker, Gretchen Blycker, LMHC, LMT, RYT, is a board-certified sex therapist in private practice and for 12 years has been teaching a Human Sexuality course at the University of Rhode Island. Her clinical work focusing on promoting sexual wellbeing, treating sexual trauma and compulsive sexual behaviours and addressing their relational impact informs her academic work and perspectives.

Borsani, Maddalena Borsani is a psychotherapist working with a systemic approach in the NHS Addiction Clinic in Milan, researcher and trainer for Sun(n)Coop GD projects in Milan. She is a member of ALEA (Association for Gambling Studies and Risky Behaviour) and GAT-P Ticino (Association for Gambling in Switzerland).

Boyer, Ms. Charlotte Boyer is a Senior Research Officer at the Centre for Social Research and Methods at the Australian National University. Having designed, implemented, and evaluated social policies and programs while working for government, NGOs, and as a consultant, she now researches a broad range of social policies and issues.

Brandt, Laura Brandt, PhD, is currently an Assistant Professor in Psychology at The City College of New York. Her professional training unfolded through theoretical and clinical psychology training at the University of Vienna, a doctoral degree in Applied Medical Science at the Medical University of Vienna and postdoctoral training in transfer and implementation science. Simultaneously, her research has evolved from observational/descriptive accounts of the psychiatric burden as well as gender-specific aspects of addiction to exploring new and improved intervention approaches and simultaneously developing implementation strategies.

Breen, Helen Breen, PhD, is an adjunct and member of the Emeritus Faculty at Southern Cross University, Australia. Her gambling expertise includes public health focused research on harm minimization, consumer protection, and promotion of social responsibility; and impacts of gambling on specific groups, including Indigenous peoples, women, victims of family violence, seniors, and tourists.

Broman, Niroshani Broman – PhD student, Faculty of Medicine, Department of Clinical Sciences Lund, Lund University, Sweden; Region Skåne, Gambling Disorder Unit, S-20502 Malmö, Sweden – is a registered nurse, specialized in psychiatry. Her research concerns excessive use of alcohol, narcotics, excessive gambling and gaming in sexual and gender minority populations.

Caillon, Julie Caillon, PhD, is a psychologist at the Mental Health Department at Nantes University Hospital and a full member of the Inserm UMR1246 SPHERE team. Her activity is mainly focused on care management of people with behavioural addiction (in particular through cognitive behavioural approaches) and on training in behavioural addictions for health and social professionals. She is also involved in clinical research, which focuses on the assessment of addicted individuals and addictive risk, therapeutic innovation for addicted patients, and prevention of risks associated with addictions.

Camacho-Barcia, Lucía Camacho-Barcia, PhD, is a registered dietitian, specialized in obesity and metabolic disorders, with a PhD in nutrition and metabolism. Currently, she is a postdoctoral researcher at the Psychoneurobiology of Eating and Addictive Disorders Group at the Biomedicine Research Institute of Bellvitge, Barcelona and a researcher at the Physiopathology of Obesity and Nutrition (CIBEROBN), Institute of Health Carlos III.

Challet-Bouju, Gaëlle Challet-Bouju (PhD/HDR) is a hospital research engineer at the Mental Health Department at the Nantes University Hospital and is a full member of the Inserm UMR1246 SPHERE team. Her research focuses on the assessment of addicted individuals and addictive risk, therapeutic innovation for addicted patients, and prevention of risks associated with addictions. More specifically, she has developed her research activity centered on behavioural addictions, especially on gambling, and is currently working on the cognitive processes involved in behavioural addictions, the prevention of online gambling disorders and the typologies of people with behavioural addiction.

Chen, Lijun Chen is a professor in the Department of Psychology, School of Humanities and Social Sciences, Fuzhou University, Fujian, China. Her research interests include problematic pornography use, hypochondria in the epidemic era, and the impact of facial dimorphism on interpersonal interaction.

Claesdotter-Knutsson, Emma Claesdotter-Knutsson – MD, PhD, Child and Adolescent Psychiatry Skånes Universitetssjukhus, Lund and the Department of Clinical Sciences, Faculty of Medicine, Lund University, Sweden – is a specialist in Child and Adolescent Psychiatry. Her research interest lies in gaming, gambling, neurodevelopmental disorders, and forensic psychiatry in a young population.

Cox, Koriann Cox, PhD, is a licensed psychologist with the University of Washington Medical Center in Seattle, Washington in the United States. She provides clinical care in inpatient and outpatient settings with a focus on addiction, trauma, and reproductive mental health. She graduated from Northeastern University in 2020 and has completed specialty training in co-occurring addiction and mental health; she previously worked within several VA hospitals and spent time training in and providing clinical care related to behavioural addictions in military veterans.

Damari, Tal Damari, MSW, works as a social worker for children at risk and their families. She completed her MA in social work at Tel Aviv University in 2020. Her dissertation deals with women's recovery experience from gambling disorder in Israel.

De Luca, Ornella De Luca is a psychologist-psychotherapist. For about 20 years she has been dealing with addiction and gambling, collaborating with the Rome Addiction Clinic as a referral for the Gambling Disorder project (Italian National Health Service). She is a member of the Regional Observatory (Lazio) on the phenomenon of gambling, and a member of the Scientific Committee of the Italian Addiction Society and of ALEA (Scientific Gambling Society).

de Vries, Linda de Vries is a senior researcher with governmental agencies and universities in South Africa as an advisor and facilitator. She served as chairperson of gambling regulatory agencies at both provincial and national levels and was part of the oversight team on research, advocacy, and regulation of gambling. In her academic role as business professor terrain she researched, supervised, and published on woman and gender in the workplace as well as on consumer behaviour and specifically on diversity in the South African context.

Della Pietà, Camilla Della Pietà is a psychologist and cognitive behavioural psychotherapist. She has been collaborating with the National Health System, Service for Addiction since 2020. She is also participating in research and development projects about gambling and published in the field of gambling.

Estévez Gutiérrez, Ana Estévez Gutiérrez is Professor of the Department of Personality, Evaluation, and Psychological Treatment of the University of Deusto, director of the Master in General Health Psychology, and senior researcher in the Clinical and Health Evaluation team responsible for non-substance addictions and associated cognitive-emotional and relational processes.

Fadeeva, Eugenia Fadeeva is a clinical psychologist and head of Department of Preventive Care in Addictions, National Research Centre on Addictions, V. Serbsky National Medical Research Centre for Psychiatry and Narcology, Ministry of Health of the Russian Federation, and Associate Professor of the Moscow State University of Psychology and Education. In my practical and scientific work, I paid attention to a number of significant vulnerable groups – children, adolescents, girls, and women who need special approaches for prevention, treatment, and rehabilitation. I conducted practical classes with students in neuropsychological and pathopsychological diagnostics, with an emphasis to biological, social, individual, and gender aspects that influence addictive behaviour. I also carried out work to evaluate activities of Russia's Regions in development and implementation of standards for addictive behaviour prevention.

Fiorin, Amelia Fiorin is a psychologist and representative of the local department for gambling of the National Health System Addictions Clinic, AULSS2 Treviso Italy. Furthermore, she is the coordinator of the scientific table for gambling in Veneto and President of the ALEA-Association for the study of gambling and risky behaviours.

Gavriel-Fried, Belle Gavriel-Fried, PhD, is a senior lecturer at the School of Social Work, Tel Aviv University. Her research interests in the past five years have centered on recovery from addictive behaviours. She implements qualitative and quantitative research methods.

Goedecke, Klara Goedecke earned her PhD in gender studies in 2018 and is a researcher at Stockholm University, Sweden. Her research focuses on men and masculinities from intersectional perspectives, including homosociality, men's friendships, postfeminism, and emotions in popular culture. In her current project she uses ethnographic methods and studies of gambling advertising to study gender constructions, affect, and class politics in Swedish gambling.

Grall-Bronnec, Marie Grall-Bronnec, PhD/HDR, is a psychiatrist-addictologist in the Mental Health Department at the Nantes University Hospital, Professor of Addictology at the Nantes Faculty of Medicine, and has been a full member of the Inserm UMR1246 team (https://sphere-inserm.fr/). Her research focuses on the assessment of addicted individuals and addictive risk, therapeutic innovation for addicted patients, and prevention of risks associated with addictions. She is also interested in mental health recovery. She joined a WHO working group on gaming disorder and conducted field testing in France regarding the category "Disorders due to substance use and addictive behaviours" for the next version of the International Classification of Diseases.

Grioni, Antonella Grioni is a clinical psychologist at the Mara Selvini School in Brescia who specializes in the systemic relational approach. She is an

Saillard, Rousselet, Thiabaud, and Leboucher, Anaïs Saillard, Morgane Rousselet, Elsa Thiabaud and Juliette Leboucher (MSc) are research assistants at the Mental Health Department at the Nantes University Hospital. Their research focuses are to understand what determines the course of behavioural addictions and compliance with care by managing recruitment of volunteers into clinical studies.

Séguin, Monique Séguin, PhD, is a psychology professor at the Université du Québec en Outaouais and a member of the McGill Group for Suicide Studies. She has conducted a number of studies on suicide trajectories.

Sim, Dr. Su Tein Sim is a psychiatrist in private practice in Malaysia. She is a co-founding member of the Malaysian Society of Internet Addiction Prevention (MYSIA). She has been actively involved in Internet addiction research since 2015.

Spångberg, Jessika Spångberg (formerly Svensson), is a public health scientist and gender researcher who conducts research on youth and gambling at Stockholm University. She also works with prevention of problem gambling at the Public Health Agency of Sweden. This chapter was partly supported by the research program REGAPS (Responding to and Reducing Gambling Problems).

Suryani, Eva Suryani is a psychiatrist and lecturer at Atma Jaya University and Hospital. In the past ten years, she has been focusing on research both in substance and behavioural addiction. She is also a member of International Technology Transfer Center (ITTC) which focuses on drug demand reduction.

Suwartono, Christiany Suwartono specializes in the field of psychology and psychometrics. Her research focuses on human interactions and how to improve human health and well-being in Indonesia. To express and sharpen her skills, she actively collaborates with other academics and professionals.

Tan, Dr. Kit-Aun Tan is a senior lecturer in developmental psychology at Universiti Putra Malaysia. Dr. Tan's research focuses on scale development and validation of psychological measures for use in internet addiction research.

Valdez, Victoria Valdez is a psychiatrist with postgraduate training at the Clinic Hospital, Barcelona University. She is a professor at the Medical School, Catholic University of Guayaquil, Ecuador, and medical staff at Kennedy General Hospital. She is the past vice treasurer of the World Federation of Societies of Biological Psychiatry (WFSBP) and secretary of the International Association for Women's Mental Health (IAWMH).

Wardle, Heather Wardle is Lord Kelvin Adam Smith Reader in Social Sciences at the University of Glasgow. She is a specialist in gambling policy, research and practice. She recently published her first book "Games without Frontiers? Socio-historical perspectives at the gaming/gambling intersection" and her PhD thesis explored female gambling behaviour. She is currently funded by Wellcome Trust, National Institute for Health Research, and the Economic and Social Research Council.

Whitty, Dr. Megan Whitty is a Research Fellow at the Australian National University's Centre for Gambling Research, Australia. Her research interests include application of program evaluation and implementation science in public health settings, particularly in relation to health promotion, addiction research, and the impacts of gambling on specific groups, such as Indigenous populations, women and affected others.

Widjaja, Eveline Widjaja, MD, is a graduate of Atma Jaya Catholic University School of Medicine. She has been a research assistant in the addiction field since 2019 and has participated in different research projects including WHO Project, the ICD-11 Field Testing in Indonesia about Disorder due to Substance Use and Addictive Behaviour.

Introduction

Why Do We Need a Female-Specific Perspective on Behavioural Addiction in Women?

Fulvia Prever, Gretchen Blycker, and Laura Brandt

For many decades, clinical researchers have prioritized men in their study samples, for various reasons, and failed to include sex differences in study design and analysis. As we slowly catch up on our knowledge about women's mental health, it becomes more and more obvious that a gendered approach to research, prevention, and treatment is highly relevant to understand and be more responsive to female-specific needs related to behavioural addiction. While publications that focus on female-specific aspects of substance-related disorders have seen an uptake in recent years, this is less so for behavioural addictions. Existing data are often not specific to women but inferred from mostly male samples. Nevertheless, more and more women are affected by gambling disorder and other non-substance related addictions.

Women have a crucial role in family and society, as the pivotal point in the family system, in child and elderly care, in many professional fields, and in interpersonal and social relationships. Therefore, their addictive behaviours, often underestimated, may have a deep impact not only on their own social and personal life but on their entire network. One key issue is that women often experience great difficulty in finding appropriate treatment services. Many health clinics are not "women friendly" and treatment programs rarely offer female-specific treatment approaches. Further, it is unclear whether diagnostic behavioural addiction diagnostic criteria are equally useful and valid in women as in men.

As female professionals working with women who are affected by behavioural addiction, it is our hope and aim to gather information about all efforts dedicated toward improving their situation. Starting from the experience of a therapy group in Milan, founded by Fulvia Prever and dedicated to women with gambling problems, we seek to investigate specific themes, informed by clinical insights, such as strategies to engage women in treatment, creating women-friendly settings, developing female-specific tools, and evaluating the applicability of diagnostic criteria for women. This vision brought together a network of female professionals with diverse cultural and professional backgrounds and high expertise in behavioural addiction among

DOI: 10.4324/9781003203476-1

women with the aim to learn from each other's experiences as researchers and clinicians, to gather data from all over the world to enrich our shared understanding of these issues, and to compare, discuss, and improve ongoing research and clinical work worldwide. This network gave birth to the book "Gambling Disorders in Women: An International Female Perspective on Treatment and Research," edited by Henrietta Bowden-Jones and Fulvia Prever, which attracted broad interest internationally by researchers and the clinical community.

With a broader focus on behavioural addiction and related themes, the current book is intended as a stylistic and thematic continuation of the first book's focus on gambling disorder. Our primary aim is to raise awareness about and interest in ongoing research efforts and clinical developments across the globe, focusing specifically on women with behavioural addictions. We offer a unique female perspective on female-specific aspects of addiction, which is generally neglected in conventional publishing media. In addition, by including contributions authored by women from all six continents, we offer insights into ongoing work from areas that are heavily underrepresented in the available literature. This is particularly true for countries that are either economically disadvantaged and thus are often unable to conform to strict (and costly) research standards, and/or those which political backdrop complicates including women in research, let alone putting them in the focus.

A female-specific perspective on research and treatment is crucial for all behavioural addictions, in all countries and cultural contexts. Our international women network is collectively working to bring this to the forefront of scientific and clinical debate – asking questions related to sex and gender differences and bringing together scientific knowledge and clinical experience from all six continents. Our ideal of pursuing research informed by clinical experience with women affected by behavioural addiction is represented in the diverse professional profiles of the authors of this book. This female transcultural perspective may provide a new point of view on research and treatment, starting from the importance of female-specific diagnostic criteria, over new therapeutic strategies, to prevention programs and harm reduction approaches. It is our hope that this book serves as a tool to inspire future research and better respond to women's health needs.

The development of this book coincided with the various stages of the COVID-19 pandemic which deeply affected our lives and existence and our physical and mental health in many ways. Addictive behaviours played an important role in the life of many women during periods of "lockdown" and social isolation. Worldwide, women paid a high price, both in their personal and professional life, and – in case we needed further proof – these trying times have shown that attention to and investment in women's health is of utmost importance. This book is a not least a reflection of the "suspended time" during the past three years and many chapters discuss the challenges many women faced from a female transcultural perspective.

We want to thank all of our international colleagues for their inspiring contributions and mutual support during these tough three years of pandemic emergency which reminded us of the importance of a women transcultural network – not only in our professional but also in our personal life. Bringing together this amazing group of women from all over the world to create a new and unique manual on behavioural addiction in women was so much more than just a book editing exercise – it was a journey during a world-wide state of emergency containing our grief and hopes, our solidarity, and our efforts in working together toward a common goal. We want to particularly thank the women who are our patients, clients and study participants for letting us get close to the complexity of their life and learn so much from them.

September 22nd 2022,
Milan, Italy/New York City and Jamestown, USA

Part I

Africa

Chapter 1

South African Women Risk-Takers

An Exploration of Risky Behaviour during Periods of Constraint

Linda de Vries

This chapter discusses risky behaviour of South African women with respect to gambling, and other possibly unhealthy risky behaviours. This chapter also describes risk and other related factors associated with these behaviours among South African women, as well as additional challenges within the current global pandemic, and how awareness programs have influenced their behaviours. The number of women who gamble has increased since the legalization of gambling in South Africa in 1996. The license conditions for infrastructure were specific around creating an environment of status and spaces of entertainment, safety as well as multi-purpose functioning that would add value to various locations across the country. The world changed substantially after these grandiose sites and great complexes where perceived and implemented, and general perceptions of gambling changed. A number of environmental factors will be discussed which may be unique to the increasing participation of women in gambling activities. These are related to factors such as more accepting attitudes toward gambling, the influence of lock down on casinos and the growth of online gambling, a new range of risky behaviours as well as the social compacts related to communities under immense new challenges.

Introduction

Women in South Africa are not a homogeneous group of people. South African women reflect the diversified groupings that were separated and shaped by racial inequalities, educational challenges, and job and career opportunities designated for certain groups. This is especially true for first generation graduands that South Africa produced 20 years post-democracy. Many of these graduands are today in a variety of careers and have come from backgrounds where they were single-parent children, in most cases raised by women, and also celebrated as many of their mothers were domestic workers, nurses, or teachers – vocations reserved for specific groups.

In 2022, 28 years post-democracy, the mothers, grandmothers, and elders still reflect a widespread pattern of difference between rural and urban sites as

DOI: 10.4324/9781003203476-3

well as among the various provinces, some being largely rural, e.g., Limpopo and the Eastern Cape as well as Mpumalanga and North West Province. Provinces such as Gauteng, Western Cape, and Kwa-Zulu Natal were regarded as more developed with urbanized population groups.

Casino sites were spread across the country and in all nine provinces. Casino and Limited Pay-out Machines (LPM) revenues as well as horse racing activities and electronic bingo were large income generators for each of the nine provinces. The National Gambling Board (NGB) statistic estimated the size of the gambling industry revenues in South Africa to be R30 billion for the financial year 2018/2019. Gross gambling revenue (GGR) for the industry was expected to rise from R26 billion in 2015 to R34.8 billion in 2020, according to NGB (2019) results.

Women's gambling participation in the more rural provinces represented a specific demographic with different educational levels and large dependence on state grants for older persons, child grants, or some form of social grants. Participation in many of the gambling modes in these rural provinces includes Ifafi/Fafi (a form of betting),[1] cards, lottery, and, possibly to a lesser extent, LPMs and casinos. The agency that records and monitors such participation in legalized gambling modes is the NGB of South Africa.

The NGB regularly conducts research studies to establish the socio-economic impact of gambling in South Africa. The latest of those studies, published in 2019, revealed that almost a third (30.6%) of respondents gambled and the most participative mode of gambling is lotteries, followed by casino gambling, betting, bingo, and LPM. Illegal gambling is also rampant with Ifafi/Fafi being the most popular. Although the gender distribution in the 18 years and older South African population is 47.2% males and 52.4% females (Statistics South Africa, 2015), the gender distribution within the study sample was slightly biased toward males (52.3% males and 47.7% females). The study confirms that males are disproportionally more inclined to gamble than females, particularly with regard to their participation in horse/sports betting, LPMs, and unlicensed gambling. Females however are more involved in casinos, lucky draws, scratch cards, and bingo as gambling modes. Table 1.1 shows participation of South African women compared to women from the United Kingdom in different gambling modes. Problem gambling was also found to be more prevalent among males than females (NGB, 2019).

The NGB's focus has been on the transformation agenda of changing ownership and employee participation from largely men to be more reflective of the demographic profile of the country. In terms of employment and ownership, there have been substantial shifts in female participation. The hidden risk of greater acceptance of gambling for women is quite present, as gambling becomes more integral as a salary or wage as part of the resources of family households. Research by the NGB does not specifically identify women's issues relating to problem gambling or their participation rate. This necessitates following the results and indications from other global studies,

Table 1.1 National gambling board research on female participation in gambling modes in comparison with UK females

Female Participation	United Kingdom	South Africa
National lottery	53.9%	46.1%
Lucky draws	48.9%	51.1%
Scratch cards	45.6%	54.4%
Horse/sports betting	76.5%	23.5%
Casinos	48.0%	52.0%
LPMs	56.5%	43.5%
Bingo	32.4%	67.6%
All unregulated/unlicensed gambling	52.3%	47.7%

Source: https://www.ngb.org.za (2019).

especially as they reflect on women's unwillingness to seek help and to access treatment protocols because of their feelings of shame and the stigma associated with problem gambling.

The COVID-19 Lock Down and Its Impact on Gambling Behaviour

The gambling industry in South Africa had a substantial setback due to the global COVID-19 pandemic and the rules and issues of lock down. As a middle-income developing country, South Africa's people responded differently to the COVID-19 context and a unified governmental response was seen by many as top-down, urban-centered, and not relevant for rural communities. While this may not be true, the community responses differed depending on the severity of cases affected COVID-19 closest to home.

Casinos as sites specifically located in areas of industrialization, such as Gauteng or urbanized hubs of provincial capital cities, were seriously impacted when South Africa's lock down started on March 27, 2020. The initial period was to be 21 days, and all were willing to assist the government in ensuring that the country is prepared for the big onslaught on access, movement, community participation and engagement, as well as community cohesion. The hard lock down included closure of casinos, and site access limits of only 50%, with no more than 100 people. The country's 2-year lock down period, implementing constraints with various levels, impacted land-based casinos, gambling sites, and bingo halls. Online betting saw substantial growth among those who are electronically savvy and have credit cards, denoting higher disposable incomes. However, the informal modes and illegal modes of gambling remain as an alternative, given their non-formalized nature and local community base.

During the COVID-19 lock down period, sites such as churches, casinos, and sports venues, and events such as funerals, where groups of people gathered and which could be seen as "super spreader events," were closed down. The large casinos were substantially impacted. The restrictions on numbers, social distancing, temperature scanning, as well as full disclosure of contact details became an infringement on privacy and anonymity, and became new imposed barriers to entry. These were especially burdensome on women, even though the regulations applied to all.

The role of gambling sites for women of single status, older women, or lonely women is often not considered in our views on gambling and its effects on a society. Issues of isolation, separation, and loneliness were experienced by many women and families, and issues of extreme poverty, hunger, and loss were experienced by many. Women whose support networks came from belonging to groups, supporting groups, and attending group activities through their various community structures carried a large part of this pandemic on their proverbial shoulders by providing care for the sick, support during loss and even through the simplistic yet effective community food parcels process.

Legalized Global Lotto Playing on the Internet

The Western Cape Gambling and Racing Board (WCGRB) licensed an operator of different lotto games with bets placed on global platforms in South Africa called Lotto Land. In this game of chance, players can place bets online and win large amounts of money. They also allow choosing a beneficiary to benefit from any individual winnings which reflects a focus on playing with good causes in mind (RSG, 2022). This form of gambling assumes that access to the Internet and smart phones is readily available.

This facility brought increased gambling revenues into the province's coffers but the nature of online gambling meant there was no access for many disenfranchised people. Furthermore, the physical participation aspect, which had been part of the gambling experience for more than 27 years since the legalization of gambling in South Africa, was curtailed as a result of the curfews and the restrictions on provincial and cross border travels as well as the denial of access to casinos during heavy lock down. As a result, a thriving illegal industry blossomed. Home card games, Fafi/Ifafi, dice, and other games continued to be played within community areas. The pictures of community cohesion and enjoyment amidst tragic deaths and mass hospitalization belie the tragic state of the economy, closing down of small businesses and myriads of people queueing for the promised R350 (30 USD) relief grant per qualified person.

Women's Stories

It was mostly women who suffered momentously during the COVID-19 lock down period and the continuous extensions. More than 60% of women whose work was located within the service sector (e.g., domestic work or small-scale enterprises such as hair salons and the beauty industry) could no longer offer their services because they were disallowed.

Women offered their care-giving skills and the number of food kitchens thrived as communities collectively took on the plight of orphans and school-going children as well as caring for the elderly.

Gambling games became a new part of the social fabric of these communities as it created togetherness and possibilities of sharing winnings in communities; however, in some cases, it led to devastation and much loss.

Diana Ferrus, the poet and social activist, reflects on how the tables in casinos and gambling houses symbolize choices in her poignant poem on slavery called "Memory of Tables" (Ferris, p. 8) which is in her collection of poems in her book *I Have Come to Take You Home* (2011). These "tables of slavery" speak to addictive behaviour to slots or gambling tables, and locate women as overwhelmed by status, their lack, their poverty, and above all their enslavement, such that they return to the comfort of gambling which eases their pain and allows them to forget and to belong to a world of potential and possibilities. It's an opportunity to escape the painful realities of abuse, oppression, and often pain and hunger. "In this world, of possibility and forgetfulness, they find their own sense of being and escapism."

Rita's Story

Rita (pseudonym), a single mother and grandmother, earning a weekly wage and visiting Grannies as her entertainment during the weekend. She is a seamstress, and a skilled textile worker and retail assistant. During the first lock down period in South Africa in 2020, Rita was asked to make only masks, no pillows, no curtains, no dresses, etc. In such a difficult and constrained environment, her only outlet seemed to be increased participation in gambling, whether legal or informal.

Binge behaviour developed with each visit to the Grannies, including drinking and gambling because she was not sure when she would have the opportunity to participate again. These sites have provided her with a sense of safety and protection from various elements and she would feel that she could safely spend a designated amount during the weekend.

The sudden and sharp restraints of lock down meant that she could not venture alone, and she was affected by the early curfews of 8 pm and then 9 pm, and being unable to travel freely. She would seek for gambling sites closer to her home where she could continue to participate in her leisurely activity which, according to her, is harmless. Due to the fear of not being able to access her favorite leisurely activities any longer, she would participate in binge gambling and in this process became more susceptible to losing larger amounts of money as she was unsure of when she would be able to access these sites in the foreseeable future.

Bossy's Story

Bossy (pseudonym) is an older widow, whose gifts and talents are closely linked to her role in community and in her workplace.

With the restrictions on her movement and the limits on her regular once a-week visit to the nearby gambling site, Bossy became extremely depressed, locked in and lonely, and found the past two years of lock down more devastating than dealing with the loneliness of losing her husband approximately 6 years ago.

After lock down, she described a sense of well-being, order, and ritual in visiting her pleasurable activity at the gambling site which has become a structure in her life. She dresses up and plans how much she will spend to play, but she often exceeds her budget. She justifies this as the cost of her entertainment and personal enjoyment.

Trudy's Story

Trudy (pseudonym) is a teacher and school principal. Gambling is her de-stress mechanism after a week of intense involvement with children and parents. She enjoys her gambling leisure activity at her favorite casino site.

She is a very proud gambling participant and she and her friends' outings are to legalized casinos. They enjoy the ritual of dressing up, eating out and gambling, as well as spending a safe weekend with all the bells and whistles as very important patrons of local casinos.

Her responsibility as a school principal has ingrained the discipline of working hard but she also knows how to play hard. Her gambling activity reflects that of many other women who are single, hard-working, and needing to be safe and yet relaxed.

Her friends are part of her social engagement and she laughs as she talks about how the friendship is also her safety net. She admits that she's had weekends pass by, where she has often had no recollection of her spending and losses. She further admits that her interest in hiking and dancing has disappeared and attributes this to her age and the need to prepare for such events carefully.

Patience' Story

Patience (pseudonym) is a gentle soul and keeps her community's activities alive. She is nostalgic about a time when bingo and card games were valued in her community. These days, such activities often receive very little support because no one is excited about the low-value prizes.

She discovered that most of her normal supporters would prefer to spend their days playing games such as Ifafi/Fafi and cards, with the possibility of winning some money or as some put it: "to be able to supplement their social grants to take care of their families."

The stokvel (savings group) is seen as a means to access larger amounts of money with which to gamble at more sophisticated sites and with much larger gains in case of a win.

Conclusion

The women whose stories are told in this chapter represent a large number of women in their respective communities. The particularities and context are of a wide spectrum of women, including well-educated women who have access and engage in online gambling, and women who are largely uneducated in the formal sense and who find solace in local community activities and in informal gambling activities such as dice or Ifafi/Fafi. Yet another group of women find that the acceptance of gambling and the allure of the sophisticated legal sites permit them to gamble safely, yet often uncontrolled, and therefore creating the potential for problem gambling.

Unhealthy gambling in South Africa is a significant health issue for families, specifically for women, and it deserves more attention. Ethnic and social inequalities are apparent and these disparities need to be considered as we explore women and gambling and related risky behaviours in South Africa. As in other times of constraint, the people of a society faced with CAVID-19 often did what they normally do. Card games, dominoes, scrabble, tile rummy, and bingo, which were already prevalent, increased during lock down. Some games were simply pure family fun played across different generations. Further, the incidences of dice, Ifafi/Fafi, and many other informal gambling modes continued as they were local and accessible, and proceeded within a framework of small rural communities. These informal modes of gambling remain unregulated and without any problem gambling protocols. The incidences of participation in these modes increased, even though the large potential sums of gain have remained low. The increase of lotto participation during this period is also notable.

More detailed discussion is needed with larger quantities of women across all orientations and backgrounds through a program of open discussion. Female support is needed in addressing issues of health (both physical and mental) as well as issues of problem gambling and uncontrolled spending. Women are open and conversationalist, and when they find safe spaces they are willing to share their experiences to benefit others. More of their stories need to be told as we learn about women and the risky behaviour they often display in the context of gambling, as they continue to make choices about their own well-being.

Note

1   Fafi or fa-fi (pronounced fah-fee), also known as mo-china, is a form of betting played mainly by black South African women and men, particularly those living in South African Townships, and is believed to have originated with South Africa's Chinese community. The game is similar to a numbers racket.

References

Books

Ferrus, D. (2011). *I've come to take you home*. UK: Xlibris Publishing.

Websites

Ngb.org.za (2019, 2021, 2022). National Gaming Board Official Website. [Online] Available at https://www.ngb.org.za/

Nlc.org.za (2021, 2022). National Lotteries Commission Website. [Online] Available at https://www nlc.org.za/

Responsiblegambling.org.za (2021, 2022). Responsible Gambling Website. [Online] Available at https://responsiblegambling.org.za/

Statssa.gov.za (2015). Statistics South Africa Website. [Online] Available at https://www.statssa.gov.za/

Wcgrb.co.za (2021, 2022). Western Cape Gambling and Racing Board Website. [Online] Available at https://www.wcgrb.co.za/

Interviews

Bekker, A., & Lotto Land Winners (2022). Radio (RSG) interview between Amore Bekker and winners of Lotto Land on assigning their personal charities.

De Vries, L. (2021, 2022). Discussions with women who shared about their lives during lock down. Cape Town.

Miller, H., & de Vries, L. (2017). Gambling patterns – A South African story. Radio (RSG) interview with Heidi Miller on her radio programme on people in gambling.

Part II

North America

Chapter 2

Women's Wellbeing

Illuminating the Harmful Impact of a Partner's Compulsive Sexual Behaviours

Gretchen Blycker

Women's sexual wellbeing is essential to public health as an important indicator of health equity and overall wellbeing. Women who are in romantic relationship with a partner with compulsive sexual behaviour (CSB), sex addiction (SA), or problematic pornography use (PPU) experience unique harms, trauma, and other negative effects due to the nature of an addiction or compulsivity operating in the sexual system of a romantic context where safety, trust, empathy, emotional intimacy, honoring of commitments, honesty, and sexual wellbeing are foundational to a healthy secure attachment bond. Theoretical conceptual models for treating women impacted by a partner's CSB/SA/PPU will be discussed as well as models for healthy relationships, sexual wellbeing, and sociocultural influences on women's sexuality. Insights from research and clinical cases will illuminate how a partner's CSB/SA/PPU may impact women's wellbeing, sexuality, and her experiences in romantic relationship.

Introduction

Sexual wellbeing has been identified as essential to public health as an indicator of health equity and wellbeing. A recommended holistic public health approach to sexuality utilizes a biopsychosocial-cultural framework that includes four main pillars, which are sexual health, sexual wellbeing, sexual pleasure, and sexual justice (Mitchell et al., 2021). Sexual health encompasses fertility management, sexual violence prevention, prevention and management of sexually transmitted infections, as well as healthy sexual functioning with desire and arousal. Sexual pleasure involves physical and psychological satisfaction during sexual experiences concurrent with key factors of self-determination, consent, safety, privacy, and healthy sexual communication. Sexual justice includes sexual rights, sexual citizenship, and a trauma-informed sex positive approach to sensual and sexual wellbeing. According to Mitchell et al.'s model, sexual wellbeing comprises seven domains. Table 2.1 shows the seven domains on sexual wellbeing (Mitchell et al., 2021) and impacts of partners' SA/CSB/PPU on women's sexual wellbeing by domain.

DOI: 10.4324/9781003203476-5

Table 2.1 The seven domains on sexual wellbeing (Mitchell et al., 2021) and impacts of partners' SA/CSB/PPU on women's sexual wellbeing by domain

	Seven Domains of Sexual Wellbeing (Mitchell et al., 2021)	Impact of Partner's SA/CSB/PPU on Women's Sexual Wellbeing (Blycker)
1.	Sexual safety, security, and relationship trust with partner.	Due to denial and secrecy, a woman's sense of safety, security and relational trust with a partner may be negatively impacted, as she may experience her partner's dishonesty, lies of omission, or gaslighting.
2.	Sexual respect comprises the perception of positive regard by others for one's sexual personhood, sexual identity with preferences being accepted by one's personal community and broader culture.	A partner's SA/CSB/PPU may interfere with a woman's felt sense of sexual respect in the relationship.
3.	Sexual self-esteem is revealed by affective appraisals of oneself as a sexual being and is associated with sexual satisfaction and mindful attention to sexual interactions, feeling good about one's body sexually as well as feeling in control of sexual thoughts and desires.	A partner's sexual compulsivity, upward comparison to pornography, preferring pornography to partnered sex, or focusing craving toward partnered sex and therefore expressing dissatisfaction or resentment of sexual frequency may all possibly interfere with a woman's sexual self-esteem and feelings about her body, sexual autonomy, and agency.
4.	Resilience in relation to sexual experiences incorporates maintaining equilibrium in response to sexual stress, dysfunctions, adversity, or trauma and involves support by having someone to talk to openly about one's sex life and long-term recovery from negative occurrences in one's sex life.	A partner's sexual compulsivity creates distress and possibly trauma and women often feel isolated and challenged in openly discussing the problems and seeking support.
5.	Forgiveness of past sexual experiences comprise practices to halt patterns of self-blame, self-stigmatization, shame, avoidance, aggression, regret, and revenge in order to reduce harm and benefit relationship quality. Effective interventions are important to support recovery from sexual trauma and improve subsequent health outcomes.	A woman with a partner with CSB/SA/PPU may be blamed for the cause of sexual or relational problems rooted in SA and may be shamed and used as a scapegoat by the SA partner to justify the sexual acting out.
6.	Self-determination in one's sexual life includes free choice or rejection of sexual partner (s), behaviours context and timing without pressure, force, or felt obligation, which directly influences sexual wellbeing, autonomous choice about only engaging in sexual activities that one really wants to do and not feeling pressure from others to do specific sexual activities.	Women with a partner in active sexual addiction or in sexual recovery may feel pressured and a sense of obligation to engage in sexuality activity.
7.	Experiencing comfort and ease with sexuality while in contemplation, communication and engagement in the flow of pleasurable sexuality, without shame or guilt are all associated with sexual wellness and healthy behaviours such as contraceptive use and facilitating discussing sexual anatomy with a health professional.	Women with a partner in denial while in active sexual addiction may be the focus of her partner's resentment, power and control dynamics, may be left out of his sexual focus or may be the target of his sexual acting out. The SA partner may experience empathy reduction and devaluation of intimate sexual communication due to PPU.

This chapter focuses on women whose wellbeing is negatively impacted by a romantic partner's sex addiction (SA), compulsive sexual behaviours (CSB), or problematic pornography use (PPU). The World Health Organization's (WHO) 11th International Classification of Diseases (ICD-11) has included compulsive sexual behaviour disorder (CSBD) as a diagnosis, which may be expressed in various ways including PPU, cybersex, masturbation, as well as sexual behaviours with others (WHO, 2022). CSBD is classified as an impulse control disorder although the diagnostic criteria are in alignment with other disorders due to addictive behaviours (Brand et al., 2020). Symptoms or consequences of SA, CSBD, or PPU may first emerge in a relational context, therefore an increased understanding of the intrapersonal and interpersonal experiences of women who have partners with SA/CSB/PPU warrants further investigation and understanding. Addictions not only impact the person suffering with the disorder, but also those they are in relationship with. However, when the addiction involves sexuality there are significantly different and unique consequences and traumatic experiences that a romantic partner suffers that sets this dynamic apart from being intimate with a person with any other addiction or compulsive behaviour.

Books written by clinicians, as resources to help partners of people struggling with sex addiction, have titles that convey the deeply personal nature of traumatic betrayal, like "Intimate Treason: Healing the Trauma for Partners Confronting Sex Addiction" (Black & Tripodi, 2012), "Deceived: Facing Sexual Betrayal, Lies, and Secrets" (Black, 2009), "Facing Heartbreak: Steps to Recovery for Partners of Sex Addicts" (Carnes et al., 2012), and "Mending a Shattered Heart: A guide for partners of sex addicts" (Carnes, 2011). Additionally, recent dissertation studies include, "Is Porn the New Mistress: A Sexual Betrayal Study" (Futrell, 2020) and "I am Enough: Therapeutic Treatment Modalities for Partners of Sex Addicts" (Lujan, 2019).

The following will focus on understanding how women's general wellbeing and sexual wellbeing, specifically, may be affected by a partner's CSBD/SA/PPU. While women who suffer with CSBD also deserve the focus of treatment and research (Blycker & Potenza, 2018; Kowalewska et al., 2020, 2022), this will not be the emphasis of study here. The intention with the language utilized centers women as the focus of their own experiences and not as peripheral to or being defined by another person's disorder or behaviours (i.e., seeking not only to identify women as *partners of sex addicts*). Evidence shows that it is necessary to "diagnose and treat the partners of sex addicts as distinct individuals, in order to address their unique needs and concerns" (Stokes et al., 2020).

A brief review of conceptual models of clinical treatment and support for women will provide insight into the evolution of understanding how this particular behavioural addiction carries unique ways of harming women who are partnered with individuals with CSBD. Examining models that assess components of relational factors that comprise healthy romantic relationships will highlight basic needs in intimate relationships that are fundamentally impacted by a partner's CSBD/SA/PPU. Exploring sociocultural factors that influence sexual socialization will identify barriers to women's sexual wellbeing, which may possibly create vulnerabilities to normalizing the problems and symptoms of CSBs, therefore masking the addiction or compulsions operating in the sexual system of a romantic relationship. Also included are suggestions to promote the process of identifying and creating safety for women with practices that manage boundaries, create a structure conducive for navigating the aftermath of discovery of a partner's CSB, help to integrate healing practices and spaces to validate their experiences, and support their own clarity by re-connecting with the wisdom of their inner guidance system.

Conceptual Models for Clinical Treatment for Women with Partners with CSB/SA/PPU

In the ever-evolving clinical and research fields focusing on promoting sexual wellbeing and treating problematic and compulsive sexual behaviours, there have been several theoretical models for treating people who have partners with SA/CSB/PPU. For decades since the 1980s, as the field was emerging, the addiction treatment model included viewing those in romantic relationship through a lens of co-addiction or codependency and considered sex addiction as a family disease in need of a systems approach for treatment and recovery (Hentsch-Cowles & Brock, 2013; Steffens & Rennie, 2006; Vogeler et al., 2018). However, there may be potential problems created by applying this lens to women who might have had experienced trauma by enduring mind/body/sexuality boundary violations and gaslighting in their romantic relationship, and therefore may be engaging in safety seeking behaviours like confirming reality, identifying truths, and working to prevent further harm. Women whose lives are disrupted by a partner's CSB/SA/PPU and who are in crisis may operate from a survival mode of hypervigilance scanning for potential threats and this and other coping behaviours might be perceived differently, depending on the model used as a lens for understanding to inform treatment considerations. For example, from the co-sex addict or codependent lens, women's behaviours have been described as controlling, such as being sexually available for their partner, expressing anger, threats, feeling anxiety,

> policing, snooping, attention/validation seeking, creating drama/chaos, self-blame, workaholism, being obsessively busy, being a super parent, rationalizing, manipulation, lying to friends and family about marriage/relationship, denial, perfectionism, self-harm, using the Internet, shopping, food, alcohol, other forms of substances to numb/act out, depression, sleeping extended hours, [and] keeping up appearances. (Hentsch-Cowles & Brock, 2013)

Findings from a review of research that examines the impact that SA has on partners show that partners experience anxiety, despair, negative perceptions of themselves as well as their partner and the relationship. In one study, 69% of wives of sexually addicted men met all, but the controversial A1 ("experienced, witnessed, or been confronted with an event that involves actual or threatened death or injury, or a threat to the physical integrity of self or others"), criteria for post-traumatic stress disorder (PTSD) (Seyed Aghamiri et al., 2022). Furthermore, regardless of whether sexual behaviours were limited to online sexual activity, the trust and relationships for couples were significantly harmed and betrayal trauma "resulted in functional impairment, difficulties fulfilling roles, preoccupation, identity loss, humiliation, and a sense of being stuck" (Seyed Aghamiri et al., 2022). In order to explore the abuse and trauma-related symptoms women were reporting, Dr. Stefanie Carnes developed the Partner Sexuality Survey (PSS) that examines the impact on the emotional wellbeing and sexuality of the partner of a person with SA. The PSS items follow a trauma model perspective and explore the presence of "(1) Feelings of victimization, (2) Intimacy impairment, (3) Shame, (4) Sexual anorexia/aversion, (5) Sexual dysfunction, (6) Body Image Issues, (7) Obligatory sex, (8) Compulsive sex, (9) Fear, and (10) Anger/ Revenge" (Carnes & O'Connor, 2016). In a confirmatory analysis of PSS data collected from a website about SA, the findings show that partners of those with SA suffer significant trauma-related consequences from the discovery or disclosure of sex addiction, and most scales were "significantly elevated for those partners who had left the relationship, suggesting that these coupleships were more distressed and the damage done by the sex addiction was more severe. The only two scales that were higher for those still in the relationship were obligatory sex and body issues" (Carnes & O'Connor, 2016). With elevated scales assessing for risk of abuse or injury, clinicians are advised to assess for the risk of intimate partner violence abuse or injury, sexual or emotional, power and control, and health consequences due to broken trust (Carnes & O'Connor, 2016).

An aspect of experience contributing to trauma is betrayal. Betrayal trauma theory was first introduced by Freyd in 1991 to describe

a betrayal of trust that produces conflict between external reality and a necessary system of social dependence ... The psychic pain involved in detecting betrayal, as in detecting a cheater, is an evolved, adaptive, motivator for changing social alliances. In general, it is not to our survival or reproductive advantage to go back for further interaction to those who have betrayed us. However, if the person who has betrayed us is someone we need to continue interacting with despite the betrayal, then it is not to our advantage to respond to the betrayal in the normal way. Instead, we essentially need to ignore the betrayal as evidenced by research that shows that betrayal in these contexts is related to avoidance and dissociative responses (Freyd, 1995). More research is needed to explore the interaction effects between the addiction enabling phenomena of denial and dishonesty operating with the SA partner with the disconnection and dissociation that might happen for women who are experiencing the impact of a partner's SA/CSB/PPU and is being lied to and told her inner senses and experience of reality are not real or true and can't be trusted (i.e., gaslighting). A measure that assesses traumatic betrayal is the Trauma Inventory for Partners of Sex Addicts (TIPSA) (Stokes et al., 2020; Vogeler et al., 2020). The TIPSA assesses for symptoms of post-traumatic stress in the setting of the discovery or being told (i.e., disclosure that is within or without a therapeutic context) about a partner's sexually addicted behaviours and includes the following focus of criteria: (1) exposure to threats of death, injury, sexual violence or sexually transmitted infection, (2) reexperiencing the event, (3) avoidance of trauma-related stimuli, (4) negative thoughts or feelings, and (5) trauma-related emotional arousal (Vogeler et al., 2020).

Changes in the formulation of conceptual frameworks for supporting recovery of women with partners with SA/CSB/PPU have been influenced by concerns and criticism within the field, by women themselves, and by the ongoing research focusing on understanding treatment needs of women. Discoveries have shown that simply using frameworks from substance abuse recovery, viewing women partners of sex addicts as co-addicts or codependent, may be unfair, inaccurate, and could possibly contribute to victim blaming that may be further traumatizing, particularly for those who have been victimized or abused by a partner. The differing perspectives between the co-addiction and trauma models have significant implications for women receiving optimal and non-harming clinical treatment, being that the co-addiction model views women who have partners with SA as having her own illness (co-addiction or codependency) that she brings into the relational dynamic, while the trauma model views her as someone who is in distress from a traumatizing experience (Steffens & Rennie, 2006; Stokes et al., 2020). Education about the traumatic impact on women is important for clinicians to provide a trauma informed approach and to avoid victim blaming.

A recent therapeutically originated alternative to codependency is the prodependence model for the clinical treatment for addicts and partners (Weiss, 2019, 2022). Another conceptual model classifies three possible primary pathways to the behaviours of SA, which are opportunity-induced, attachment-induced, or trauma-induced (Hall, 2013). The OAT (opportunity, attachment, trauma) model is purported to be beneficial for supporting therapists and partners of sex addicts to better understand possible contributors to the formation of SA or PPU and it offers an alternative to the codependency model. Informed by survey data and clinical experience, the OAT model identifies that addiction is not always an intimacy or attachment disorder and that the isolation, relational damage, and intimacy problems experienced may be a consequence of SA/CSB/PPU and not necessarily the cause. The digital world is impacting human sexuality with the prevalence of Internet pornography, cybersex, and the increased opportunity to become dependent on sexual acting out behaviours for a physical release due to the accessibility, affordability, and anonymity of focusing sexual energy and attention toward impersonal expressions of sexuality.

Qualitative research exploring which kinds of support women use to cope when dealing with a spouse's SA/CSB, conceptualized support broadly to include therapy, support groups, medical attention, talking to friends, self-help books, helpful beliefs, narratives, or metaphors that enhanced one's resiliency and facilitated an expanded perspective to problems (Manning & Watson, 2008). Sixty-eight percent of participants experienced isolation and other forms of coping that made things worse, such as self-blaming (45%), enabling spouse (18%), and drinking alcohol (9%). The two forms support identified to be most beneficial were coping support and change-oriented support, and included five common factors: (1) connection, (2) advocacy, (3) validation, (4) education, and (5) direction (C.A.V.E.D Theory) (Manning & Watson, 2008). Connection to family, friends, God (higher power), and others with similar experiences reduced isolation and had a normalizing effect. Advocacy gave access to resources and reconnection to inner power and agency to make decisions. Validation provided reassurance and diminished self-blame, self-doubt, and insecurity. Education was shown to be essential in depersonalizing the problems and identifying choices for next steps. Direction facilitated informed action with confidence (Manning & Watson, 2008).

Relational Health, Love, and Intimacy

In order to understand the impact of SA/CSB/PPU operating in a romantic relationship, it is helpful to identify the components of a healthy romantic relationship. A recent study across 25 countries examined and validated the cultural universality of Sternberg's Triangular Theory of Love Scale (STLS), based on a theoretical model of sexual and romantic love that has been prominent for the last 35 years (Sorokowski et al., 2021). The STLS has three domains which are passion, commitment, and intimacy. Intimacy is part of the "warm" component of love and is not used as a euphemism for sex nor is it exclusive to romantic relationships, but rather refers to feelings of closeness, caring, healthy communication, and emotional investment, while passion refers to the "hot" component of sexual excitement and attraction (Sorokowski et al., 2021). A deeper analysis of intimacy is incorporated in Reis and Shaver's interpersonal process model of intimacy, which theorizes that feelings of closeness and connectedness between romantic partners is created and strengthened with bi-directional emotional disclosure and sharing of thoughts between partners, with perceived empathic partner responsiveness including demonstrations of understanding, validation and caring

(Laurenceau et al., 1998). A study exploring how these three components of intimacy (self-disclosure, perceived partner disclosure, and perceived partner responsiveness) might mediate the relationship between history of childhood maltreatment and dyadic sexual and relationship satisfaction found that perception of a partner's empathic responsiveness was positively associated with their own sexual satisfaction as well as relationship satisfaction for each person (Vaillancourt-Morel et al., 2019).

These findings point toward the essential component of perceptive experience of a partner's empathy in the evaluation of intimacy, sexual satisfaction, and relationship satisfaction. A recent study investigating men with PPU, showed that PPU is associated with reductions in empathy (Kor et al., 2022). The findings about empathy impairment are relevant to the impact on partners of people with PPU and deeper understanding about the implications on how this may affect women and relational health necessitate further investigation.

Pornography, Sexually Explicit Material, Sexual Violence as a Sexual Script, and Classifying Problematic Sexual Behaviours

Problems associated with pornography, sexually explicit material, and the impact on sexual behaviours and abuse go beyond the context of sexual addiction and compulsivity. For example, impersonal approaches to sex, which are absent of emotional intimacy, have been associated with a higher degree of sexual aggression in men, lower sexual satisfaction, and decreased mental health (Tokunaga et al., 2019; Wright et al., 2021). A meta-analysis including data from over 70 reports from the last 40 years from 13 countries revealed that pornography consumption was associated with impersonal approaches to sex for men and women and the results provided support for identifying impersonal sexual attitudes as a mediating link between pornography consumption and impersonal sexual behaviour (Tokunaga et al., 2019). A review of research investigating the effect of pornography use (i.e., non-compulsive pornography use) on romantic relationship and sexual satisfaction by Bennett-Brown and Wright reports that for men, pornography use and sexual and relationship satisfaction are negatively related and mediated by men's devaluation of intimate sexual communication, preference for pornographic over partnered sexual excitement, decrease of dyadic sex due to masturbation displacement, and experience of an upward comparison between one's own sex life to pornography while finding sex in pornography to be better than one's own sex life (Bennett-Brown & Wright, 2022).

Understanding contributing factors to problematic sexuality is essential for effective treatment. Identifying sources that contribute to the formulation of one's sexual arousal template is a fundamental component of sexual recovery. Sexual script theory is valuable in understanding cultural effects on sexual beliefs, attitudes, expected roles, and behaviours that influence sexuality. Wright's $_3$AM model describes components of how sexual mass media exerts a causal influence on sexual socialization by acquisition of a sexual script from sexual media, activation of the sexual script during sexual arousal or exposure to sexual cues, and application of the script in sexual situations (Wright, 2011). Recent research that explored pornography's social function in influencing normative sexual scripts analyzed the content describing titles of 131,738 pornographic videos advertised to first time users from the landing pages of three mainstream pornography websites and found that one out of eight titles described sexual violence (Vera-gray et al., 2021). The four common categories of sexual violence depicted include sexual activities between family members as the most common followed by physical aggression and sexual assault, image-based sexual abuse, and coercion and exploitation (Vera-gray et al., 2021). These findings that show mainstream pornography is placing sexual violence as a normative sexual script add a greater complexity and severity to the meaning of problematic pornography use.

A review of image-based sexual abuse (also referred to as "nonconsensual sharing of sexual imagery" or "revenge porn") research and its social, legal, and clinical implications identifies how this gendered sexualized violence is used to punish, abuse, and control women (DeKeseredy, 2021). Hidden camera images or videos, upskirting, nonconsensual sharing of consensually photographed or filmed images are being posted, shared, viewed online with at least 3,000 "revenge porn" websites dedicated to images uploaded by men without the consent of the women portrayed. One study of 6,109 survey participants (ages 16–64) revealed that 1 in 3 respondents was victimized by image based-sexual abuse and 1 in 6 respondents perpetrated image-base abuse (DeKeseredy, 2021). Given the normalization of sexualized violence depicted in online material people use for masturbation and the prevalence of image-based sexual abuse victimization and offending, there is a need for further research to understand the relationship between image-based-abuse and pornography consumption, as well as treatment needs for those who are victimized and those who offend. For research and clinical purposes, it has been identified that for accurate data about sexual behaviours and sexually explicit material that people use for sexual arousal purposes, the content and context need to be assessed (Mestre-Bach et al., 2021). Clinical assessments would also benefit from the operational definition of pornography proposed by social science researchers as "material deemed sexual, given the context, that has the primary intention of sexually arousing the consumer, and is produced and distributed with the consent of all persons involved" (Ashton et al., 2019). Consent to the *production and distribution* is a critically important component of this definition that differentiates legal and non-abusive from illegal and offending behaviours. Clinical measures, assessments, and research questions that omit this differentiation risk failing to identify crucial problematic factors of sexual behaviours as well as "avoid the inadvertent appearance of endorsing sexual assault through the connotations of the language used" (Ashton et al., 2019).

To address the necessity of classifying problematic sexual behaviours in order to assess and treat sexual functioning concerns, sexual addiction/compulsivity, PPU as well as nonconsensual, illegal or offending sexual behaviours, a four-quadrant model has been proposed by Delmonico and Griffin (2002). This model conceptualizes characteristics of the person and the problematic sexual behaviours along with individualized treatment to target the specified problems. The four distinct groups are (1) sex addiction with sex offending, (2) sex offending (without sex addiction), (3) sex addiction (without sex offending), and (4) sexual concerns (without offending or addiction). Having thorough clinical assessments to identify which quadrant a person belongs in is imperative for effective treatment for the identified patient as well as for understanding the impact on and the treatment needs of the partner.

Data show that men with PPU may experience a sense of loss of agency or power, or feelings of helplessness due to the addiction operating in their relationship to pornography (Taylor & Jackson, 2018). More research is needed to further understand how this experience of helplessness or loss of agency might interact or operate with power and control dynamics in romantic relationships. It has been recommended that clinicians working with individuals and couples in sexual addiction recovery to assess for the risk of intimate partner violence abuse or injury involving sexual or emotional harm and for power and control dynamics (Carnes & O'Connor, 2016). In West's review of the research on Black, Indigenous, People of Color consumers of pornography, the many problems identified include racist films and marketing practices contributing to amplifying racism and discrimination, creation of a sexual script of higher levels of aggression against Black women leading to a sociocultural "context of devaluing Black female bodies," associations of adolescent dating abuse victimization, and exploitation of female partners (West, 2022).

Sociocultural Considerations Impacting Sexual Wellbeing for Women

Sociocultural contributions and determinants of women's experience and expression of sexuality may impact beliefs, expectations, and influence what is accepted as normative. One such prevalent gendered attitude informing different standards of sexual permissiveness for men and women is the sexual double standard, whereby women's sexual behaviours (in some contexts or expressions like sex outside of marriage or being sexually liberal) may be stigmatized and men's may be expected and rewarded (Crawford & Popp, 2003). Other gendered messaging focuses on sex in relationships and identifies whose pleasure in important and whose sexual agency is respected. Some contemporary sex manuals problematically advise women in romantic relationships to "just do it" and describe the disciplinary or performative "work" required for women to prepare themselves for sex out of obligation or commitment, and advise women to be warm and responsive to their partners' desires, regardless of if they are feeling sexual desire or not (Gupta & Cacchioni, 2013). This approach has detrimental effects on women's sexual pleasure and desire for sex, as clinical reports show that women who feel duty bound to be available for sex and engage in consistently "forcing oneself to be sexual without willingness can result in low sexual desire or even sexual aversion in the long term" (Robinson et al., 2011). One may wonder if this contributes to cultural grooming, where a woman may not necessarily be physically forced by a partner, but she may be enculturated to follow a script whereby she is expected to force herself to be sexual.

A heteronormative theory of low sexual desire in women partnered with men identifies four sources contributing to low sexual desire for women: the inequitable division of labor, the caregiver-mother role to partner, gender norms about sexual initiation, and objectification whereby women are socialized to focus on their sexual appearance rather than their own sexual pleasure (van Anders et al., 2022). A substantial body of research describes a gendered orgasm and pleasure gap that is influenced by men's sense of entitlement to sexual pleasure and the phallocentric imperatives of heterosexual sexuality (Klein & Conley, 2021; Mahar et al., 2020; Willis et al., 2018). Studies show that this gendered discrepancy is not due to differences in anatomical or physiological capacity for sexual pleasure or responsivity to conducive conditions for sexual arousal (Laan et al., 2021). In fact, a study investigating traits and behaviours correlating with orgasm frequency found that heterosexual women were the least likely (65%) to experience orgasm during partnered sex and heterosexual men were the most likely (95%) to report orgasm, followed by gay men (89%), bisexual men (88%), lesbian women (86%), and bisexual women (66%) (Frederick et al., 2018).

There are many sociocultural and relational factors that may contribute to conditions that limit women's sexual pleasure who are partnered with men. Given this reality, clinicians and researchers need to be aware of assessing for the presence of these barriers so as not to pathologize women with a sexual dysfunction diagnosis when she may be experiencing a natural and appropriate physiological response, i.e., lack of sexual arousal or absence of orgasm when not experiencing conducive conditions relationally and with insufficient physical stimulation (Mestre-Bach et al., 2022).

Insights from a Clinical Practice Focusing on Promoting Sexual Wellbeing and Treating Compulsive Sexual Behaviours and Sexual Trauma

Despite variable challenging sociocultural circumstances women are enculturated with, a significant motivation for engaging in a sexual experience with a partner is the reward of emotional intimacy, involving "feelings of closeness connectedness and bonding" (van Lankveld et al., 2021). When a woman is in relationship with a partner with SA/CSB/PPU, there are additional factors that complicate the possibility of experiencing emotional intimacy during partnered sex, as PPU is associated with reductions in the empathy system (Kor et al., 2022). For women, there may be conflicting needs – sexual desire motivated by the hopeful reward of emotional intimacy, and the need to protect oneself from the effects of their partner's sexuality being distorted through the addiction or compulsivity.

In clinical treatment, a woman in recovery from the trauma of being the target of her husband's sex addiction and offending behaviours, described how before discovery of his SA she would try to manage her husband's "consumption of her" in ways that reminded her of how she tried to deal with his out-of-control alcohol consumption before he went into recovery for his substance use disorder. Her relational desire to feel close to her husband conflicted with the reality of the addiction and power and control dynamics operating in their sexual relationship. Body dissociation during partnered sex, alcohol use to cope, and relapse of her eating disorder and body dysmorphic disorder seemed to be connected to experiencing her husband's undiagnosed and untreated SA and video voyeurism. Her discovery of the hidden camera in her home was the excruciatingly painful beginning of her recovery and healing journey. As the therapeutic process supported her clarity, self-compassion, and repairing the trust in herself she identified that ...

> the truth is that for the entirety of our relationship there have been addictions, manipulation, coercion, violation, gaslighting, deflection, lying, abandonment, neglect, power and control. So why did I stay? That's the tricky part about addiction. There is also so much else going on. For one, I loved him and the family we created together. With a therapeutic separation and engaging in my support group and individual therapy, I kept putting one foot in front of the other and you know what happened? Eventually I turned around and realized how far I had gone. That not only was I still alive, but in this process, I had finally found myself. I had connected with myself and my spirituality for maybe the first time in my entire life. When that happened, I was able to fully embrace boundaries that kept me safe because I was clear in my values, how I deserved to be treated, and what I would under no circumstances ever tolerate again.

In addition to individual therapy focusing on healing from trauma and the impact of sex addiction, sex offending, and power and control dynamics in her relationship, she also participated in Compassion-Based Resilience Training (CBRT). CBRT facilitated the integration of the skills and practices of embodied mindful awareness, emotion regulation, compassion, and resiliency to manage trauma reactivity and create boundaries for safety while increasing empathy, self-respect and reconnection to herself and her inner guidance system to support her healing and recovery journey.

Clinical Case Examples: In His Own Words

In a flash of insight during a couple's therapy meeting, a wide-eyed man gazed into his wife's eyes and remarked, "there is a soul inside your body," during an "aha" moment while describing a shift in acknowledging his wife's inner being and sovereignty that he had not been acknowledging or considering during sexual experiences together. She had initiated the desire for therapy to address the lack of connection she felt with sexual and emotional intimacy with her husband in their sexual relationship. Although neither partner had any moral discomfort with pornography use, he seemed to have been unaware of how his masturbating while viewing pornography integrated sexual objectification into his sexual arousal template. This contributed to a lack of attunement to his partner and the objectification "may foster feelings of dehumanization, which, in turn, may make it more difficult to communicate with a sexual partner—inhibiting women's sexual satisfaction" (Holland et al., 2021).

After working in individual therapy with a male client in recovery from PPU for two years, he continued to uncover and dismantle the addiction operating system impacting his sexual relationship with his wife. During one session he gained further insight and owned how his addict mind made his wife "not enough."

> I hate to say this, verbally it is very hard to acknowledge ... If I am honest, I MADE her "not enough." I expected her to play out a part from my fantasies, that I would talk to her and tell her about. I treated her like she wasn't even important in sexual experiences. I treated her like she was a thing to project my fantasies on. When you tell yourself and another person a lie long enough, it becomes a kind of truth to you. I would tell her that she is enough. Though now looking deeper into it, I wanted her to be the porn. I don't like admitting this. Knowing that I have thought those things about my wife, shows me that she knew me better than I knew myself. Whenever she would question me and say she felt that I believed she wasn't enough, I would tell her she was wrong, that she was enough. The truth is I treated her as less than, not as an equal partner, but rather more as a participant in what I wanted. I haven't wanted to see these things for a long time, it is painful, and I don't feel good about myself that I did this to the person I love. The reality is that it wasn't loving. In recovery now, when I have learned to be present and truly be with her, I feel like I am falling in love with her again.

Another male client in recovery from PPU identified how he had been impacted by the compartmentalization that happens when sexuality develops disconnected from emotional intimacy. In his therapeutic disclosure letter he wrote to his wife and later read to her in a therapy appointment he shared:

In retrospect, I grew up feeling unwanted by peers, male and female. I was afraid of hurting women and being hurt by women, which led to sub-consciously keeping women at a distance, even those that I have dated. I was afraid of rejection, failure, and disappointment. Masturbation and porn use were a safe way for me to experience sexual pleasure without the risks involved with an emotional relationship. Developing my sexual behavior without another person, enabled my sexual desires to evolve disconnected from my or other people's emotions. I now see how this has been harmful and contributed to my PPU and problems in our relationship. My fear of rejection, failure, and disappointment has been a huge driving force in many aspects of my life. I think this is also part of the fundamental problem, which has bled into so many other areas of our relationship. Your requests for courage and honesty are not only what you need, but what I need as well. I need to trust your persevering love for me and stop acting out of fear of rejection, failure, and disappointment. This fear is a huge obstacle inhibiting our deeper emotional and physical connection. Sharing all of this with you is very scary for me because I'm afraid you may be even more disappointed in me, as a result of what I share. But I now understand that you are more disappointed when I am unable to share. It's this vulnerability, this willingness to go out on a limb and show you my deepest self, that will allow for our greatest capability to connect. I will also work on showing you daily attention and loving affection, if you are open to and wanting physical affection. I will commit to sharing more deeply what is going on inside my head and heart, as well as my intimate desires. I want my sexual behavior and desires to be intimately connected with my and your emotions. I want to understand you better, your desires, your emotions. I want our intimate relationship to be an exploration, together; an extension and deepening of our emotional connection.

Clinical Case Examples: In Her Own Words

In recovery from the harms of a partner's SA/CSB/PPU, it is essential for women to experience validation, support, and to be trusted in being the authority and source of information about her own experiences. The following is an impact letter written by a woman that she read to her partner who was in PPU recovery during a therapy session.

I am writing this letter so you will have a better understanding of how your pornography use has affected me. My deepest hope is that you will understand this connection of why I have struggled with body image, self-worth, depression, and anxiety in our relationship. For me, the worst part of all of it was your denial. I know now that you are working to understand the issues your behavior has caused. There have been many consequences of your betrayal that have greatly affected me emotionally, physically, sexually, and personally. I feel the sexual wounds may be the deepest. The trauma of the years leading up to the therapeutic disclosure of your pornography addiction was painful. I felt ashamed of our issues and found it hard to talk to friends about real-life updates. The background noise of our broken connection distracts almost every aspect of my life. Our relationship as a whole has suffered from this betrayal as well. I question your judgment and wonder what you're keeping from me on a near-daily basis. I felt crazy wondering what on earth was happening in our relationship. I had wondered if you were questioning your sexuality or if you might be having an affair. I have had a hard time learning the extent of your denial and your compulsive behaviors with pornography.

The disclosure of your pornography use was traumatic for me. Both the staggered disclosures of half-truths about where your sexual energy was going. When you told me that using pornography "is just easier," I felt very sad and worried that my needs were too much. Before you acknowledged your porn problem, I blamed myself for the problems in our relationship. I thought if I were skinnier, prettier, more feminine, wore sexier lingerie, styled my hair the way you like, cooked more, needed less, asked for less, talked less or had fewer opinions ... maybe I could attract your attention back to me. It felt lonely and sad to be in bed with you. I cried myself to sleep feeling deep sorrow for our lack of connection on a weekly basis. I was sure that if I could just be better, you would come around. I realize now that I am not and never was at fault. When I think about the worries I had about our disconnection being all my fault I feel terribly sad. I feel angry that I wasted those years feeling terrible and negative about myself rather than appreciating my body and acknowledging my self-worth. I have come to realize that this story is part of my lineage (of how women have been viewed in my family) and part of our culture's history. The narrative is "if your man is not happy, it is your fault or if your man is not happy, change yourself until he is." This is the story I intend to end with me, so it doesn't get passed on in our family.

Your porn use made me feel alone and like I was left out of your expression of your sexuality. I feel porn has influenced your conceptualizations about sex, while conveniently being ignorant if in porn a women may be forced to fill a role to appear pleasured. Our sex life has been affected by your porn use. I feel a lack of desire of being sexually intimate with you in order to avoid the pain all this has caused. Then I also have wondered if you were thinking of other women when we were together. To me, porn is a form of sexuality where real life is left out and a patriarchal fantasy world designed for male pleasure takes over. I was not aware that the sexual functioning issues you were experiencing with me were related to Porn-Induced Erectile Dysfunction (PIED). I had felt compassion for you and would consistently focus on supporting your pleasure over my own, because I knew you felt anxiety and embarrassment. So, I stopped asking for what would be pleasurable for me, because it seemed to trigger erection problems for you. Now I realize that was another way my desires and needs were left out of our sexual relationship entirely, another way I was disregarded. I have also felt isolated socially in my pain in facing how this has impacted me. I appreciated that you have encouraged me to talk with my close friends for support. I know my friends will hold space for me, yet I also worry that they will judge you and maybe think less of me. I also worry that they might feel I am overreacting because of how common porn use is, and they might not understand how much pain your behaviors have caused me. I want to feel a sense of trust and safety with you again. I want to work together to restore these important aspects of relationships. I also fear that your habits of justification, defensiveness, and your ability to fail to see the problems (denial) might arise again. I ask for your courageous vulnerability and continuing self-reflection into the future. I will continue to practice my self-care, the boundaries I need, and asking for the support I need. I need you to recognize that I am riding an emotional roller coaster that isn't my fault. Overwhelm happens for me now, like I have never in my life have known before. My sense of self-worth has hit an all-time low. This process of writing this letter to you has been difficult as well as healing for me. I hope this helps you better understand my experience and my part of this story. I understand that this may be challenging for you to hear and I thank you for listening.

In Her Own Words: Insight for Clinicians

A woman in recovery from the trauma of her husband's SA/PPU sought both individual and couples' treatment from several clinicians over many years, without her husband's SA/PPU ever being identified. Her whole family would have benefited from earlier intervention and harm prevention, which seemed like a failure of the clinicians who unwittingly participated in the gaslighting of her that her husband had started.

When I discovered my husband was viewing rape and abuse porn, it validated the feelings and experiences I had in our sexual relationship. The harm and trauma I experienced was difficult to put into words. I wished therapists had asked about the content of my husband's porn use. I wish they had asked what happens sexually between us as a couple. I wish the clinicians that were treating him individually as well as the couples therapists we worked with, would have explored what things (like his use of sexually violent porn) meant. I couldn't initiate talking about the sexual part, I didn't have words or language to describe or understand. Later, itbecame clearer to me that sex for him was about power, control and winning. I didn't feel safe. I was seeking safety. I had symptoms. His gaslighting created confusion which led to a disconnection within myself and the ability to put language to my experiences.

Like with other diagnoses, if you experience symptoms without knowing the cause, you might continue to suffer or treat the symptoms in ways that do not address the cause. When you have a diagnosis or understand the cause, you have language and an understanding of how to treat the problem. There is power and clarity in naming something to describe it. Who do you talk to about sex addiction and abuse of power and control in a sexual relationship? Friends? Even therapists missed it and they didn't understand.

How do you bring this out to the light without making the whole family suffer? In many ways I helped to preserve this veneer of normalcy in our relationship and family. I don't want to feel guilty about that because I needed things to feel ok. In our household, we all did this adaptation. Sometimes I was rewarded for it, things got better in other parts of the relationship when I did what he wanted sexually. But the whole relationship ended up being one big punishment. As a kid I learned you can protect yourself if you take the blame. I had worked my whole life to feel like I didn't deserve punishment. I worked hard to appreciate aspects of myself. It has required a significant amount of resiliency for me to hold onto myself and fight to overcome that. I also feel a lot of sadness and anger. I want for mychildren to be aware and want to find safe ways to talk about this without it being a secret. I don't want to pathologize sex when addressing these problems with my adolescent daughter and son. I want them to identify safety for themselves. To know what safety feels like. And to know when things don't feel safe and what they can do to find and create safety.

Discussion

Research and clinical data show that women's general and sexual wellbeing are impacted by a partner's SA/CSB/PPU. Referencing the seven domains of sexual wellbeing proposed by Mitchell et al. (2021), a partner's SA/CSB/PPU may create barriers to women's sexual wellbeing in following ways according to the respective domains. (1) As addictions often operate in denial and secrecy, a woman's sense of safety, security, and relational trust with a partner may be negatively impacted, as she may experience her partner's dishonesty, lies of omission, or gaslighting. (2) A partner's SA/CSB/PPU may interfere with a woman's felt sense of sexual respect in the relationship. (3) A partner's sexual compulsivity, upward comparison between own sex life and sex depicted pornography, preferring pornographic over partnered sexual excitement, or focusing craving toward partnered sex and therefore expressing dissatisfaction or resentment of sexual frequency may all possibly interfere with a woman's sexual self-esteem and feelings about her body and sexual autonomy. (4) A partner's sexual compulsivity creates distress and possibly trauma and women often feel isolated and challenged in openly discussing the problems and seeking support. (5) A woman with a partner with CSB/SA/PPU may be blamed for the cause of sexual or relational problems caused by SA and may be shamed and used as a scapegoat by the SA partner to justify the sexual acting out. (6) Women with a partner in active sexual addiction or in sexual recovery may feel pressured and a sense of obligation to engage in sexuality activity. (7) Women with a partner in denial while in active sexual addiction may be the focus of her partner's resentment, power, and control dynamics may be left out of his sexual focus or may be the target of his sexual acting out. The SA partner may experience empathy reduction and devaluation of intimate sexual communication due to PPU.

There is evidence that the source of harmful effects to women's sexual self-esteem are not only due to her own body dissatisfaction and negative body image that are associated with exposure to or consumption of pornography (Paslakis et al., 2022), but also may be impacted by men's non-compulsive pornography use that contributes to an upward comparison perceiving sex in pornography to be better than one's own sex life and devaluing intimate sexual communication (Bennett-Brown & Wright, 2022). While a woman's healthy positive sexual self-esteem may contribute to her resiliency against the impact of upward comparison in non-SA/CSB/PPU relationships, with addiction and compulsivity where consumption is never enough, there may be additional complexities that warrant further investigation. For example, when SA/CSB/PPU is impacting a relational system where sexual comparison, sexual compulsion, and sexual consuming are all co-occurring, there may be many negative effects. It has been said that comparison is the thief of joy, perhaps in addition in these cases, it may also be the thief of peace, sexual pleasure, a healthy relationship and perhaps much worse. Here, if there is compulsive consuming, as addiction operating through sexuality may be conceptualized, then, unlike with a substance or other behavioural addictions like gambling, gaming, or shopping, a female partner may be the focus of compulsive consumption or alternatively may be disregarded as not enough. The implicit or explicit messaging to her may be that she is not enough, the sex frequency is not enough, the kind of sexual activity happening is not enough. She may get the message in a painful and powerful way, "*you* are not enough."

More research is needed to explore the interaction effects between the addiction enabling phenomena of denial and dishonesty operating with the SA partner with the disconnection and dissociation that might happen for women who are experiencing the impact of a partner's SA/CSB/PPU and are being lied to, told that her inner senses and experience of reality are not real or true and can't be trusted (i.e., gaslighting). A particularly confusing and brutal aspect of this experience may be that the partner with the addiction may not be aware of how his denial has been operating and therefore not be consciously aware that he has been engaging in gaslighting his romantic partner. Having seen this time and time again working with men in SA recovery, this can be a deeply painful reality for men to allow themselves to see, yet without this inner work relational healing does not happen.

From clinical case work, common experiences among women in relationship with a partner with SA/CSB/PPU include gaslighting, confusion, tensions in relationship while struggling to get clear at causes, being blamed for problems, partner's defensiveness, justifications, excuses, secrets, and a sexual relationship that was deficient of experiences of emotional intimacy and sexual empathy. When women experienced the positive effects of their own recovery and healing and their partner's sexual recovery in their relationship, they felt their partner's presence which contributed to feelings of closeness, increased sexual satisfaction which was created from the safety of boundaries, attunement to themselves, and attunement from their partner.

Conclusion

Women who have partners with SA/CSB/PPU experience unique harmful effects to their overall and sexual wellbeing. Their romantic relationships may also be negatively impacted in all three essential domains of passion, intimacy, and commitment identified in Sternberg's Triangular Theory of Love. There are problematic sociocultural influences which may contribute to the normalization of self-objectification, self-subjugation, male sexual entitlement, phallocentric imperatives, sexual double standards, and gendered pleasure and orgasm gaps for women who have sex with men. Women with partners with SA/CSB/PPU may be isolated without proper support. Education about the traumatic impact on women is important for clinicians in order to provide a trauma informed approach to treatment and to avoid victim blaming. More is needed in the research and clinical fields to advance understanding and knowledge to inform evidence-based treatment needed by women impacted by their partner's SA/CSB/PPU. Without this and having clarity and language to identify the root causes of problems, the risk is that many women may be in pain while not having the important language to elucidate and give voice to the indelible inner experiences that can seem ineffable. Its challenging to heal the deep-rooted pain when the experiences are ineffable or invalidated.

There is power and clarity in naming something to describe it.

References

Ashton, S., McDonald, K., & Kirkman, M. (2019). What does 'pornography' mean in the digital age? Revisiting a definition for social science researchers. *Porn Studies*, 6(2), 144–168. 10.1080/23268743.2018.1544096

Bennett-Brown, M., & Wright, P.J. (2022). Pornography consumption and partnered sex: A review of pornography use and satisfaction in romantic relationships. *Current Addiction Reports*. 10.1007/s40429-022-00412-z

Blycker, G.R., & Potenza, M.N. (2018). A mindful model of sexual health: A review and implications of the model for the treatment of individuals with compulsive sexual behavior disorder. *Journal of Behavioral Addictions, 7*(4), 917–929. 10.1556/2 006.7.2018.127

Brand, M., Rumpf, H.-Jü., Demetrovics, Z., MÜller, A., Stark, R., King, D.L., Goudriaan, A.E., Mann, K., Trotzke, P., Fineberg, N.A., Chamberlain, S.R., Kraus, S.W., Wegmann, E., Billieux, J., & Potenza, M.N. (2020). Which conditions should be considered as disorders in the international classification of diseases (ICD-11) designation of "other specified disorders due to addictive behaviors"? *Journal of Behavioral Addictions.* 10.1556/2006.2020.00035

Carnes, S., & O'Connor, S. (2016). Confirmatory analysis of the partner sexuality survey. *Sexual Addiction and Compulsivity, 23*(1), 141–153. 10.1080/10720162.2015.1039151

Crawford, M., & Popp, D. (2003). Sexual double standards: A review and methodological critique of two decades of research. *Journal of Sex Research, 40*(1), 13–26. 10.1080/00224490309552163

DeKeseredy, W.S. (2021). Image-based sexual abuse: Social and legal implications. *Current Addiction Reports.* 10.1007/s40429-021-00363-x

Delmonico, D., Griffin, E., & St Louis Park, M.N. (2002). Classifying problematic sexual behavior: A working model revisited. In *Clinical Management of Sex Addiction,* Edited by Patrick J. Carnes, Kenneth M. Adams, 1st Edition. New York: Routledge, 361–376.

Frederick, D.A., John, H.K.S., Garcia, J.R., & Lloyd, E.A. (2018). Differences in orgasm frequency among gay, lesbian, bisexual, and heterosexual men and women in a U.S. National sample. *Archives of Sexual Behavior, 47*(1), 273–288. 10.1007/s10508-017-0939-z

Freyd, J.J., & Definitions, S. (1995). What is a betrayal trauma? What is betrayal trauma theory? *Short Definitions.* https://dynamic.uoregon.edu/jjf/defineBT.html

Futrell, L. (2020). Is porn the new mistress?: A sexual betrayal study.(Order No. 28409982). Available from ProQuest Dissertations & Theses Global; ProQuest One Academic; Publicly Available Content Database. (2539485385). Retrieved from https://www.proquest.com/dissertations-theses/is-porn-new-mistress-sexual-betrayal-study/docview/2539485385/se-2

Gupta, K., & Cacchioni, T. (2013). Sexual improvement as if your health depends on it: An analysis of contemporary sex manuals. *Feminism and Psychology, 23*(4), 442–458. 10.1177/0959353513498070

Hall, P. (2013). A new classification model for sex addiction. *Sexual Addiction and Compulsivity, 20*(4), 279–291. 10.1080/10720162.2013.807484

Hentsch-Cowles, G., & Brock, L.J. (2013). A systemic review of the literature on the role of the partner of the sex addict, treatment models, and a call for research for systems theory model in treating the partner. *Sexual Addiction and Compulsivity, 20*(4), 323–335. 10.1080/10720162.2013.845864

Holland, K.J., Silver, K.E., Cipriano, A.E., & Brock, R.L. (2021). Young women's body attitudes and sexual satisfaction: Examining dehumanization and communication as serial multiple mediators. *Psychology of Women Quarterly, 45*(2), 255–266. 10.1177/0361 684321994295

Klein, V., & Conley, T.D. (2021). The role of gendered entitlement in understanding inequality in the bedroom. *Social Psychological and Personality Science.* 10.1177/ 19485506211053564

Kor, A., Djalovski, A., Potenza, M., Zagoory-Sharon, O., & Feldman, R. (2022). Alterations in oxytocin and vasopressin in men with problematic pornography use: The role of empathy. *Journal of Behavioral Addictions*. 10.1556/2006.2021.00089

Kowalewska, E., Gola, M., Kraus, S.W., & Lew-Starowicz, M. (2020). Spotlight on compulsive sexual behavior disorder: A systematic review of research on women. *Neuropsychiatric Disease and Treatment, 16*, 2025–2043. 10.2147/NDT.S221540

Kowalewska, E., Gola, M., Lew-Starowicz, M., & Kraus, S.W. (2022). Predictors of compulsive sexual behavior among treatment-seeking women. *Sexual Medicine, 10*(4), 100525. 10.1016/j.esxm.2022.100525

Laan, E.T.M., Klein, V., Werner, M.A., van Lunsen, R.H.W., & Janssen, E. (2021). In pursuit of pleasure: A biopsychosocial perspective on sexual pleasure and gender. *International Journal of Sexual Health, 33*(4), 516–536. 10.1080/19317611.2021.1965689

Laurenceau, J.-P., Feldman Barrett, L., Pietromonaco, P.R., Reis, H.T., & Shaver, P. (1998). Intimacy as an interpersonal process: The importance of self-disclosure, partner disclosure, and perceived partner responsiveness in interpersonal exchanges. *Journal of Personality and Social Psychology, 74*(5), 1238–1257.

Lujan, K. (2019). I am enough: Therapeutic treatment modalities for partners of sex addicts.(Order No. 13427311). Available from ProQuest Dissertations & Theses Global; ProQuest One Academic. (2207600914). Retrieved from https://www.proquest.com/dissertations-theses/i-am-enough-therapeutic-treatment-modalities/docview/2207600914/se-2

Mahar, E.A., Mintz, L.B., & Akers, B.M. (2020). Orgasm equality: Scientific findings and societal implications. *Current Sexual Health Reports, 12*(1), 24–32. 10.1007/s11930-020-00237-9

Manning, J.C., & Watson, W.L. (2008). Common factors in Christian women's preferences for support when dealing with a spouse's sexually addictive or compulsive behaviors: The C.A.V.E.D. theory. *Sexual Addiction and Compulsivity, 15*(3), 233–249. 10.1080/10720160802288886

Mestre-Bach, G., Blycker, G.R., Actis, C.C., Brand, M., & Potenza, M.N. (2021). Religion, morality, ethics, and problematic pornography use. *In Current Addiction Reports, 8*(4), 568–577. 10.1007/s40429-021-00388-2

Mestre-Bach, G., Blycker, G.R., & Potenza, M.N. (2022). Behavioral therapies for treating female sexual dysfunctions: A state-of-the-art review. *Journal of Clinical Medicine, 11*(10), 2794. 10.3390/jcm11102794

Mitchell, K.R., Lewis, R., O'Sullivan, L.F., & Fortenberry, J.D. (2021). What is sexual wellbeing and why does it matter for public health? *The Lancet Public Health, 6*(8), e608–e613. 10.1016/S2468-2667(21)00099-2

Paslakis, G., Chiclana Actis, C., & Mestre-Bach, G. (2022). Associations between pornography exposure, body image and sexual body image: A systematic review. *Journal of Health Psychology, 27*(3), 743–760. 10.1177/1359105320967085

Robinson, B.B.E., Munns, R.A., Weber-Main, A.M., Lowe, M.A., & Raymond, N.C. (2011). Application of the sexual health model in the long-term treatment of hypoactive sexual desire and female orgasmic disorder. *Archives of Sexual Behavior, 40*(2), 469–478. 10.1007/s10508-010-9673-5

Seyed Aghamiri, F., Luetz, J.M., & Hills, K. (2022). Impacts of sexual addiction on intimate female partners—The state of the art. *Sexual Health & Compulsivity*, 1–37. 10.1080/26929953.2022.2050862

Sorokowski, P., Sorokowska, A., Karwowski, M., Groyecka, A., Aavik, T., Akello, G., Alm, C., Amjad, N., Anjum, A., Asao, K., Atama, C.S., Atamtürk Duyar, D., Ayebare, R., Batres, C., Bendixen, M., Bensafia, A., Bizumic, B., Boussena, M., Buss, D.M., ...Sternberg, R.J. (2021). Universality of the triangular theory of love: Adaptation and psychometric properties of the triangular love scale in 25 countries. *Journal of Sex Research, 58*(1), 106–115. 10.1080/00224499.2020.1787318

Steffens, B.A., & Rennie, R.L. (2006). The traumatic nature of disclosure for wives of sexual addicts. *Sexual Addiction and Compulsivity, 13*(2–3), 247–267. 10.1080/1072 0160600870802

Stokes, S.S., Moulton, S., Sudweeks, R.R., & Fischer, L. (2020). An item analysis of the trauma inventory for partners of sex addicts. *Sexual Addiction and Compulsivity, 27*(1–2), 65–89. 10.1080/10720162.2020.1751362

Taylor, K., & Jackson, S. (2018). 'I want that power back': Discourses of masculinity within an online pornography abstinence forum. *Sexualities, 21*(4), 621–639. 10.11 77/1363460717740248

Tokunaga, R.S., Wright, P.J., & Roskos, J.E. (2019). Pornography and impersonal sex. *Human Communication Research, 45*(1), 78–118. 10.1093/hcr/hqy014

Vaillancourt-Morel, M.P., Rellini, A.H., Godbout, N., Sabourin, S., & Bergeron, S. (2019). Intimacy mediates the relation between maltreatment in childhood and sexual and relationship satisfaction in adulthood: A dyadic longitudinal analysis. *Archives of Sexual Behavior, 48*(3), 803–814. 10.1007/s10508-018-1309-1

van Anders, S.M., Herbenick, D., Brotto, L.A., Harris, E.A., & Chadwick, S.B. (2022). The heteronormativity theory of low sexual desire in women partnered with men. *Archives of Sexual Behavior, 51*(1), 391–415. 10.1007/s10508-021-02100-x

van Lankveld, J.J.D.M., Dewitte, M., Verboon, P., & van Hooren, S.A.H. (2021). Associations of intimacy, partner responsiveness, and attachment-related emotional needs with sexual desire. *Frontiers in Psychology, 12.* 10.3389/fpsyg.2021.665967

Vera-gray, F., Mcglynn, C., Kureshi, I., & Butterby, K. (2021). Sexual violence as a sexual script in mainstream online pornography. *British Journal Of Criminology*, April, 1–18. 10.1093/bjc/azab035

Vogeler, H.A., Fischer, L., Bingham, J.L., Hansen, K.S.W., Heath, M.A., Jackson, A.P., & Skinner, K.B. (2020). Assessing the validity of the Trauma inventory for partners of sex addicts (TIPSA). *Sexual Addiction and Compulsivity, 27*(1–2), 90–111. 10.1080/10720162.2020.1772158

Vogeler, H.A., Fischer, L., Sudweeks, R.R., & Skinner, K.B. (2018). An examination of the factor structure of the trauma inventory for partners of sex addicts (TIPSA). *Sexual Addiction and Compulsivity, 25*(1), 46–64. 10.1080/10720162.2018.1452086

Weiss, R. (2019). Prodependence vs. codependency: Would a new model (prodependence) for treating loved ones of sex addicts be more effective than the model we've got (codependency)? *Sexual Addiction & Compulsivity, 26*(3-4), 177–190.

Weiss, R. (2022). *Prodependence: Beyond the myth of codependency.* Simon and Schuster.

West, C.M. (2022). Pornography consumers of color and problematic pornography use: Clinical implications. *Current Addiction Reports.* 10.1007/s40429-022-00410-1

Willis, M., Jozkowski, K.N., Lo, W.J., & Sanders, S.A. (2018). Are women's orgasms hindered by phallocentric imperatives? *Archives of Sexual Behavior, 47*(6), 1565–1576. 10.1007/s10508-018-1149-z

World Health Organization (WHO) (2022). 6C72 Compulsive sexual behaviour disorder. Retrieved from https://icd.who.int/dev11/l-m/en#/http://id.who.int/icd/entity/1630268048

Wright, P.J. (2011). Mass media effects on youth sexual behavior assessing the claim for causality. *Annals of the International Communication Association*, *35*(1), 343–385. 10.1080/23808985.2011.11679121

Wright, P.J., Paul, B., & Herbenick, D. (2021). Pornography, impersonal sex, and sexual aggression: A test of the confluence model in a national probability sample of men in the U.S. *Aggressive Behavior*, *47*(5), 593–602. 10.1002/ab.21978

Chapter 3

Clinical Perspectives of Love Addiction & Compulsive Sexual Behaviour

Rebecca J. Jacobson and Koriann Cox

Compulsive sexual behaviour (CSB) and love addiction are behavioural addictions that may be intertwined. Historically, CSB has been considered a disorder impacting mostly men, and it may be underreported in women due to shame and cultural norms. Compulsive sexual behaviour and love addiction are often comorbid, with approximately 50% of individuals reporting both. Though both conditions have been studied for a number of years, there has been little research conducted on the direct impact on women who have been diagnosed with one or both. This chapter will provide an overview of overlap, gaps, and areas for future research.

Clinical Perspectives of Love Addiction & Compulsive Sexual Behaviour

Attitudes toward sexuality in the United States are more conservative compared to other western cultures due to the influence of Puritan heritage, though views about sex and sexuality have become more flexible over the years. The United States has a robust double standard between men and women when it comes to sexual behaviours – while men are often celebrated and described as "experienced" when they engage in casual sexual relationships, women who engage in multiple emotional or sexual relationships are often labeled with derogatory terms. When sexual or emotional behaviour crosses over from "all in good fun" to behaviours that are part of an addiction, individuals may struggle to report it due to fear of stigma or judgment. Compulsive sexual behaviour is most often attributed to men, though there is a strong possibility that American women are underreporting sexual compulsive behaviours due to cultural norms and a concern that the reporting of these behaviours may not be taken seriously by clinicians. A woman's participation in casual sexual behaviour collides with our abiding sociocultural beliefs on how a woman should behave and when a woman is engaging in that behaviour compulsively, she may experience both internal and external shame. In contrast, a woman suffering from love addiction may receive less judgment, as this behaviour may be seen as more in alignment

DOI: 10.4324/9781003203476-6

with the American cultural norm that a woman should be loving and nurturing. In this chapter, we will examine the differences and overlap of compulsive sexual behaviour versus hypersexuality in female trauma survivors and look at the emerging topic of love addiction in American women.

Compulsive Sexual Behaviour in Female Trauma Survivors

Compulsive sexual behaviour (CSB) is defined as an intense, persisting pattern of uncontrollable, repetitive sexual impulses that cause distress and impairment in personal, family, social, educational, occupational, or other important areas of functioning (Kraus et al., 2018). In a nationally representative study performed in the United States, 7% of women reported that they have experienced a feeling at some point that their sexual behaviour was out-of-control (Dickinson et al., 2018), and prevalence estimates of Compulsive Sexual Behaviour Disorder (CBSD) range from 1–6% in both men and women (Kraus et al., 2018). Some problems reported by women who have engaged in CSB are the acquisition of sexually transmitted infections, unwanted pregnancies, legal consequences related to sex work, as well as perceived stigmatization through the violation of societal norms (Kalichman & Cain, 2004).

Although CSB has not been recognized as a mental disorder diagnosis in the DSM-5, it has been conceptualized as a behaviour addiction disorder among some researchers. Brain imaging studies have shown that similar regions are activated in individuals with behavioural addictions as are typically associated with drug use including the ventral striatum, dorsal anterior cingulate cortex (DaCC), and the amygdala being activated. A study on explicit material viewing subjects showed these same areas activated (Voon et al., 2014).

One common factor that is found in many women who abuse substances and who engage in CSB is the experience of trauma. Adverse childhood experiences in form of physical, emotional, sexual abuse and neglect are thought to perpetuate symptoms of CSB (Vaillancourt-Morel et al., 2014), with childhood sexual abuse being the most prevalent casual factor (Kurbitz, 2021; Slavin, 2020). Shame often arises following the experience of a traumatic event and this shame has been theorized as a mediating factor for CSB in women (Dhuffar & Griffiths 2014). Engaging in CSB has been reported by trauma survivors to avert feelings of shame, a way to avoid the processing of painful feelings (Derbyshire & Grant, 2015; Gilliland et al., 2011). The experience of shame may be a barrier to seeking treatment for CSB (Brem et al., 2018).

Clinicians working with women who are engaging in sexual behaviours following the experience of a traumatic event may want to consider the differences and similarities of compulsive sexual behaviour as a diagnosable disorder and the experience of hypersexuality as a response to the trauma. These behaviours may be similar in presentation (e.g., a woman engages in frequent sexual intercourse with one or multiple partners) but the purpose of this behaviour may be different: in one case, a woman may feel compelled to engage in CSB even though it does not provide pleasure (though it may provide relief) and in another, a woman may engage in the behaviour without pleasure because it helps her to feel in control of her body and sexual experience. Women seeking treatment (either for "real" or perceived CSB or for a comorbid condition such as posttraumatic stress disorder) may benefit from conversations with providers to better understand the etiology of their behaviours. Just as a prescriber would want to confirm what type of medication would work best for treating a specific medical condition, so too would a clinician want to understand if they should be addressing CSB from the lens of addiction or as a component of trauma sequelae.

Shame does seem to be perpetuated in American society with clinicians viewing patients that were in non-monogamous relationships more negatively (Reddick et al., 2017). To best support women with CSB, it is paramount that providers offer non-judgmental, trauma-informed care. Such care should include strategies that incorporate ways to reduce shame, regulate effect, and assist the woman in implementing appropriate and healthy boundaries relating to sexual behaviours. Research has shown that individuals with behavioural addictions respond similarly to treatments as individuals with substance use disorders (Kraus et al., 2021), including cognitive behavioural therapy and 12-step programs. Women with CSB may also benefit from medication management for mood and behavioural regulation and for reducing cravings, though the specific research on medications for CSB is in its naissance.

Love Addiction in Women

Humans are evolutionarily hardwired for the pursuit of connections with others. While a physical connection for the purpose of reproduction is essential to the survival of the species, an emotional connection and loving bond may enrich the relationship between two people. Some theorists believe that this romantic love can cross the normal boundary of healthy love and can turn into love addiction (Burkett & Young, 2012; Fisher et al., 2016). Love addiction has been defined as behaviours that can become extremely maladaptive such as repeatedly seeking physical, emotional, or psychological contact with another individual despite negative consequences to relieve obsessive thought patterns about the desired person (Fisher et al., 2016). The behaviours and characteristics of love addiction may parallel those of other addictions including being compulsive, chronic in nature, and leading to negative social, psychological, financial, and legal consequences (Fisher et al., 2016). Though love addiction has not been widely studied, some prevalence estimates for the general population in the United States are about 3–11% (Sussman et al., 2010). One theory suggests that women experience love addiction more frequently than men because they are more interested in securing satisfactory relationships (Ferree, 2010). In the United States, as with many countries, it is a social construct to marry and have children; many women may measure their worth on securing a mate. Literature on co-dependence provides a clinical explanation of the perplexities of love addiction—women may perpetuate an identity based on caretaking and romantic relationships (Melody & Freundlich, 2003).

In a study on the outcomes of romantic relationships based on attachment style, there were notable differences in women who were identified as having an anxious-ambivalent attachment style when compared to individuals with other attachment styles (Feeney & Noller, 1990). Attachment theory posits that the bond between the child and caregiver influences later bonding and attachment for an individual and their romantic partner; someone with an anxious-ambivalent style would likely tend to be anxious, overly needy, and demonstrate low self-esteem in relationships (Feeney & Noller, 1990). Attachment theory may be the basis of why more women are thought to experience more infatuation or obsession with another person characterized by frenzied passion and intrusive thoughts in relationships known as limerence (Feeney & Noller, 1990). The anxious-ambivalent subjects in Feeney and Noller's (1990) study were characterized by higher scores on mania, emotional dependence, and reliance on their partner and scored higher on obsessive preoccupation. Melody and Freundlich (2003) hypothesized that love addiction may be the result of an adult attachment style based on learning to survive or tolerate feelings of abandonment and/or neglect from the attachment figures (e.g., parents, early romantic partners, etc). Those suffering with love addiction may possibly engage in negative and maladaptive patterns because it feels familiar to them.

When someone falls in love, their brain releases the neurotransmitters oxytocin and vasopressin, resulting in euphoric feelings that have been compared to the experience of a cocaine high (Sanches & John, 2019). Affectionately called the "cuddle drug," oxytocin is released during hugging, touching, massage, nipple stimulation, and orgasm as well as in childbirth. The release of oxytocin in the brain has been shown to correlate with pair bonding behaviour in women (Burkett & Young, 2012). This neuro-transmitter may be responsible for the stronger attachment that women feel when being in a romantic relationship. In studies using functional magnetic resonance imaging (fMRI) to examine the brain activity of individuals who self-reported experiencing love addiction, the researchers found that the areas of the brain that were activated when the subject was shown photographs of romantic partners and reported "intense romantic love" were the same regions active in individuals with substance or behavioural addictions who reported experiencing cravings and withdrawal (Burkett & Young, 2012; Fisher et al., 2010). Additionally, those who had experienced a romantic rejection also had activity in the ventral pallidum (which is associated with feelings of attachment), the insular cortex and the anterior cingulate (which are associated with physical pain), the nucleus accumbens and orbitofrontal/prefrontal cortex (which are responsible for calculating one's gains and losses and are also involved in craving and addiction; Fisher et al., 2010).

Love can be rewarding, but unrequited love can be a painful experience. In individuals with love addiction if the feeling of love is left unreciprocated it may cause extreme emotional suffering. The withdrawal symptoms reported by individuals with love addiction who have experienced romantic rejection are similar to some of the common symptoms associated with drug withdrawal including lethargy, anxiety, insomnia or hypersomnia, loss of appetite or binge eating, and irritability (Fisher et al., 2016). The intensive obsessive thoughts about the desired partner can lead to impulsive behaviours and may begin to manifest as stalking and other crimes of passion (Fisher et al., 2016). These behaviours are often performed to relieve stress (Sussman, 2010) and individuals report experiencing relief similar to individuals who have just consumed a substance of choice. Stalking is one of the most common outward behaviours associated with love addiction (Sussman, 2010) and some research has found that women engage in 75% more stalking behaviours than men (Purcell et al., 2001). Although the Purcell and colleagues (2001) study did not address love addiction, one could potentially hypothesize that some participants who exhibited stalking behaviours may have been experiencing symptoms related to love addiction.

Interventions that have shown promise in treating love addiction include psychotherapy such as psychodynamic therapy, cognitive behavioural therapy, and self-help groups such as Sex and Love Addicts Anonymous (Reynaud et al., 2010). According to Reynaud and colleagues (2010), men have the tendency to attend Sex and Love Addicts Anonymous for sex addiction while women attend for love addiction. According to a review by Sussman and colleagues (2011), love and sex addiction are often overlapping, with approximately 50% of those who are attending primarily for sex addiction also reporting symptoms of love addiction and vice versa. In addition to psychotherapy and/or attendance of 12-Step meetings, clinicians should direct the patient with symptoms of love addiction to remove any photos, memoirs, and refrain from any contact with the love interest as these reinforce the brain circuits to be wired for attachment (Fisher et al., 2016). Another helpful approach may be diverting one's attention by engaging in other activities. Exercise has been found to be beneficial for the mind and is suggested to achieve more harmony (Fisher et al., 2016). Although not widely studied, some pharmacological treatments have been implemented, including antidepressants, mood stabilizers, exogenous neuropeptides, and naltrexone (Redcay and Simonetti, 2018).

Love addiction is not currently recognized by the Diagnostic and Statistical Manual, 5th edition (DSM-5) or the International Classification of Disease (ICD) as an accepted diagnosis. The concept has been studied since 1975 and many studies (e.g., Fisher et al., 2016; Sussman, 2010; Zou et al., 2016) support its classification as a mental health disorder. Given the lack of widespread study, the full impact on individuals and society at large is unknown. Further research is needed in order to understand the diagnosis to consider it for inclusion in future versions of the ICD and the DSM. It is imperative that clinicians are able to identify this condition and be able to intervene with a client that is afflicted with love addiction so that proper treatment can be provided to reduce suffering and the potential for harm.

References

Brem, M. J., Shorey, R. C., Anderson, S., & Stuart, G. L. (2018). Does experiential avoidance explain the relationships between shame, PTSD symptoms, and compulsive sexual behaviour among women in substance use treatment? *Clinical Psychology & Psychotherapy*, 25, 692–70010.1002/cpp.2300.

Burkett, J. P., & Young, L. J. (2012). The behavioral, anatomical, and pharmacological parallels between social attachment, love and addiction. *Psychopharmacology*, *224*(1), 1–26. 10.1007/s00213-012-2794-x

Derbyshire, K. L., & Grant, J. E. (2015). Compulsive sexual behavior: A review of the literature. *Journal of Behavioral Addictions*, *4*(2), 37–43. 10.1016/j.cpr.2020.101925

Dhuffar, M. K., & Griffiths, M. D. (2014). Understanding the role of shame and its consequences in female hypersexual behaviours: A pilot study. *Journal of Behavioural Addictions*, *3*(4), 231–237. 10.1556/JBA.3.2014.4.4

Dickenson, J. A., Gleason, N., Coleman, E., & Miner, M. H. (2018). Prevalence of distress associated with difficulty controlling sexual urges, feelings, and behaviors in the United States. *JAMA Network Open*, 1, e18446810.1001/jamanetworkopen.2018.4468.

Ferree, M. (2010). *No Stones: Women Redeemed from Sexual Addiction*(2nd ed.) Downers Grove, IL: InterVarsity Press.

Feeney, J. A., & Noller, P. (1990). Attachment style as a predictor of adult romantic relationships. *Journal of Personality and Social Psychology*, 58, 281–29110.1037/0022-3514.58.2.281.

Fisher, H. E., Brown, L. L., Aron, A., Strong, G., & Mashek, D. (2010). Reward, addiction, and emotion regulation systems associated with rejection in love. *Journal of Neurophysiology*, *104*, 51–60. http://jn.physiology.org/content/104/1/51

Fisher, H. E., Xu, X., Aron, A., & Brown, L. L. (2016). Intense, passionate, romantic love: A natural addiction? How the fields that investigate romance and substance abuse can inform each other. *Frontiers in Psychology*, 7. https://doiorg.ezproxy.library.unlv.edu/10.3389/fpsyg.2016.00687

Gilliland, R., South, M., Carpenter, B. N., & Hardy, S. A. (2011). The roles of shame and guilt in hypersexual behavior. *Sexual Addiction and Compulsivity: The Journal of Treatment & Prevention*, *18*(1), 12–29. 10.1080/10720162.2011.551182

Kalichman, S. C. & Cain, D. (2004). The relationship between indicators of sexual compulsivity and high-risk sexual practices among men and women receiving services from a sexually transmitted infection clinic. *Journal of Sex Research*, *41*(3), 235–241. 10.1080/00224490409552231

Kraus, S. W., Krueger, R. B., & Briken P. (2018). Compulsive sexual behaviour disorder in the ICD-11. *World Psychiatry*,*17*(1), 109–110. 10.1002/wps.20499

Kraus, S. W., Popat-Jain, A., & Potenza, M. N. (2021). Compulsive sexual behavior and substance use disorders. In R. Balon & P. Broken (Eds.), *Compulsive Sexual Behavior Disorder: Understanding, assessment, and treatment* (pp.22–34). American Psychiatric Association Publishing.

Kürbitz, L. I., & Briken, P. (2021). Is compulsive sexual behavior different in women compared to men? *Journal of Clinical Medicine, 10*(15), 3205. 10.3390/jcm10153205

Melody, P., & Freundlich, L. (2003) The intimacy factor: The boundaries of love. *The Meadows*

Purcell, R., Pathé, M., & Mullen, P. E. (2001). A study of women who stalk. *American Journal of Psychiatry, 158*(12), 2056–2060.

Redcay, A., & Simonetti, C. (2018). Criteria for love and relationship addiction: Distinguishing love addiction from other substance and behavioral addictions. *Sexual Addiction & Compulsivity, 25*(1), 80–95. https://doiorg.ezproxy.library.unlv.edu/10.1080/10720162.2017.1403984

Reddick, G. T., Heiden-Rootes, K. M., & Brimhall, A. S. (2017). Therapists' assessments in treating "sex addiction" and their relationship to clients' gender, relationship status, and exclusivity status. *Journal of Marital Family Therapy, 43*(3), 537–553. 10.1111/jmft.12210.

Reynaud, M., Karila, L., Blecha, L., & Benyamina, A. (2010). Is love passion an addictive disorder? *The American Journal of Drug and Alcohol Abuse, 36*(5), 261–267. 10.3109/00952990.2010.495183

Sanches, M., & John, V. P. (2019). Treatment of love addiction: Current status and perspectives. *The European Journal of Psychiatry, 33*(1), 38–44. https://doi.org.ezproxy.library.unlv.edu/10.1016/j.ejpsy.2018.07.002

Slavin, M. N., Blycker, G. R., Potenza, M. N., Bo the, B., Demetrovics, Z., & Kraus, S. W. (2020). Gender-related differences in associations between sexual abuse and hypersexuality. *Journal of Sexual Medicine, 17*, 2029–2038. 10.1016/j.jsxm.2020.07.008

Sussman, S. (2010). Love addiction: Definition, etiology, treatment. *Sexual Addiction & Compulsivity, 17*(1), 31–45. 10.1080/10720161003604095

Sussman, S., Lisha, N., & Griffiths, M. (2011). Prevalence of the addictions: A problem of the majority or the minority? *Evaluation & the Health Professions, 34*(1), 3–56. 10.1177/0163278710380124

Vaillancourt-Morel, M.-P., Godbout, N., Labadie, C., Runtz, M., Lussier, Y., & Sabourin, S. (2014). Avoidant and compulsive sexual behaviors in male and female survivors of childhood sexual abuse. *Child Abuse & Neglect, 40*, 48–59. 10.1016/j.chiabu.2014.10.024

Voon, V., Mole, T. B., & Banca P. (2014). Neural correlates of sexual cue reactivity in individuals with and without compulsive sexual behaviours. *PLoS One, 9*(7): e102419. 10.1371/journal. pone.0102419

Zou, Z., Song, H., Zhang, Y., & Zhang, X. (2016). Romantic love vs. drug addiction may inspire a new treatment for addiction. *Frontiers in Psychology, 7*, 1436–1436. 10.3389/fpsyg.2016.01436

Chapter 4

Clinical Considerations of Behavioural Addiction in Pregnancy

Koriann Cox

There are currently no published studies examining the impact of behavioural addictions during pregnancy in the United States. The United States is one of the global leaders in rates of caesarean births and maternal mortality among developed countries and offers the worst availability of paid parental leave. Even without addiction, pregnant women in the United States can experience a variety of difficulties. This chapter provides a comparison between behavioural addictions and substance addiction, reports on some of the negative consequences of substance use disorders during pregnancy, and proposes potential clinical considerations for and areas of future research on behavioural addiction in pregnancy.

Clinical Considerations of Behavioural Addiction in Pregnancy

To date, there have been no nationally representative studies in the United States that have examined the impact of behavioural addictions during pregnancy. Without this research, it is difficult to impossible to ascertain the impact of behavioural addictions (e.g., gambling, compulsive sexual behaviour, or food addiction) on pregnant women and their children. The purpose of this chapter is to present comparisons between behavioural addictions and substance addictions and to highlight potential clinical considerations of behavioural addiction in pregnancy.

In the United States, the rate of birth in 2019 was 11.4 per 1,000; 31.7% of these births were via caesarean section (Center for Disease Control [CDC], 2021). According to the Commonwealth Fund (2020), the United States also has the highest rate of maternal mortality compared to other developed countries (17.4 per every 100,000 births compared to the next closest, France, at 8.7 per 100,000; New Zealand reported 1.7 deaths per 100,000 births). The United States is the only developed nation that does not offer paid parental leave (Pew Research Center, 2019). Clearly, the United States is lacking in supporting pregnant individuals; it is no surprise then that there is no research exploring the impact of behavioural addiction during pregnancy.

DOI: 10.4324/9781003203476-7

Behavioural addictions and substance addictions share many similarities in etiologies and experiences; individuals with both types of addiction report similar course (chronic, relapse history, and origin prior to adulthood), symptomatology (e.g., cravings, experience of a "high," tolerance, comorbidities), and even similar brain reactivity (e.g., involvement of the serotonergic and/or dopaminergic systems; Alavi et al., 2012; Grant et al., 2010). Both behavioural and substance addictions also respond to similar treatment approaches, such as Cognitive Behavioural Therapy or 12-Step Meetings (Alavi et al., 2012). In a comparison between behavioural addiction (specifically food addiction) and substance addiction in women, Hardy et al. (2017) noted that there are many overlapping components of cause and course between substance addictions and behavioural addictions. These include trauma exposure, a comorbid mental health condition such as depression, and emotional dysregulation. In Hardy's study, comparisons were made between women who had experienced trauma and had no addiction, experienced trauma and had a substance addiction, and experienced trauma and had a food addiction. In the sample, the women who had a substance addiction and those who endorsed the behavioural addiction were more similar in their posttraumatic stress disorder symptom severity, depression severity, and emotional dysregulation compared to the women who had no addiction concerns (Hardy et al., 2017). Given these similarities, it seems likely that at least some of the challenges and consequences of substance addiction during pregnancy could translate to the experience of behavioural addiction during pregnancy.

More than a decade ago, it was estimated that approximately 225,000 infants per year may have been exposed to illicit substances in utero (Keegan et al., 2010), and there is evidence that substance use in pregnancy is on the rise in the United States. In the 2019 National Survey of Drug Use and Health (NSDUH) conducted by the Substance Abuse and Mental Health Services Administration (SAMHSA), 12.6% of pregnant women reported that they had used alcohol or illicit drugs in the past month. When tobacco was included, that percentage went up to 18.4% (SAMHSA, 2020). The use of substances during pregnancy can have an impact on both the fetus and the pregnant woman; some consequences include spontaneous abortion, birth defects, and developmental delays (Keegan et al., 2010). Approximately 12–15% of people continue to smoke during pregnancy and the likelihood of spontaneous abortion in these individuals is approximately 20–80% higher when compared to those who do not smoke during pregnancy (Keegan et al., 2010). Consider the impact of direct and second-hand smoke on the fetus and pregnant woman, particularly in those who may be engaging in gambling within settings such as casinos. According to a summary report from the CDC, 50% of casinos (where smoking was permitted) included in an air sample study had pollution at levels known to put one at risk for cardiovascular disease after 2 hours (CDC, n.d.). The average person gambling (in Las Vegas) spends approximately 2–4 hours in the casino during any given visit which could be putting pregnant gamblers at risk for cardiovascular disease in addition to the other risks of first- and/or second-hand smoke (Las Vegas Convention and Visitors Association, n.d.).

Even with the potential negative consequences of drug use during pregnancy, some women struggle to abstain from their use while pregnant. Women have reported ambivalence – both related to their pregnancy and toward abstinence from their addiction (Soderstrom, 2012). One theory posited for this was related to an attachment-like relationship; that in times of stress or pain, an individual may turn toward their addiction for relief or numbing and this may not be an available option when one is pregnant and/or parenting a newborn. In speaking with a group of women about the reasons why they have previously continued or had currently discontinued their use of substances during their pregnancies, Latuskie et al. (2019) reported that ongoing stressors and a desire for escapism (particularly for numbing) were reasons the women continued using. Another qualitative study with pregnant women highlighted another difficulty with discontinuation of the use of substances: the women lost a key component of their social network (Soderstrom, 2012). They felt alone and without social support. This lack of support left some of the pregnant women considering returning to use just so they would not feel so alone.

According to Konkoly Thege et al. (2016), addiction-related problems often have comorbidities with other problems, such as mental health diagnoses and other addictions. Within the study sample of 1,382 females, 61.8% reported having a single substance and/or behavioural addiction problem, 25.3% reported struggling with two addictions, and 13.3% reported struggling with three or more addiction-related problems (Konoly Thege et al., 2016). This highlights the importance of screening for both substance and behavioural addictions in women based on the prevalence of multiple problems. While obstetric providers may be screening for drug or alcohol use in pregnancy, it is unlikely that they are screening for behavioural addictions unless a specific concern has been raised during a medical visit. Without appropriate screening and identification, specific treatments to address the addiction-related problems cannot be implemented.

When a pregnant woman is struggling with behavioural addiction or a substance addiction (or both), it is important for providers to understand the nuances that accompany these comorbidities. Many of the women included in Soderstrom's (2012) study reported that their journey toward motherhood did not always feel safe or exciting and several reported that they feared what would happen when they gave birth. A common reason cited for this was that they had older children who had been removed from their custody. While this might not be as common of an occurrence in individuals who solely experience behavioural addictions (versus substance addictions), a fear of consequences related to their addiction and impact on the person's life is understandable. Jansson et al. (1996) summarize it well: "one cannot address pregnancy needs without considering the woman's drug abuse, as she would be more at risk for sexually transmitted diseases, premature delivery, etc." (p. 323). This holds true regardless of type of addiction; while the individual may not be directly exposing the fetus to substances such as cocaine or alcohol, the actions of the woman engaging in behavioural addictions (such as compulsive sex or gambling) may still have an impact on that woman's health and the health of the fetus. The fetus may still be exposed to nicotine via second-hand smoke if the pregnant woman is in a casino or may experience effects related to a sexually transmitted infection obtained by the pregnant woman during a compulsive sexual encounter. Both the pregnant woman and the fetus can experience medical problems secondary to gestational diabetes should that pregnant woman also be struggling with a food addiction which causes their gestational diabetes to be poorly controlled. Consider another potential commonality: the financial cost of maintaining an addiction (be it something like opioids or gambling), which may lead in turn to housing, food, or other related insecurity. Soderstrom found a similar theme when she interviewed pregnant women, "Pregnancy and early motherhood provide a unique opportunity for change. However, the mother-to-be is not helped unless the interventions manage to combine the best interests of the woman with the well-being of the child" (2012, p. 465).

A goal of obstetric care is to establish open and non-threatening communication between the care team and the woman giving birth; this is especially true in woman with an addiction, as these individuals may have preconceived mistrust or fear of providers involved in their care (related to fear of consequences to them or to their infant). Women who are pregnant and who have an addiction may also experience barriers to care. The woman may have medical or mental health concerns independent of their pregnancy and they may be experiencing some difficulties including poor self-esteem, body image issues, and challenges forming secure/stable relationships with close others (Jansson et al., 1996). They may also experience logistical concerns including lack of access to adequate food, shelter, and childcare for existing children as well as transportation issues getting to/from appointments (Jansson et al., 1996). The women in Latuskie et al.'s (2019) study suggested that self-efficacy and positive, non-judgmental relationships with care providers were key to helping them discontinue and maintain abstinence from their addiction. These women were also asked what they would recommend to providers to help other pregnant people and they suggested screening and easy-to-access resources (or knowledge of resources, such as a pamphlet with treatment information; Latuskie et al., 2019). These are easily translatable to behavioural addictions and could play a key role in improving the knowledge about the prevalence and impact of behavioural addiction during pregnancy.

It may be possible that behavioural addictions do not have a direct impact on pregnancy, pregnant individuals, and infants. Given the information on substance addiction and pregnancy and the parallels between substance and behavioural addictions, this is unlikely. Future research that either specifically samples or seeks to include pregnant women is important to understand the overall impact of behavioural addictions during pregnancy. Additionally, it is important to acknowledge that topics covered in this chapter may apply to those who are pregnant and who do not identify as women; such individuals are likely even more overlooked than pregnant women. Future research should include and address the concerns of all pregnant individuals who may be experiencing the impact of behavioural addictions. With an increase in knowledge, treatments may be developed and implemented to best support those individuals who struggle with a behavioural addiction during pregnancy. Without more information about the potential risks and consequences of behavioural addictions during pregnancy, providers cannot offer the best possible care to their struggling pregnant clients. As the women in Latuskie et al.'s (2019) study requested, we must be able to offer appropriate support and resources to support pregnant individuals and their children.

References

Alavi, S.S., Ferdosi, M., Jannatifard, F., Eslami, M., Alaghemandan, H., & Setare, M. (2012). Behavioral addiction versus substance addiction: Correspondence of psychiatric and psychological views. *International Journal of Preventive Medicine, 3*(4), 290–294.

Center for Disease Control(n.d.). STATE system. Retrieved from https://www.cdc.gov/statesystem/factsheets/gaming/Gaming.html

Center for Disease Control (2021). National vital statistics reports, *3*(2). Retrieved from https://www.cdc.gov/nchs/data/nvsr/nvsr70/nvsr70-02-508.pdf

Commonwealth Fund (2020). Maternal mortality and maternity care in the United States compared to 10 other developed countries. Retrieved from https://www.commonwealthfund.org/publications/issue-briefs/2020/nov/maternal-mortality-maternity-care-us-compared-10-countries

Grant, J.E., Potenza, M.N., Weinstein, A., & Gorelick, D.A. (2010). Introduction to behavioral addictions. *The American Journal of Drug and Alcohol Abuse, 36*(5), 233–241. doi:10.3109/00952990.2010.491884.

Hardy, R., Fani, N., Jovanovic, T., & Michopoulos, V. (2017). Food addiction and substance addiction in women: Common clinical characteristics. *Appetite, 120*, 367–373. doi:10.1016/j.appet.2017.09.026

Jansson, L. M., Svikis, D., Lee, J., Paluzzi, P., Rutigliano, P., & Hackerman, F. (1996). Pregnancy and addiction: A comprehensive care model. *Journal of Substance Abuse Treatment, 13*(4), 321–329.

Keegan, J. K., Parva, M., Finnegan, M., Gerson, A., & Belden, M. (2010). Addiction in pregnancy. *Journal of Addictive Diseases, 29*(2), 175–191. doi:10.1080/10550881003684723

Konkoly Thege, B., Hodgins, D.C., & Wild, C. (2016). Co-occurring substance-related and behavioral addiction problems: A person-centered, lay epidemiology approach. *Journal of Behavioral Addictions, 5*(4), 614–622. doi:10.1556/20065.2016.079.

Las Vegas Convention and Visitors Authority(n.d.). *Facts about Las Vegas*. Retrieved from https://www.lvcva.com/.

Latuskie, K.A., Andrews, N.C.Z., Motz, M., Leibson, T., Austin, T., Ito, S., & Pepler, D.J. (2019). Reasons for substance use continuation and discontinuation during pregnancy: a qualitative study. *Women and Birth*, *32*, e57–e64. doi:10.1016/j.wombi.2018.04.001

Pew Research Center (2019). Among 41 countries, only the U.S. lacks paid parental leave. Retrieved from https://www.pewresearch.org/fact-tank/2019/12/16/u-s-lacks-mandated-paid-parental-leave/

Soderstrom, K. (2012). Mental preparation during pregnancy in women with substance addiction: A qualitative interview-study. *Child & Family Social Work*, *17*, 458–467. doi:10.1111/j.1365-2206.2011.00803.x

Substance Abuse and Mental Health Services Administration [SAMHSA] (2020). National Survey on Drug Use and Health 2019. Retrieved from https://datafiles.samhsa.gov

Part III

South America

Chapter 5

COVID-19 and What Was Not Grieved in the Woman Addicted to Gambling

Deborah Blanca

Through storytelling, this chapter will articulate theory about and clinical aspects of gambling addiction among Argentinian women. This "tour" will include some reflections on the effects of the COVID-19 pandemic, quarantine, the closure of gambling venues, and their subsequent reopening.

Introduction

In Argentina, gambling venues are inhabited by many solitary women. "Solitary" does not mean that they do not have family or friends. They are women with a strong feeling of emptiness, renouncement, depression, dissatisfaction, and rejection from everyone. Frequently, they are women who feel disappointed and betrayed (for example, by a partner's infidelity), and an unconscious thirst for revenge pushes them toward the slot machine.

In gambling, we should not talk about the gambling venue but rather about the *Kingdom of Oblivion*. Addicted gamblers seek to erase what they feel is their source of suffering – a powerful forgetfulness under the effects of the machine, only resulting in a ravaged resolution.

Aided by lights, noises, and all the rituals related to gambling, and dissociated through magical beliefs, the feeling of guilt and the unconscious need for punishment, those women bear their life – more and more devitalized, but they endure. Gambling offers them a "solution," but at the same time alienates and makes them sick.

They are the *Queens of Oblivion*. They are queens, but also subordinates who are suffering the dependence on a significant other in their life, a dependence displaced in gambling. With each bet, some of the tension resulting from a memory full of bitterness and dissatisfaction is released.

In Argentina, there are many great women, grandmothers, who spend hours and hours in front of a slot machine or bingo cards in the community gambling space. Many of them were housewives, and following common life changes, such as children gaining independence or becoming widowed, they began to gamble. Others are not widowed, but their husbands are very ill and

DOI: 10.4324/9781003203476-9

deteriorate in their house or in a nursing home. In gambling, they find a powerful distractor from anguish, loneliness, and guilt.

Some women have worked their entire lives, are now retired, and don't know what to do with their time. Others suffered illnesses of their own or in their loved ones (children, grandchildren) – illnesses that could not be processed, getting stuck in the middle of an emotional process.

Other women are very lonely because they never nurtured their ties, either because they belong to a generation that prioritized the endogamous over the exogamous, or because their personality did not favor the formation and maintenance of friendship ties.

All these women find in the *Kingdom of Oblivion* a place of belonging, the only place for which they embellish when they leave their home.

Elena's Story

At the beginning of the chapter, I mentioned that I would articulate theoretical and clinical aspects of gambling addiction in women through storytelling. Many years ago, I wrote a story with the lead character Elena, a great woman, grandmother, and *Queen of Oblivion*. I will repeat parts of this story here, and I will tell an end adapted to the current COVID-19 times to illustrate some of Elena's ups and downs: her abstinence, her stumbles, and relapses; her bond with her children, her dreams, and nightmares; her "non-grieved" losses and the beginning of therapy; the pandemic, the forced isolation, and her efforts to adapt.

Let's start with the story then:

There are no doubts, Elena had lied to Ernesto and Camilo, her children, in these latest years, more precisely, after Alberto, her husband, died.

She claimed that the tenants of Almagro's apartment owed her three months' rent and she was falling behind with paying off her debts. And she was helping Paulina, her best friend, pay for her alcoholic son's treatment. Or she had less food in the fridge because she preferred going out to grab a bite.

Neither the tenants were late, nor did Paulina ask for money for the treatment of her son, and nor was she eating out. Although, the last one was not entirely a lie, but it was a particular "out." The restaurant was always the same, inside the Bingo Hall.

When they discovered the lies on November 2, 2018, they could not believe it. Elena told them, trying to make the matter sound less dramatic, she sometimes went to the slot machines, she did it some afternoons when she was bored, but that was not so bad.

Ernesto and Camilo looked at her without recognizing her. Their look distressed Elena, and she then went from an unemotional story to a sobbing one.

"I miss dad, you can't imagine how I miss him. I am lost, I feel very lonely! I'm alone. A-L-O-N-E!" Elena yelled. "You barely come to visit me, the boys hardly ever call me on the phone, and when I visit, they hang out with those filthy little gadgets that make them look like idiots."

"Like the machines you gamble on, right?" Camilo said ironically as he glanced at her.

"Yes, like the machines, but I'm not an idiot all the time. I realize it takes money from me, I even get bored sometimes ... ."

"Are you bored?" Ernesto interrupted, surprised. "Really? If you get bored, you lose money, now you also lie, then, why do you go?"

Ernesto, I'm going because I'm alone. My brother Silvio is in the nursing home, he hardly recognizes me anymore. Every time I go to visit him, I go out cursing against god. He always was a brilliant man, now he repeats four or five sentences: 'Is it hot outside?', 'That haircut looks nice on you.', 'Nobody touches the books in my library, right?' And a couple more. Your dad died like that, suddenly, I didn't even have time to say goodbye. He entered the clinic, he told me 'Here they operated on my old father and he died, why the hell did they send me here? Bingo!'. You two, with your lives, your families ... .

There was a pause; it was necessary to breathe deeply and stop talking. A stage inhabited by absences, pain, and loneliness had been installed. The opacity of loneliness shone like a razor's edge.

Elena had lied to Ernesto and Camilo for some time, and she did it to continue gambling, and to not be questioned, to have a secret.

She lied, like all addicts. Nothing interested her anymore, she had isolating herself from her affections. She was furious about the unwanted absences: Alberto's death, Silvio's dementia.

Elena felt a victim of her destiny. Destiny was taking revenge on her, or so she believed, by introducing her to her accomplice: the slot machine. And while she was losing money, she was gaining meaning in life. The adrenaline of not being detected, of making up stories. Dressing up and combing her hair to gamble, talking to the neighbors, to the waitresses, of whom she memorized the names, their children's names, and even their Zodiac sign. And the waitresses smiled at her when they saw her come in and asked her about her grandchildren and the recipe for *empanadas*,[1] which, according to Elena, were so delicious.

But one day what had to happen at some point, happened: she was exposed. And after some time of never-before-spoken angry words, and rebukes, and acceptance of Ernesto helping her manage her retirement money, things began to get better.

After 2 months, one night Elena dreamed about Alberto. Her dream was this: he called her with that loving voice as he used to. She was looking for him and looking for him and where did she find him? Yes, in the Bingo Hall, right next to her usual slot machine. She awoke upset, distraught. She cried for a long time, and without having breakfast and barely combing her hair, she went to gamble. She lost the little money she had with her, which she found in the kitchen box. She returned to her house extremely anguished and ashamed, especially ashamed. After thinking about it for a while, she called Ernesto. She asked him about that psychologist whom he had told her about, a friend of a friend of his wife, "the one who attends to those who gamble."

They arranged for a first meeting. Ernesto escorted Elena to the door, but for the second session, he came along with her and Camilo. And they talked. They began treatment with Alma, the psychologist. Elena went to see her every week. And they also had family sessions.

Sharing each of their versions of different family moments, putting words to what had been mute and loaded with hostility and guilt, was healing. Alma offered Elena tenderness, she tucked her in, and she also pointed out some repetitions in her story, those rocks she had stumbled over more than once. But she did it with a balance between sweet and challenging, and with a sense of humor she made Elena, who had never discussed her things with a therapist, want to come back the following week. In some sessions, she cried a lot; in others, she got angry. In several she laughed.

One day Elena gambled again, and she had severe headaches afterward, accompanied by vomiting. She canceled a session, but upon Alma's insistence and the effect of an analgesic that Camilo gave her, she returned. She didn't tell her about her relapse right away, she tried to hide it, disguise it, but she was finally able to talk about it. With shame, regret, and she was angry too, but she did it. Alma restrained her, helped her think about some things, and reminded her that stopping gambling is not magic, but that she is on the right track and should stop punishing herself. Relieved, Elena followed her sessions continuously. And she also decided that, facing a nearing family reunion for the New Year 2019, she would cook the *vitel-tonné*[2] her grandchildren enjoyed so much.

One morning in February 2020, while preparing *mate,*[3] Elena watched the news. She heard something strange was happening in Europe, a virus called *Coronavirus* was killing so many people. Masks, confinement, terror; Elena frowned. She could not stop watching the news, and she was not surprised when in March, when the country faced the first cases of infection, the government decided on quarantine. Life became unimaginable. Elena was very scared, scared to death of catching it and dying alone in a hospital.

Two months after that, her fear turned to anger and rebellion against the measures that had left her locked up. Her isolation made her feel bad, she missed hugging her children, her grandchildren, visiting Silvio at the nursing home, for whom she was also very worried. She couldn't go to Alma's office neither. She proposed to have the sessions by video call, but Elena did not want it that way; she resisted saying it was useless, that she was going to be able to do it by herself. And once again, after Alma's tender insistence and Ernesto's and Camilo's request, she accepted. They taught her how to make video calls on WhatsApp (Elena was a quick learner), and they also resumed the bonding sessions. She was relieved, even though she didn't say it.

Another study conducted among women in the Peruvian highlands identified, through references from health professionals, "a high consumption of alcohol among women, which led to deaths from liver cirrhosis or aspiration pneumonia."

In Lima, in 2002, 1.4% of 145 women reported sexual violence by a coworker, while in Cuzco, 5.3% of 207 women reported this type of violence. Pregnant women do not escape situations of violence, which aggravates the situation, if we consider that violence against a pregnant woman can have serious consequences for the mother and the fetus.

Some studies show that abused women use drugs (alcohol, sedatives, marijuana, etc.), both at home and at work, which causes headaches, insomnia, gastrointestinal disturbances, and psychological suffering. The use of drugs, especially tranquillizers, sedatives, and relaxants, is often an escape mechanism.

The use and abuse of alcohol and illicit drugs among nonviolent people is prevalent. However, these substances are also present in many situations of violence – used by aggressors and victims. Some studies have shown that there is an association between drug use and violence experienced both at home and at work.

There is evidence of a growing prevalence of violence associated with drug use in Latin America. The phenomenon of economic globalization may be aggravating the problem by facilitating increased access to the drug market, diversifying production sources, and increasing demand among different population groups, including women.

Many women are initiated into drug use by their partners, as a way of maintaining their relationship or because they were forced to do so, and if they start treatment, this is often boycotted by their abusive partner. Immersed in a relationship of relational dependence, women often justify their abuse by their consumption behaviour or relapses.

On the other hand, there are independent women who, because of hypercompetitive work environments, begin to consume substances to tolerate the stress of having to manage multiple roles in a society that does not make room for them. In both cases, the situation is complex (UNODC, 2005, 2016).

Drug use in women can be triggered by different situations: coping with a problem, relaxing, combating boredom, frustration, unsatisfactory sexual relations, trying to achieve weight loss, dysfunctional families, economic difficulties, and many others. Violence and drug use often go hand in hand. Experiences of violence usually begin in childhood, with child sexual abuse (CSA), traumas that later configure Post Traumatic Stress Disorders (PTSD), and other mental health pathologies. In most Latin American countries there are agreements dedicated to preventing violence against women and drug abuse, but the governments do not comply with them because they do not guarantee a life free of violence for women.

Conclusions

Although progress has been made in terms of equal opportunities for genders, the gap is still wide. Gender stereotypes and prejudices circulate both among patients and clients themselves and among mental health professionals. There is a need for shelters and addiction treatment centers, and specific programs for battered drug users.

IPV is a health problem with a high prevalence, and numerous acute and chronic mental and physical health conditions are associated with it. Future studies are needed to better describe the prevalence of IPV, its distribution across major racial/ethnic and economic groups, and societal factors that promote or protect against violence, especially in underdeveloped countries.

References

Boira, S., et al. (2016). Fear, conformity and silence. Intimate partner violence in rural areas of Ecuador. *Psychosocial Intervention, 25*(2016), 9–17

Caldentey, C. et al. (2017). Intimate partner violence among female drug users admitted to the general hospital; screening and prevalence. *Adicciones, 29*(3), 172–179.

DEMUS (2022). *Study For The Defense Of The Women S Rights.* PERU

Llopis, J. (2005). Use of drugs and gender violence in addict women in Europe. Keys for the comprehension and intervention. *Revista Salud y Drogas, 5*(2), 137–158.

Martínez, V.T., & Marín, Y.H. (2009). The gender psychological violence is a hidden way of aggression. *Revista Cubana de Medicina General Integral.*

Najavits, L.M. et al (2002). "Seeking safety": Outcome of a new cognitive behavioral psychotherapy for women with posttraumatic stress disorder and substance dependence. *J T J Trauma Stress*, 1998 Jul.

Pontón Cevallos, J. (2009). Femicidio en el Ecuador: realidad latente e ignorada. [Femicide in Ecuador: latent and ignored reality]. FLACSO sede Ecuador. *Programa de Estudios de la Ciudad*, 4–9.

Rivas-Rivero, B., Algovia, E., & Vasquez, J.J. (2020). Risk factors associated with drug abuse and women o victims of violence in a poverty context. *Annals of Psichology, 36* (1 Jan), 173–180.

Sirvent, C. (2005). Gender differences in. Revista Salud y Drogas. Addiction and therapeutics implications. *Revista Salud y Drogas, 5*(2), 81–98.

Tenorio, J. & Marcos, J. (2000). Dual disorders; tratamiento and coordination. *Revista Papeles del Psicologo, 2000*(77), 7758'63

United Nations Office on Drugs and Crime, UNODC (2005, 2016). Peru, Ecuador and the southern subregion cone. *Global Program Treatment and Attention for Drug Abuse.*

Part IV

Asia

Chapter 7

Family and Social Relationships during Recovery – Perspectives of Israeli Women Overcoming Gambling Disorder

Belle Gavriel-Fried and Tal Damari

Women with gambling disorder (GD) cope with many challenges during their recovery including shame, guilt, and the social stigma attached to them as women who betrayed their traditional gender roles. This chapter shows how women who have recovered from GD depict and re-establish their relationships in recovery. Twelve Israeli women aged 45–71 were interviewed. They described how they actively repositioned themselves in family relationships as spouses and mothers, changed their communication patterns and interactions with their loved ones, and developed friendships with members of support groups. These findings are interpreted through two theoretical lenses: social capital and self-in-relation.

Introduction

Recovery from addictive disorders is a holistic multistage process of change that includes re-gaining voluntarily sustained control over addictive behaviours, and improving and maximizing physical health and well-being (Ashford et al., 2019; Inanlou et al., 2020). An individual's community, family, and social relationships are crucial parts of this process as well (Cloud & Granfield, 2008). As is the case for other addictive behaviours, recovery from gambling disorder (GD) is a difficult process during which individuals encounter obstacles while also experiencing personal growth and re-integrating into society (Gavriel-Fried & Lev-el, 2020, 2021; Pickering et al., 2020).

Women who have recovered from addictive disorders face different challenges and have different needs than men (Andersson et al., 2020; Neale et al., 2014). Previous studies on recovery of women with GD indicate they deal with feelings of shame and guilt, public gendered stigma, and fear of losing custody of their children (Brandt & Wöhr, 2017; Iliff, 2009; Kushnir et al., 2016; Rogers et al., 2020).

Social support, including family and friends, is perceived as one of the key recovery capital resources that help people recover from addiction (Cloud & Granfield, 2008). Social recovery capital provides valuable resources to the

DOI: 10.4324/9781003203476-12

individual through participation in social networks (Boeri et al., 2016). Previous studies have shown that during recovery, individuals tend to restore their conflictual relationships with their families (Binde, 2012). The few studies on recovery processes of women with GD show that these women tend to use informal support systems such as Gamblers' Anonymous (GA) (Avery & Davis, 2008; Davis & Avery, 2004; McGowan, 2003). They are motivated to stop gambling to be able to resume their traditional gender roles as caregivers (Avery & Davis, 2008). Karter (2014) highlighted mutual aid, and connections between women as basic elements that help women to recover. In a study on recovery capital resources in 91 Israelis who recovered from GD (22 were women) a high percentage (62.64%) mentioned family support as an important recovery capital resource (Gavriel-Fried & Lev-el, 2020).

Aim and Context of This Study

This chapter examines the social relationships formed by Israeli women during their recovery, based on a broader qualitative study conducted in Israel from 2018–2019, which included 12 women with lifetime GD ranging in age from 45–71 (M = 58). They had been in recovery for a year to ten years. The women were recruited through rehabilitation centers, and gave their written informed consent before engaging in in-depth interviews. All names in this chapter are pseudonyms. This study was approved by the Institutional Review Board of Tel Aviv University.

Women's expected gender roles in Israel are still constructed around being wives and mothers (Fogiel-Bijaoui & Rutlinger-Reiner, 2013). According to the Global Gender Gap Index for 2020, Israel was ranked 64 out of 153 countries. This inequality may derive from the combination of traditional and modern features of Israeli society (Bystrov, 2012) where many recent laws protecting women's rights relate to institutional disparities and not to personal equality (Pershitz, 2019). The social expectation that women should fulfill their gender roles as mothers and wives in addition to the social stigma attached to women with gambling disorder (Lesieur & Blume, 1991) is likely to impact their motivation to apply for treatment and may hinder their recovery process (Baxter et al., 2016). On the other hand, Israeli society is characterized by its strong pro-family orientation (Gavriel-Fried & Shilo, 2017) which may facilitate family closeness and support in recovery.

Findings

This chapter focuses on the relationships built by women who have recovered from GD, and re-established with their surroundings during their recovery. Content analysis showed that the relationships they formed during recovery were continually compared to their relationships during the period of addiction in terms of couplehood, motherhood, and relations with their expanded social circles.

For the women in recovery, couplehood was characterized by changing patterns of communication with their partners. This was reflected in the transition from a communication pattern characterized by lies, concealment of gambling, and broken promises to stop gambling, to a pattern of sharing and open communication during the recovery period.

Ruth (53, married) described the period of addiction:

I deceived my husband [...] even though he realized that I was exaggerating, he didn't have any idea about the financial disaster. I managed the bank account. He only knew that our financial situation was not good. He always said, "I don't understand why we are always in a crazy overdraft. Why is the bank calling all the time?" And I told him, "Sweetheart, you don't earn enough, you are not good enough." ... and he believed it. I managed to persuade him of that too.

The transition from concealment to sharing occurred when she closed off the possibility of returning to gambling: "I told my husband on my one-year milestone that I had finally stopped gambling. I knew that if he found out that I had gone back [to gambling] I would be lost ..."

Motherhood during the period of addiction was linked to daily care routines enacted at an emotional distance. In contrast, motherhood during the period of recovery was described as present and involved, and full of interest and emotion. Efrat (71, married) described her motherhood during the addiction period:

One way or another, I fell into serious gambling and I did not know how to cover my debts, and my children became very angry with me ... Suddenly, I didn't relate to the children in their new situations, such as the army or engagements.

In contrast, Ella (46, married) described motherhood in recovery:

... Once I was very selfish. Today I understand that this is the disease of gambling; nothing was under my control. Today I take responsibility for my family. I cook, I go to parent-teacher meetings. I am patient; a mother that listens.

Ruth (53, married) said she gradually became more present in her children's lives:

The children are my whole life. When I was gambling, I wasn't there at all. When I was in recovery I wasn't there either because physically I wasn't there. I was focused on my recovery, on the fear that I would return to gambling. But my children slowly started to feel a change; although I am very busy, I feed them, I am patient, I see them and their problems.

All the women described motherhood as a source of protection and support that helped them in the recovery process. Dana (69, widow) said that women in recovery are unique in their ability as mothers to fulfill their duties which also apply to recovery:

> *Women persist. [...]. Motherhood strengthens you. You are always thinking, giving to the children or the grandchildren. You mature and you say "wow", look at the treasures I have. What have I done in my life – good children; they were unfortunate to have to go through crises, but we must go on because they see me as a figure that keeps going, that smiles, that moves forward, initiates.*

Orna (53, married) stated frankly that she maintains her recovery by looking after her household: "I try very hard to preserve a full recovery. I try because I have to maintain my home, my children, my family. I am a grandmother."

The two women in the study who did not have children also related to motherhood, stating that if they had been mothers this gender role would have supported them in recovery:

> *Look, couplehood and children provide you with an anchor. You have obligations. I tell myself that if I had had a child perhaps I wouldn't have gotten into a situation in which I gamble. (Yael, 63, single)*

Relationships connected to the period of gambling were contrasted with decisions to make a fresh start in a new social environment in recovery. This new environment included belonging to support groups as part of the recovery process. An important step involved withdrawing from the social environment they had as gamblers in order to distance themselves from the triggers that led to their gambling in the first place or that reminded them of gambling. Michal (46, divorced) described her decision to avoid family members and the social environment that had encouraged her to gamble: "I cut myself off from the 'trash', I got rid of everything negative in my life. Even it was one of the people closest to me. [...] I had to made a clean break ... ."

The components of their social lives that supported recovery included relatives and friends from the past but also new social relationships cultivated during recovery. These relationships developed out of participation in Gamblers Anonymous (GA) groups, individual therapy, group therapy, rehab centers, rehabilitation communities, and others. Yael (age 63, single) who is a member of various support groups said that the friends she has in these groups helped her to overcome the temptation to gamble:

> *I say "thank God" that I go to the GA groups and that I have managed to overcome all of the little temptations. They are constantly telling and writing to me that they love me and friends send words of encouragement – that helps.*

Anat (age 57, widow) had to deal with cancer and the loss of her husband in addition to being addicted and recovering from gambling. She described how taking part in a psychodrama group helped her:

I am constantly looking for some group I can draw strength and energy from and then radiate them outwards – that keeps me going. It's like – what are you going to accomplish alone? Yoga? Dance Pasodoble? It's enough if I tell someone to be strong. Two words! That gives her a lift. That is the strength of […]. Today I am in a psychodrama group. I go home after the workshop and suddenly all of my chakras are open. […]. You aren't flying on drugs or on gambling. You are flying on your spirit, your body and that opens you up.

Discussion

This chapter illustrated how women who have recovered from GD depict and re-establish their relationships in recovery. This involves actively re-positioning themselves in family relationships as spouses and mothers, changing their communication patterns and actual presence with their loved ones, and developing friendships with members of support groups. These relationships, whether with family members or new friends from their wider social circle, start a new chapter in their lives.

The participants compared their present relationships in the period of recovery to acquaintances and friends they had during their gambling period. This comparison enabled them to process the past and gain strengths from their relationships today, thus laying the foundation for recovery. In order to promote the recovery, therapists should work with patients to narratively connect the past and the present to help them avoid alienation from both their pasts and their recovery (McConnell, 2016).

More broadly, the findings here can be interpreted through two theoretical lenses. The first is the concept of social capital, which suggests that forming new relationships and contacts with other people is critical to sustained recovery (Boeri et al., 2016). At the same time, repairing previous ones is necessary, as shown in the current findings, especially with spouses and children. Beyond the support these relationships give to the women, they reported finding strength in their roles as mothers and related to this as a protective factor that enhances their motivation to recover. On the broader social level, this gender role may help women overcome the stigma of "women who gamble," which views them as having abandoned their traditional gender roles as mothers (Lesieur & Blume, 1991). Hence, motherhood is an important element in the recovery process that serves as a bridging capital to society at large.

The participants also described the new relationships they formed in support groups, mainly in GA. Previous studies have highlighted the advantages of GA self-help groups (Schuler et al., 2016), and the fact that women who overcome the barriers to treatment and attend GA do so intensively and frequently (Rogers et al., 2020). Thus, therapists should encourage women to form social relations with people without a background of addictions, given their potential to serve as a bridging recovery capital to society at large (Lyons & Lurigio, 2010).

The concept of self-in-relation (Miller, 1976; Surrey, 1985) provides another theoretical lens. This concept is based on the feminist model of developmental psychology which suggests that a woman's main motivation throughout her life is to establish a basic sense of connection with the other, where the self organizes and develops in the context of meaningful relationships. These relationships can only develop in cases of healthy relationships. This perspective has been validated by studies that probed women with a range of addictions and showed that peer support helps in recovery (Mendoza et al., 2016). Thus, during the recovery period in which the woman is reflecting and healing, social relationships are critically important.

Overall, this chapter shows how relationships in the family and social circles can support women's recovery. It highlights the importance of the gender role of motherhood for recovery. Therapists should thus encourage women in recovery to develop connections with people in society at large.

References

Andersson, C., Wincup, E., Best, D., & Irving, J. (2020). Gender and recovery pathways in the UK. *Drugs: Education, Prevention and Policy*, 1–11.

Ashford, R.D., Brown, A., Brown, T., Callis, J., Cleveland, H.H., Eisenhart, E., ... & Whitney, J. (2019). Defining and operationalizing the phenomena of recovery: A working definition from the recovery science research collaborative. *Addiction Research & Theory*, 27(3), 179–188.

Avery, L., & Davis, D.R. (2008). Women's recovery from compulsive gambling: Formal and informal supports. *Journal of Social Work Practice in the Addictions*, 8(2), 171–191.

Baxter, A., Salmon, C., Dufresne, K., Carasco-Lee, A., & Matheson, F.I. (2016). Gender differences in felt stigma and barriers to help-seeking for problem gambling. *Addictive Behaviors Reports*, 3, 1–8.

Binde, P. (2012). A Swedish mutual support society of problem gamblers. *International Journal of Mental Health and Addiction*, 10, 512–523.

Boeri, M., Gardner, M., Gerken, E., Ross, M., & Wheeler, J. (2016). "I don't know what fun is": Examining the intersection of social capital, social networks, and social recovery. *Drugs and Alcohol Today*.

Brandt, L., & Wöhr, A. (2017). Factors influencing treatment-seeking behavior in female pathological gamblers. *Gambling Disorders in Women: An International Female Perspective on Treatment and Research*, 99, 99–112.

Bystrov, E. (2012). Religion, demography and attitudes toward civil marriage in Israel 1969–2009. *Current Sociology*, 60(6), 751–770.

Cloud, W., & Granfield, R. (2008). Conceptualizing recovery capital: Expansion of a theoretical construct. *Substance Use & Misuse*, 43(12–13), 1971–1986.

Davis, D.R., & Avery, L. (2004). Women who have taken their lives back from compulsive gambling: Results from an online survey. *Journal of Social Work Practice in the Addictions*, *4*(1), 61–80.

Fogiel-Bijaoui, S., & Rutlinger-Reiner, R. (2013). Guest editors' introduction: Rethinking the family in Israel. *Israel Studies Review*, *28*(2), vii–xii.

Gavriel-Fried, B., & Lev-el, N. (2020). Mapping and conceptualizing recovery capital of recovered gamblers. *American Journal of Orthopsychiatry*, *90*(1), 22.

Gavriel-Fried, B., & Lev-el, N. (2021). Negative recovery capital in gambling disorder: A conceptual model of barriers to recovery. *Journal of gambling studies*. 10.1007/s1 0899-021-10016-3

Gavriel-Fried, B., & Shilo, G. (2017). The perception of family in Israel and the United States: Similarities and differences. *Journal of Family Issues*, *38*(4), 480–499.

Iliff, B. (2009). *A womans guide to recovery*. *Simon and Schuster*.

Inanlou, M., Bahmani, B., Farhoudian, A., & Rafiee, F. (2020). Addiction recovery: A systematized review. *Iranian Journal of Psychiatry*, *15*(2), 172.

Karter, L. (2014). *Working with women's groups for problem gambling: Treating gambling addiction through relationship*. London: Routledge.

Kushnir, V., Godinho, A., Hodgins, D.C., Hendershot, C.S., & Cunningham, J.A. (2016). Gender differences in self-conscious emotions and motivation to quit gambling. *Journal of Gambling Studies*, *32*(3), 969–983.

Lesieur, H.R., & Blume, S.B. (1991). *When Lady Luck loses: Women and Compulsive Gambling*.

Lyons, T., & Lurigio, A.J. (2010). The role of recovery capital in the community reentry of prisoners with substance use disorders. *Journal of Offender Rehabilitation*, *49*(7), 445–455.

McConnell, D. (2016). Narrative self-constitution and recovery from addiction. *American Philosophical Quarterly*, 307–322.

McGowan, V. (2003). Counter-story, resistance and reconciliation in online narratives of women in recovery from problem gambling. *International Gambling Studies*, *3*(2), 115–131.

Mendoza, N.S., Resko, S., Wohlert, B., & Baldwin, A. (2016). "We have to help each other heal": The path to recovery and becoming a professional peer support. *Journal of Human Behavior in the Social Environment*, *26*(2), 137–148.

Miller, J.B. (1976). *Toward a new psychology of women*. Boston: Beacon Press.

Neale, J., Nettleton, S., & Pickering, L. (2014). Gender sameness and difference in recovery from heroin dependence: A qualitative exploration. *International Journal of Drug Policy*, *25*(1), 3–12.

Pershitz, A. (2019). The prospective status of women in Israel following a clash between the feminist and religious revolutions in the Israeli army. *Studia Europaea Gnesnensia*, (19), 289–302.

Pickering, D., Spoelma, M.J., Dawczyk, A., Gainsbury, S.M., & Blaszczynski, A. (2020). What does it mean to recover from a gambling disorder? Perspectives of gambling help service users. *Addiction Research & Theory*, *28*(2), 132–143.

Rogers, J., Landon, J., Sharman, S., & Roberts, A. (2020). Anonymous women? A scoping review of the experiences of women in Gamblers Anonymous (GA). *International Journal of Mental Health and Addiction*, *18*(4), 1008–1024.

Schuler, A., Ferentzy, P., Turner, N.E., Skinner, W., McIsaac, K.E., Ziegler, C.P., & Matheson, F.I. (2016). Gamblers anonymous as a recovery pathway: A scoping review. *Journal of Gambling Studies*, *32*(4), 1261–1278.

Surrey, J.L. (1985). *The "self-in-relation": A theory of women's development.* Wellesley College, MA: Stone Center for Developmental Services and Studies.

Chapter 8

Women, Love, and Sexuality in Saudi Arabia

A Window to Our World

Nora Sahly

In this chapter, I share lived personal and clinical experience within my culture with regards to different aspects throughout a woman's daily life, love and sexuality. Together, we will walk in her footsteps way back from where it all started, venture into her encounters, share her thoughts, and face her fears. This comprehensive review delves into challenges toward a healthy, authentic, and safe female sexual health ... A basic human right!

"إِنِّي قَدْ رُزِقْتُ حُبَّهَا "

"Her love had been nurtured in my heart by Allah Himself."
    – Prophet Mohammed Peace Be Upon Him (Sahih Muslim #2435)

Background

Saudi Arabia is located in the Middle East, in the continent of Asia. It embraces a family-based system regulated mainly by the Islamic religion and cultural norms. Our society is divided between traditional Bedouin tribes, desert dwelling nomadic-pastoralists, and the more modernized Urban socialites.

Women had a prominent place in society in the Ancient Arab World. In addition to homemaking and raising children, they were farmers, influencers, teachers, preachers, merchants, rulers, and lovers. In the Arabian Peninsula during the Pre-Islamic era, female infanticide was practiced (وَأَد البنات); fathers consciously burying female newborns to their death. Till date, pinpointing the origin and actual reason behind such an unfortunate practice remains unknown. Proposed reasons mainly circulate around the fear of poverty, shame, and humiliation this "female" may bring upon her family (*AlWatan*, 2020). However, it was when Islam was embraced that these horrendous killings were forbidden and finally ceased.

DOI: 10.4324/9781003203476-13

Islam Honored Women – Then Cultural Takeover

She was granted her rights, privileges, status, and equality. She had freedom over herself and her body. She was given a voice to state her opinion, choose her mate, and work for a living.

Nevertheless, with time cultural shifts predominated. Women became conditioned to be deemed as overprotected objects, property to their men. She merely exists to serve and not be heard, be grateful and not complain. If she needed surgery, she was not allowed to sign for herself, use birth control, nor leave her house to seek treatment without permission of her male legal guardian. The woman still remains a symbol of the "Ultimate Sacrifice." Nowadays, with more awareness, many women have re-claimed their individuality and self-rights, and are empowered toward equality and equity.

Love Is Sustenance

Love was mainly platonic in the Arab world. Expression of love took forms of songs and poems. In the ideal world, a successful fairy tale love story ended in marriage. It would be interesting to look at what is perceived as love in our society. I have translated the 25-item Love Addiction Self-Assessment (LASA) questionnaire – adapted from Patrick Carnes, PhD, Pia Mellody, and Sex and Love Addicts Anonymous' "40 Questions for Self Diagnosis" – to explore the presence and awareness of love addiction in a forthcoming study. To get as much participation and honest answers as possible, it was prepared in a non-identifying digital form.

What about Sex? Opening Pandora's Box

"All that is Prohibited is Desired" – a well-known Arabic proverb. Curiosity is one of the most basic biological drives of our behaviors. With something unfamiliar to us, our brain becomes dopamine-charged with the "Desire" hormone. This lights up certain areas in the brain and brings up a feeling of deprivation and a desire to explore. This excitement continues till the secret is learned (Gruber et al., 2014; Jepma et al., 2012).

Sex is a taboo in the Arab world. It is portrayed mainly as a reproductive function and is delineated in Islam as an expression of feelings and emotions through connected bodies. Culturally, it is also described as an outlet for a man's energy. Elderly and widowed women perceive themselves as "too old for sex." Some elect surgical closure of their vagina (Colpocleisis) to address its prolapse. The views and attitudes of women toward sex across different age groups and martial statuses are highly variable.

Fantasy and Seduction

Feminine seduction is universal, and her modesty was viewed as most seductive. In the Middle East, women's sensuality is stereotyped as enticement with the whole lavish 1001 Arabian night theme. Today with worldwide traveling and widespread media, Arabs fantasize about various TV stars, living a love story, having passionate sex, and some with kink involved; specifically, consensual binding, humiliation, and spanking. However, it is vital to educate that porn, despite its wide variety, is somewhat exaggerated and leads to unrealistic expectations.

What do women perceive as attractive and sexy in their partner? This would be another interesting topic to explore, using sexual fantasy scales. This may provide leeway for sensual cosplay and other methods to bridge differences and create varying states of mystery and adventure.

Sex Education

Information about sex is considered "forbidden knowledge" that opens a girl's eyes to a tarnished world. Most of the information is acquired from peers, TV, social media, and porn. It is important to note that the Saudi Arabian cyberspace is filtered by a nationwide firewall that blocks users from directly entering porn sites. Therefore, analytics concerning statistics of porn site use are inaccurate. Problematic porn use among women here remains unknown.

Most parents are uncomfortable discussing sex. In my opinion, sex education taught in schools was "Sex Horrification." There is no structured curriculum discussing inappropriate touch, safe sex, birth control, and vetting a partner. This is not advocating promiscuity but rather safeguarding and promoting responsibility.

Virginity and Chastity "The Hidden Pearl"

Women are analogous to "The Hidden Pearl" (اللؤلؤ المكنون) pampered and protected in her shell. Virtuosity is a burden placed on the family from the moment a female is born. In some communities, honor killings are carried out to "cleanse" the shame.

It is important to be very cautious when approaching virgin patients. Never perform an internal vaginal examination nor take internal samples in the clinic, even if the patient insists or yells, beware of getting emotional when a mother is bringing her young daughter to your clinic to "check her," and ALWAYS have a chaperone. Examination of virgins may be performed, under general anesthesia for specific indications, such as intersex condition, with specific consents in place for medico-legal purposes, as a breached virginity complaint comes with serious detrimental social and legal consequences. Having said that, rectal examinations may be performed in cases of bleeding to check for any lacerations resulting from sodomization, and referral to authorities and forensic specialists.

Forbidden Fruit Is the Sweetest

In our society, any pregnancy outside marriage deems her life and reputation over. Elective abortions are forbidden and illegal but are permitted with extremely narrow indications. The doctor will be faced with a large fine, jail time, and be stripped of their license. Some resort to cover ups, dumpster babies, or infanticides. However, any lady in the reproductive age, even single, presenting with acute lower pelvic pain or going for any elective surgery is to have a pregnancy test. It is pertinent to inform and explain this in a non-stigmatizing way as it is for her safety. An undiagnosed ruptured ectopic pregnancy is a lethal condition which is treatable once diagnosed. Dealing with the aftermath socially is another issue.

Female Genital Cutting/Mutilation

Female genital cutting/mutilation (FGC/M) is performed in certain Arab countries as means to chastity. A woman is deemed inappropriate for marriage unless she has this done. She lives her life unaware of what a usual vulva looks like. There are several types of FGC/M, mild (type 1) seen in women from the Southern region, and a more severe Pharonic (type 3) in women of African origin. Those who remember share details of being taken to a circumcision party by someone they trusted at around 7 years of age, treated with a lot of presents, a new party dress, brightly colored balloons right before being pinned down and botched without any anesthesia. This leads to long-term struggles with post-traumatic stress disorder (PTSD), female sexual dysfunction, particularly sexual pain and lack of orgasm, along with other physical complications. A young 16-year-old (Figure 8.1) presented to us with urinary retention and found to have a completely closed vaginal opening, which was surgically addressed (defibulation) (Rouzi et al., 2014).

Marriage

Marriage is the gateway to sex. This is mostly achieved via arranged marriage. The ideal wife is viewed as a young, virgin lady, who is a first-degree cousin. A woman is deemed suitable to wed once she gets her period at puberty even at the age of 9 – a child with no knowledge of what to expect other than the sole purpose to please and serve. It does not matter what the age of the man is, or how long they remain married. Fortunately, a law was

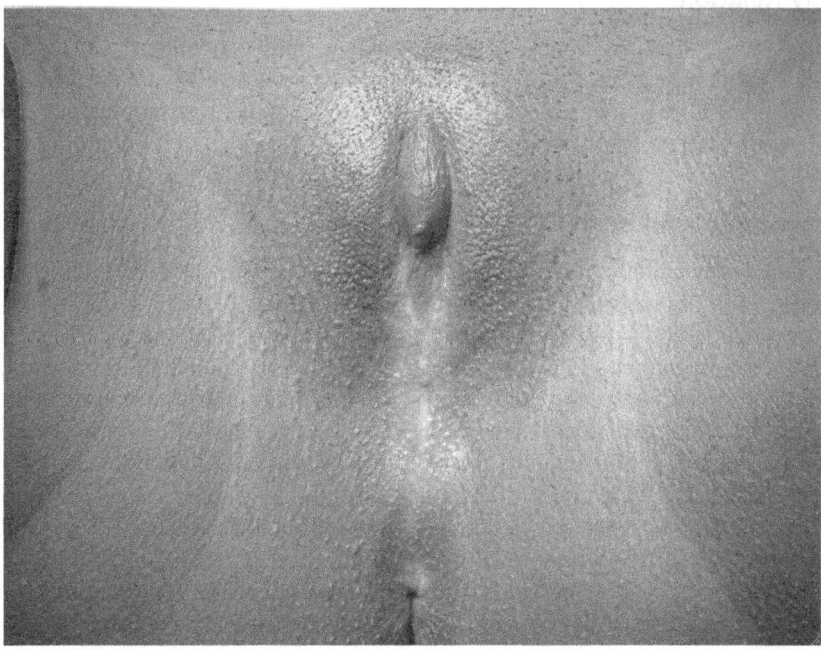

Figure 8.1 The vagina is completely obliterated by the scar resulting from the female genital mutilation procedure.

implemented that bans child marriage and regulates marriages between ages 15 and 18 years through legal courts (Arab News, 2019). When evaluating a couple, it is very important to enquire about consanguinity, inherited diseases, and offer genetic counseling.

Consummation

The sense of establishing virginity is a culture-wide obsession. Traditional (indigenous) consummation (دخلة بلدي) is predominant in some Arabian cultures which also serves the groom's performance anxiety. It involves restraining the bride by a group of women from her family, parting her legs, ferociously penetrating her using the finger of the village midwife or the husband, and staining a white handkerchief or gauze with her blood. After that, it is proudly presented to the whole village as a proof of her virtue and his manhood. Difficulty in consummation due to vaginismus is falsely attributed to having a "thick hymen." This leads some couples to seek consummation within a hospital using sedatives, or surgically. Controversially, non-virgins seek illegal practices which offer re-virginiation procedures.

Poly Relations

In the past, men had many wives, sex slaves, and concubines. Currently, polygamy is restricted to four wives maximum, simultaneously married to the same man. Threesomes are unreported due to religious restrictions, but the fantasy is interesting to explore.

Procreation and Birth Control

Bearing many children is desirable and women are very much attached to their uterus. It symbolizes their fertility and femininity, and women avoid hysterectomy while enduring many years of pain or heavy bleeding. The highest number of pregnancies I have ever seen was 36 total pregnancies in a one lady, and another with 11 caesarean sections. Many women still believe myths that birth control pills will affect their fertility, and they prefer natural options such as outer-course. Unfortunately, men here do not like to use condoms and in their perspective, vasectomy is absolutely out of the question. Aghast was a woman I routinely offered family planning options after her 13th vaginal delivery. Internalized within older generations, a real woman should be quick to get pregnant, have natural pains, unassisted vaginal delivery, no epidural nor painkillers, and breastfeed her child. This, of course, has changed dramatically.

Genital Hygiene and Vulvar Care

Pubic hair removal starts around adolescence. It is done mainly for hygienic and aesthetic reasons. Shaving is the most common method but nowadays laser hair removal is preferred. "Not being ready" by hair removal is one of the most common reasons a woman may refuse or feel uncomfortable to be examined, even by female physicians. Reassurance and release of shame help them get past this, but they are never forced of course.

During menses, a couple may become intimate as long as no period sex is carried out. After bleeding cessation, women are to perform ritual purification showers (Ghusl). It is also customary for women to fumigate their vagina using incense and apply musk. Herbal preparations and folk remedies have a strong place in our culture, especially myrrh and honey for postpartum perineal healing. However, as a medical professional, I am in no position to recommend such practice without high-quality scientific evidence.

Sexual Pleasure

"هُنَّ لِبَاسٌ لَكُمْ وَأَنْتُمْ لِبَاسٌ لَهُنَّ" سورة البقرة (آية ١٨٧)

"Women are enfolding as a garment to you as you are to them."
(Holy Quran, Surat Al-Baraqa, verse 187)

Sexual relations within the vicinity of the marriage are "Sacred." A man and his wife are blessed when they enjoy and satisfy each other in privacy. Initiation is usually by the husband, yet women express desires with suggestive cues. It is customary to start the process with "Bismillah" (in the name of God-Allah). Sex can be in any position as long as it involves vaginal penetration. Furthermore, oral sex is permitted but anal sex is not. Anal sex is resorted to in intersex conditions or single women. Also, some wives present with torn and weak anal sphincter muscles from forceful sodomy by their husbands. Marital rape is not officially recognized in our culture and is not accepted in the Islamic religion. Women have a right to file for divorce if they are abused or not sexually gratified.

Female Sexual Dysfunction

It is customary for women to seek help from female gynecologists, especially for sexual issues. Anonymity and utmost secrecy are important, and clients are reminded of confidentiality. Conflicted, she drags herself carrying considerable shame, guilt, and self-blame to save her marriage, so it is crucial to ask her directly about any issues. Many do not want their husbands to know they came for consultation, and especially that she is the one needing "fixing"!

Most common sexual dysfunctions in the female population include arousal, orgasmic, and genital pain disorders. Arousal issues are due to insufficient clitoral stimulation. Apart from lubricants, women are advised to communicate their desires to their husbands using verbal or tactile methods. Generally, women are reluctant to pleasure themselves. Moreover, sex toys are strictly prohibited in the Kingdom. Suggested by male spouses, some couples utilize porn with the intent to help stimulation. Internalized guilt and shame with underlying Madonna/Whore complex are main reasons behind orgasmic issues. Perceived fear of sex and trauma is behind genital pain. Vaginismus is a major reason for marital frustration, delayed conception, and divorce. One of the major challenges is the ambition for an unrealistic quick fix. Also, special needs and disability populations deserve more attention.

Additionally, sexual compulsion in women is yet to be explored. I have translated the 25-item Women's Sexual Addiction Screening Test (SAST-W)® (copyright of Dr. Patrick Carnes) for this purpose, and seek appropriate permissions to carry out this survey in the future.

Genital Procedures

A large and full vulva is appreciated in our culture and vulvar augmentation is frequently sought. One notable consultation was "To puff it up just like sex movies"! Nonetheless, the most common requested procedure is vaginal tightening, followed by genital and perianal lightening. The "daddy's stitch" (putting in an extra stitch when repairing episiotomies or tearing from birth) is requested by many women electively during a vaginal birth. Recently, there is more awareness in the newer generations with regards to the female pelvic floor, leading to requests of elective cesarean section.

Rising Divorce Rates

Women comprise about 50% of the population in which a third are divorced. There has been a steady rise in the divorce rates all over the Kingdom notably over the last 5 years; seven divorces per hour as illustrated by the most recent national statistical 2020 report by the General Authority for Statistics of Kingdom of Saudi Arabia (2020) and Al-Medina (2020). Reasons behind it include disparities in many economical, educational, social, and sexual aspects. Other reasons are infidelity, abuse, and substance abuse.

Research in Female Sexuality

With limited scientific evidence, there is much to learn. As mentioned earlier, I seek to explore the presence and awareness of love addiction using the LASA in a non-identifying digital form in addition to sexual compulsion using the SAST-W in forthcoming studies. Obtaining approvals and social acceptance for structured research on issues related to female sexuality are more challenging yet vital to provide more clarity and insight to sort out covert issues.

References

Al-Saad M. (2020, September 20). The reality of female infanticide in the pre-Islamic era. *AlWatan Newspaper* [Online]. https://www.alwatan.com.sa/article/1056415.

Divorce is a phenomenon in the Kingdom, 7 cases per hour. (2020, January 28). *Al-Medina*, Article 670129 [Online]. https://www.al-madina.com/article/670129

General Authority for Statistics of Kingdom of Saudi Arabia. (2020). Social statistics; marriage and divorce. https://www.stats.gov.sa/ (English Online) Retrieved July 3, 2021. https://www.stats.gov.sa/sites/default/files/Marriage%20and%20Divorce%20Statistics%202020%20EN.pdf

Gruber, M.J., Gelman, B.D., & Ranganath, C. (2014). States of curiosity modulate hippocampus-dependent learning via the dopaminergic circuit. *Neuron, 84*(2), 486–496. doi:10.1016/j.neuron.2014.08.060.

The Holy Quran. (n.d.). Surat Al-Baraqa, verse 187.

Jepma, M., Verdonschot, R.G., van Steenbergen, H., Rombouts, S.A., & Nieuwenhuis, S. (2012). Neural mechanisms underlying the induction and relief of perceptual curiosity. *Frontiers in Behavioral Neuroscience, 6*, 5. doi:10.3389/fnbeh.2012.00005.

Rouzi, A.A., Sahly, N., Alhachim, E., & Abduljabbar, H. (2014). Type 1 female genital mutilation: A cause of completely closed vagina. *Journal of Sexual Medicine, 11*(9), 2351–2353. doi:10.1111/jsm.12605. Supplemental video: https://onlinelibrary.wiley.com/action/downloadSupplement?doi=10.1111%2Fjsm.12605&file=jsm12605-sup-0001-si.m4v

Sahih Muslim. (n.d.). Book 44: The book of the merits of the companions, Chapter 12: The virtues of Khadijah, the mother of the believers (RA), Hadith 108. Translated version (online) Sunnah.com online, Hadith 2435, https://sunnah.com/muslim:2435b

Saudi Justice Minister Vows Against Underage Marriages. (2019, December 24). *Arab News*, https://arab.news/5vs9h

Chapter 9

Women's Pornography Use in China

Lijun Chen

In this chapter, we described pornography use motivation and prevalence in Chinese men and women, and screening scales for PPU. More than 50% percent women reported use of porn. As for types of online sexual activities, the largest gender difference was observed in "found sexual partners online" and the smallest difference in "flirting and maintaining a relationship." During the COVID-19 pandemic, people's porn use motivations were stress reduction, self-exploration, and fantasy, but men had a stronger motivation to use porn than women. Although existing PPU screening scales weren't originally developed in Chinese samples, several scales were confirmed valid for Chinese women.

Women's Pornography Use in China

Over the past two decades, the revolution in information and communication technology has altered sexual behaviours. The Internet is characterized by a seemingly endless supply of free sexual materials unprecedented in its variety, and especially the arrival of smartphones in 2007 allowed consumers to have greater, more flexible access to pornography (Wood, 2011). In most cases, pornography use is not associated with negative consequences, however, it can become problematic and have a range of negative effects, such as interpersonal difficulties, depression, and sexual functioning problems (Engel et al., 2019; Harper & Hodgins, 2016). With a growing number of individuals involved in excessive porn use who are becoming dysfunctional and developing addiction symptoms (e.g., withdrawal, tolerance), excessive sexual behaviours have been discussed as a clinically significant mental disorder which emerged as a potentially important form of compulsive sexual behaviour disorder (CSBD) (Kafka, 2010; Kraus et al., 2018). The World Health Organization (WHO) has included the diagnosis of CSBD as an impulse control disorder in the International Classification of Diseases (ICD-11). The use of Internet pornography, especially problematic pornography use (PPU), has attracted academic and the public's attention.

The sociocultural context may play an important role in influencing people's attitudes toward sexual behaviours (Griffiths, 2012; Meston et al., 1996) and females' sexual expression (Guo, 2019). Compared with other countries,

DOI: 10.4324/9781003203476-14

sociosexuality was restricted in both sexes in China (Zheng et al., 2014). Although conservative cultures stipulate sexual restriction for both men and women, female sexuality is typically more restricted, especially for girls and unmarried women (Kim, 2009). However, as other researchers proposed, our current understanding of pornography and PPU has cultural limitations since previous studies mainly took place in Western, industrialized countries with predominately Christian samples (Kraus & Sweeney, 2019). It is necessary to understand PPU in China, particularly the use by women, which may reflect the influence of a conservative culture on pornography use.

As for the quantity of pornography use (i.e., usage time and frequency) of Chinese women, they typically consume less pornography than men (Chen et al., 2018a, 2018c; Chi et al., 2012; Zheng & Zheng, 2014), consistent with studies from other countries (Martyniuk et al., 2016). Only 12.2% of women watched no pornography at all in a sample of German women (Kraus et al., 2018) and several studies reported that more than 90% of men reported viewing pornography (Fernandez & Griffiths, 2021; Kafka, 2010; Wéry & Billieux, 2017). In China, according to a survey among college students in 2019, 88.8% of men (350/466) and 67.0% of women (160/342) reported participating in at least one type of online sexual activities in the past 12 months. In this survey, online sexual activities were defined as four types: (1) viewing sexually explicit materials, (2) seeking out sexual partners, (3) cybersex, and (4) flirting and relationship maintaining. Men reported a higher frequency in all online sexual activities. The biggest gender gap was observed in "found sexual partners online" and the smallest difference in "flirting and maintaining a relationship" (Chen et al., 2019). Another survey in an adult community sample showed similar gender differences, but the smallest difference in "viewing sexual explicit materials" (Zheng et al., 2014).

Examining the motivations of pornography use may result in a more detailed understanding of pornography-viewing behaviours including PPU. According to a survey conducted nearly 20 years ago, Chinese college students used pornography for four motivations: freshness and curiosity, satisfaction of sensory stimulation (30.6%); eliminate loneliness, relieve pressure and sexual distress (27.4%); recreation and sex education (32.3%); satisfying psychological sexual needs and improving sexual desire (9.7%) (Yuan, 2004). These findings are similar to more recent results from western permissive cultures (Grubbs et al., 2019).

In 2020, during the outbreak of COVID-19, a Network Comparison Test showed that the characteristics of pornography use motivation in both Chinese men and women were stress reduction, self-exploration, and fantasy, but men have a stronger motivation to use porn than women (Jiang et al., 2022). The fear of COVID-19 may have contributed to this change, because these participants had a high fear of COVID-19 when they watching news and stories about COVID-19 on social media. During the home quarantine restrictions, the Anonymity, Convenience, and Escape (ACE) characteristics of internet pornography promoted the public use of internet porn as a coping strategy, to alleviate the stress caused by the uncertainty of life and anxiety about the epidemic's threat to health (Mestre-Bach et al., 2020). This finding supports the hypothesis that problematic internet pornography use has a unique psychological mechanism based on the characteristics of the internet. On the other hand, this survey indicated that men and women encountered the same stress, but women still demonstrated a lower frequency of pornography use.

In general, pornography use is the consequence of an increased sex desire which is stronger in men than in women because historically an increased sex desire would have promoted men's opportunity of reproducing (Buss, 1995). Furthermore, casual sex (less emotional investment) benefited our ancestors by facilitating their reproductive success (Buss, 2008). China is considerably more conservative and traditional than the West in sexual attitudes and behaviour (Tong, 2013), and a conservative sexual cultural context may contribute to discrepancies. In more conservative cultures, non-marital or recreational sexual activities are often stigmatized, members' sexuality is controlled and the sexuality of an individual, especially a woman's, is tied to family honor (Guo, 2019).

There are two ways for individuals to become exposed to Internet pornography: unintentional exposure (such as "pop-up" advertising Windows containing pornographic pictures) and intentional exposure (such as seeking and browsing pornographic websites on purpose). There is a significant gender difference in the two ways of exposure to pornography. For intentional exposure, male adolescents reported more exposure than females, however, for unintentional exposure, there were no significant differences (Sevcikova et al., 2014). Similar results were found in Taiwan: boys reported more intentional exposure to online pornography than girls, and spent more time on pornography use (Chen et al., 2013). Respondents in more permissive areas reported more intentional exposure, and there were smaller gender differences in intentional exposure; but cultural permissiveness didn't influence the unintentional exposure (Sevcikova et al., 2014).

In the conservative country China, pornography is seen as a difficult issue to talk about, studies on PPU are lacking and there aren't any original screeners/scales to assess PPU. In order to understand the PPU situation in China, researchers have translated several scales, including the Short Internet Addiction Test Adapted to OSAs (s-IAT-sex) (Chen et al., 2018a), the Problematic Pornography Use Scale (PPUS) (Chen et al., 2018c), the Problematic Pornography Consumption Scale (PPCS-18) (Chen et al., 2021), and the Brief Pornography Screener (BPS) (Chen & Jiang, 2020). These screeners were confirmed valid in the Chinese context. In comparison with PPUS and s-IAT-sex, the PPC-18 demonstrated stronger reliability and validity, including criterion validity, as well as greater sensitivity and acceptable specificity (Chen & Jiang, 2020). Moreover, these screeners appeared invariant in the Chinese community of men and women (Chen et al., 2018b, 2021); in other words, these screeners can be used to screen PPU in Chinese women.

Pornography use is prevalent, but the PPU rate varies widely. The PPU prevalence rates range from 0.1% to 13% (Wéry & Billieux, 2017). In a Chinese community sample screened with the PPCS-18, about 9.1% of adult users are prone to PPU (Chen & Jiang, 2020). Consistent with other studies from western cultures (Kafka, 2010; Kraus et al., 2015, 2016), men are more engaged in online pornography than women (Chen et al., 2019) and have higher PPU scores (Chen et al., 2018b). Chinese men are more prone to problematic use, and score higher than women on distress and functional problems, excessive use, self-control difficulties, and use to escape or avoid negative emotions, suggesting that men are more likely to overuse pornography, leading to compulsive use. A multiple mode was used to explore this gender difference. Men showed higher sexual sensation seeking, and they tend to pursue more varied sexual experiences to meet their desire. They also report more sexual arousal, sexual excitement, and masturbation when browsing pornographic materials online with females reporting more avoidance, disgust, or worries. Therefore, males and particularly those high in sexual sensation seeking, may be more likely to seek novel sexual stimulation online which may in turn lead to PPU (Chen et al., 2018c).

References

Buss, D.M. (1995). Psychological sex differences: Origins through sexual selection. *American Psychologist, 50*, 164–168. 10.1037/0003-066X.50.3.164

Buss, D.M. (2008). Human nature and individual differences: Evolution of human personality. In R. W. R. In O.P. John, & L.A. Pervin (Ed.), *Handbook of Personality: Theory and Research* (pp. 29–60). The Guilford Press.

Chen, A.S., Leung, M., Chen, C.H., & Yang, S.C. (2013). Exposure to internet pornography among Taiwanese adolescents. *Social Behavior and Personality: An International Journal, 41*(1), 157–164. 10.2224/sbp.2013.41.1.157

Chen, L., & Jiang, X. (2020). The assessment of problematic internet pornography use: A comparison of three scales with mixed methods. *International Journal of Environmental Research and Public Health, 17*(2), 488. 10.3390/ijerph17020488

Chen, L., Ding, C., Jiang, X., & Potenza, M.N. (2018a). Frequency and duration of use, craving and negative emotions in problematic online sexual activities. *Sexual Addiction & Compulsivity, 25*(4), 396–414. 10.1080/10720162.2018.1547234.

Chen, L., Wang, X., & Chen, S. (2018b). Reliability and validity of the problematic Internet pornography use scale-Chinese version among college students. *Chinese Journal of Public Health, 34*(7), 1034–1038. 10.11847/zgggwslll5589

Chen, L., Yang, Y., Su, W., Zheng, L., Ding, C., & Potenza, M.N. (2018c). The relationship between sexual sensation seeking and problematic Internet pornography use: A moderated mediation model examining roles of online sexual activities and the third-person effect. *Journal of Behavioral Addictions, 7*(3), 565–573. 10.1556/2006.7.2018.77

Chen, L., Jiang, X., & Su, W. (2019). Effect of sexual sensation seeking, the third person effect and gender on online sexual activity among university students. *Chinese Journal of Public Health, 35*(11), 1552–1556. 10.11847/zgggws1119696

Chen, L., Luo, X., Bőthe, B., Jiang, X., Demetrovics, Z., & Potenza, M.N. (2021). Properties of the problematic pornography consumption scale (PPCS-18) in community and subclinical samples in China and Hungary. *Addictive Behaviors, 112,* 106591. 10.1016/j.addbeh.2020.106591.

Chi, X., Yu, L., & Winter, S. (2012). Prevalence and correlates of sexual behaviors among university students: A study in Hefei, China. *BMC Public Health, 12*(1), 1–10. 10.1186/1471-2458-12-972

Engel, J., Kessler, A., Veit, M., Sinke, C., Heitland, I., Kneer, J., ...Kruger, T.H. (2019). Hypersexual behavior in a large online sample: Individual characteristics and signs of coercive sexual behavior. *Journal of Behavioral Addictions, 8*(2), 213–222. 10.1556/2006.8.2019.16.

Fernandez, D.P., & Griffiths, M.D. (2021). Psychometric instruments for problematic pornography use: A systematic review. *Evaluation & the Health Professions, 44*(2), 111–141. 10.1177/0163278719861688.

Griffiths, M.D. (2012). Internet sex addiction: A review of empirical research. *Addiction Research & Theory, 20*(2), 111–124. 10.3109/16066359.2011.588351

Grubbs, J.B., Wright, P.J., Braden, A.L., Wilt, J.A., & Kraus, S.W. (2019). Internet pornography use and sexual motivation: A systematic review and integration. *Annals of the International Communication Association, 43*(2), 117–155. 10.1080/23808985.2019.1584045.

Guo, Y. (2019). Sexual double standards in white and Asian Americans: Ethnicity, gender, and acculturation. *Sexuality & Culture, 23*(1), 57–95. 10.1007/s12119-018-9543-1.

Harper, C., & Hodgins, D.C. (2016). Examining correlates of problematic internet pornography use among university students. *Journal of Behavioral Addictions, 5*(2), 179–191. 10.1556/2006.5.2016.022.

Jiang, X., Lu, Y., Hong, Y., Zhang, Y., & Chen, L. (2022). A network comparison of motives behind online sexual activities and problematic pornography use during the COVID-19 outbreak and the post-pandemic period. *International Journal of Environmental Research and Public Health, 19*(10), 5870. 10.3390/ijerph19105870.

Kafka, M.P. (2010). Hypersexual disorder: A proposed diagnosis for DSM-V. *Archives of Sexual Behavior, 39*(2), 377–400. 10.1007/s10508-009-9574-7.

Kim, J. (2009). Asian American women's retrospective reports of their sexual socialization. *Psychology of Women Quarterly, 33*(3), 334–350. 10.1111/j.1471-6402.2009.01505.x

Kraus, S.W., & Sweeney, P.J. (2019). Hitting the target: Considerations for differential diagnosis when treating individuals for problematic use of pornography. *Archives of Sexual Behavior, 48*(2), 431–435. 10.1007/s10508-018-1301-9.

Kraus, S.W., Potenza, M.N., Martino, S., & Grant, J.E. (2015). Examining the psychometric properties of the Yale–Brown Obsessive–Compulsive Scale in a sample of compulsive pornography users. *Comprehensive Psychiatry, 59,* 117–122. 10.1016/j.comppsych.2015.02.007

Kraus, S.W., Martino, S., & Potenza, M.N. (2016). Clinical characteristics of men interested in seeking treatment for use of pornography. *Journal of Behavioral Addictions, 5*(2), 169–178. 10.1556/2006.5.2016.036

Kraus, S.W., Krueger, R.B., Briken, P., First, M.B., Stein, D.J., Kaplan, M.S., ...Atalla, E. (2018). Compulsive sexual behaviour disorder in the ICD-11. *World Psychiatry, 17*(1), 109. 10.1002/wps.20499.

Martyniuk, U., Briken, P., Sehner, S., Richter-Appelt, H., & Dekker, A. (2016). Pornography use and sexual behavior among Polish and German university students. *Journal of Sex Marital Therapy*, *42*(6), 494–514. 10.1080/0092623X.2015.1072119

Meston, C.M., Trapnell, P.D., & Gorzalka, B.B. (1996). Ethnic and gender differences in sexuality: Variations in sexual behavior between Asian and non-Asian university students. *Archives of Sexual Behavior*, *25*(1), 33–72. 10.1007/BF02437906

Mestre-Bach, G., Blycker, G.R., & Potenza, M.N. (2020). Pornography use in the setting of the COVID-19 pandemic. *Journal of Behavioral Addictions*, *9*(2), 181–183. 10.1556/2006.2020.00015

Sevcikova, A., Serek, J., Barbovschi, M., & Daneback, K. (2014). The roles of individual characteristics and liberalism in intentional and unintentional exposure to online sexual material among European Youth: A multilevel approach. *Sexuality Research and Social Policy*, *11*(2), 104–115. 10.1007/s13178-013-0141-6

Tong, Y. (2013). Acculturation, gender disparity, and the sexual behavior of Asian American youth. *Journal of Sex Research*, *50*(6), 560–573. 10.1080/00224499.2012.668976.

Wéry, A., & Billieux, J. (2017). Problematic cybersex: Conceptualization, assessment, and treatment. *Addictive Behaviors*, *64*, 238–246. 10.1016/j.addbeh.2015.11.007.

Wood, H. (2011). The internet and its role in the escalation of sexually compulsive behaviour. *Psychoanalytic Psychotherapy*, *25*(2), 127–142. 10.1080/02668734.2011.576492.

Yuan, D. (2004). *The study for Cybersex behavior and Cybersex addiction of the college student[D]*. Hunan: Hunan Normal University. 格式改了一下 不确定对不对）

Zheng, L., & Zheng, Y. (2014). Online sexual activity in mainland China: Relationship to sexual sensation seeking and sociosexuality. *Computers in Human Behavior*, *36*, 323–329. 10.1016/j.chb.2014.03.062

Zheng, W., Zhou, X., Wang, X., & Hesketh, T. (2014). Sociosexuality in mainland China. *Archives of Sexual Behavior*, *43*(3), 621–629. 10.1007/s10508013-0097-x.

Chapter 10

Understanding Repetitive Non-Suicidal Self-Injury and Recovery among Chinese Women

A Qualitative Study

Artemis Leung

Previous literature has suggested that non-suicidal self-injury (NSSI) could be conceptualized as a behavioural addiction as they share common characteristics. While NSSI continues to be a problem among the Chinese female population, help-seeking rates remain low. There has been little research into the psychosocial factors and cultural influence contributing to NSSI and help-seeking behaviour. This research presents an up-to-date background and prevalence rate of NSSI behaviour in Hong Kong. It seeks to explore the subjective experiences of NSSI as an addictive behaviour through a qualitative analysis of interviews with 13 Chinese female participants who are in recovery from NSSI. Interviews were transcribed and analyzed for understanding the shared themes across participants' accounts in deliberate self-injurious behaviour. Alexithymia was found to be a trait that may contribute to their NSSI. Participants' self-wounding habits met some addictive criteria included in DSM-V. The implications of these findings for treatment of and interventions for Chinese women engaged in NSSI are discussed.

Introduction

Non-Suicidal Self-Injury (NSSI) is regarded as the act of an individual purposely harming or distracting their body without suicide intention (Nock et al., 2006). It is also known as deliberate self-harm, self-destruction, and self-mutilation. Self-harm behaviour is more widespread among teenagers. According to the clinical reference of Hong Kong in the previous 14 years, 127,801 self-harm episodes were reported by 99,116 people; 7.36% to 28.71% repetitive self-mutilative acts were reported (Forrester et al., 2017). The risk of self-harm repetition within one year of the index event was 14.25%. The rate of committing self-harm behaviour among local secondary school students engaged in self-harm behaviour in the previous 12 months was approximately 23.5% of secondary students (Shek & Law, 2013). Across the studies, women were more likely to report NSSI than men. Many of these

DOI: 10.4324/9781003203476-15

self-injurers reported that multiple methods of self-injury were used, such as cutting, burning, scratching, and hitting.

As suggested in the preceding literature, NSSI and suicidal behaviour (SB) may be conceived as behavioural addictions because they share some similarities in neurobiological and psychological mechanisms with substance use (Blasco-Fontecilla et al., 2016). According to behavioural scientists, anything that can stimulate an individual might be addictive and if a route becomes obligatory, addiction may develop. Therefore, an object's (e.g., a drug's) ability to induce tolerance and withdrawal symptoms is often used to assess "addictiveness". NSSI behaviour typically includes features such as lack of control and social consequences, preoccupation with the behaviour, the inability to reduce the behaviour, and participation in the behaviour despite knowledge of the behaviour's adverse consequences. These criteria are consistent with the DSM-IV criteria for Substance Dependence and Impulse Control Disorders, including pathological gambling. Hence, some researchers adopted these criteria in their studies as no psychological measure scales were available. It has been proposed that comparing the individual behaviour with the clinical criteria established for a "typical" or drug-related addiction is the best approach to determine whether it may be classified as an addiction.

Nixon et al. (2002) explored whether NSSI among adolescents could be explained as a behavioural addiction by adapting the DSM-IV criteria for Substance Dependence. Nixon's team substituted the term "substance" with "NSSI",' and an individual had to meet at least three of the seven criteria to be considered having NSSI with addictive features. The authors developed a self-report measure adapted from the DSM-IV criteria for substance dependence and reported that 80% of their sample endorsed over five criteria. In DSM-V, substance abuse and substance dependence were combined to create a single diagnostic category of substance use disorder. NSSI behaviours were separately categorized within categories of conditions for further study since suicidal ideation and the relationship between NSSI and suicidal behaviours remained unclear (Zetterqvist, 2015).

In the past decades, much research about NSSI behaviour has focused on the classification, prevalence, correlates, forms, and functions of self-mutilation. Few researchers have addressed the roles of NSSI in psychosocial and cultural perspectives among Asian communities, which are strongly influenced by Confucian values. The present chapter aims to investigate the relationship between personality traits of Chinese women, their cultural values, and the inability of disguising emotion and self-harming behaviours through the qualitative lens. The participants' accounts of their self-destructive habits and addictive behaviours were also included.

The Hong Kong Situation

The demographic and cultural background of Hong Kong contributed to how young Chinese women in Hong Kong view self-harm. Hong Kong is one of the most heavily populated cities in the world. A skewed gender demographic is found in the city, with 839 men per 1,000 women. More women are encouraged to actively engage in social activities in recent decades. Because of the enhancement in education levels and expanding training opportunities, the percentage of women aged 15+ who have received tertiary education or higher has risen in the previous ten years.

Although youngsters are reported to have satisfactory academic performance, they also suffer from the most significant stress level compared to other students in the world. Many parents and students are oriented toward high academic achievement because they believe that grades determine future success. Parents frequently stress students' university entrance examination performance since they believe receiving tertiary education is the only way to a promising future. Students revealed they are suffering from mounting pressure regarding their academic results. A local survey included 15,560 secondary school students in Hong Kong and found that 53% exhibited symptoms of depression. Among these youths, senior high school students are more vulnerable as they experience fierce competition for university spots, and only 30% of the candidates receive post-secondary education offers. Another survey (Yau, 2017) found that more than one in three pupils from primary and secondary schools had experienced distress and more than half of them revealed they had suicidal ideation.

With the rise of Hong Kong young females' social status in society, their psychological health is of growing concern. Research on mental health morbidity in Hong Kong reported that among the 5719 Chinese participants aged 16 to 75, the weighted prevalence estimate for Common Mental Disorders for the past seven days was 13.3% (Chang et al., 2017; Cheung et al., 2012). The most common diagnoses were anxiety disorder and depression, and these are highly associated with female gender. It is believed that Confucian values might contribute to Chinese views on the social environment and their own mental health. Confucianism is a social and moral philosophy originating from Confucius in the 6th–5th century BCE. Its virtues include humaneness and kindness, trustworthiness and righteousness, loyalty and earnestness, respectability and rightness, and wisdom that guides the social responsibility and order of the society. The Confucian values permeated Chinese culture and maintain significant influence in Asian countries. In Chinese culture, women are still considered to be the primary caregivers for their families. Hence, women in Hong Kong play different roles in their daily life. Apart from workplace stresses, women are struggling in their personal, career, and family life. A study shows that women are more easily triggered by negative events which are related to their family, relationships, and physical health-related issues (Ni et al., 2020), yet they are prone to suppress their feelings.

Alexithymia is a psychological condition in which one's ability to express and control one's own emotion is limited or hindered. The phrase was coined by Peter Emanuel Sifnéos (1973) to characterize individuals with psychosomatic issues who are unable to find the word to explain thoughts and feelings. Clinical patients who experienced this difficulty have mental functioning impairments, and constricted imaginal processes, and are more likely to encounter difficulties in interpersonal relationships since they prefer using action to prevent conflicting situations. The alexithymia rate among Chinese adolescents remains high, compared to other adolescents in the world. They tend not to discuss their mental health sufferings with their close family members, due to the influence of traits of low expressiveness. Research also found that over 75% of females with mental distress had not sought professional help in the past year (Cheung et al., 2012). These results highlight the need of investigations on the function of keeping face in Confucian communities. Chinese society is characterized by a strong emphasis on authority and interpersonal relationships, discussing negative events such as stress and failures in life may be regarded as "face losing" behaviours that make the social situation embarrassing and impacts the sense of equilibrium. Hence, individuals will endeavor to prevent or reduce the chance of losing face, personally and regarding one's family. Even though families show support for women who have emotional issues, self-blaming, and self-labeling are common as women believe they are the black sheep of their families. Thus, these unique cultural perspectives on self, family, and groups create "pull factors" of the help-seeking behaviours for mental distress.

Methodology

This research sought to explore the subjective experiences of repetitive non-suicidal self-injury as an addictive behaviour through a qualitative analysis of interviews with 13 Chinese young female participants who are in recovery from NSSI. Participants were recruited through a snowball sampling approach. Participants who met the criteria for the study were referred and invited to take part in this study. Interviews were transcribed and analyzed with a thematic analysis approach for understanding the shared themes across participants' accounts of deliberate self-injurious behaviour.

Result

Thirteen in-depth interviews were conducted during the first quarter of 2021, and the duration of each interview was 30-90 minutes. The characteristics of the participants, including socio-demographic data, are summarized in Table 10.1 along with quotes from the interviews. The findings indicate that female participants were suffering from different levels of mental illness and distress in daily life. Several major themes were recognized in the interviews.

Table 10.1 Sample description and themes, subthemes, and quotes from the semi-structured interviews

Participant	Age	Occupation	Theme	Subtheme	Opinion of NSSI
P1	18	Student (Secondary School)	(a) Negative social self-efficacy perception (b) Alexithymia is a trait of Chinese females (c) NSSI as an emotion regulation strategy	Negative help seeking experience	" … I think I am introverted and stubborn and do not have many friends. I do not enjoy going out because I have no special hobbies. I do not enjoy going to school … ." (P1) " … Whenever I have a problem, my father and aunt will say I am useless and leave me with the problem. That will be the time that I unconsciously pinch or cut myself until I bleed. I think it is not useful to find social workers to talk about my problem. She is not me, and she cannot understand how I feel. I think no one cares about me, and I did not think about the future. The adults are not willing to listen to me. (P1) " … I always think about the past. I cried at night and scratched myself. When I woke up in the morning, I found some scratching marks on my arm but I didn't feel pain at all at that moment … ." (P1)
P2	29	Teacher (Kindergarten)	(a) Negative social self-efficacy perception (c) NSSI as an emotion regulation strategy (f) Gaining new perspectives on emotional distress	negative self-image due to trauma	" … I was raised in a low-income family. My father enjoyed gambling with his coworker. I remember when I was small; he returned home late. Even when my brothers or I were sick, he did not bring us money to see the doctor … In my secondary school time, I think my teachers discriminated against me because of my height. My classmates sometimes bullied and made fun of me because of my height, so I sometimes cut the inner side of my arm to relieve stress … ." (P2) " … I felt miserable because I lost both my job and the boyfriend which I treasured the most. I did not want to see anybody, and I felt scared to go out. At night, I stayed in my bedroom. I wept secretly when I read the old messages. Gradually, my self-harm behaviour has become more serious. I scratched myself and banged my head against the wall … ." (P2) " … my brother-in-law found a counsellor to see me. I learnt I should not be self-blaming. The counsellor was very kind. She introduced me to WRAP (Wellness Recovery Action Plan) and Mental Health First Aid,

ID	Age	Occupation			Quote
P3	24	Teacher (Secondary School)	and developing emotional sobriety as core factors of recovery		she encouraged me to go for a walk and do handicrafts as a wellness tool to release stress. She also introduced me to some community centres to get some social support. Although I still feel sad and not able to work now, I have faith that I will be better …" (P2)
			(b) Alexithymia is a trait of Chinese females	NSSI as a negative emotional regulation tools	"… As a teacher It is shameful to harm yourselves like this. I am afraid of gossiping, so I tried to cover them up by wearing long sleeves. I guess some of my colleagues who are close to me know about this, but they dare not to ask. They will also avoid inviting me to join students' suiciding prevention programmes. It is not convincing for a teacher who cut herself to teach the students not to kill themselves, right? …" (P3)
			(b) Alexithymia is a trait of Chinese females	Negative help seeking experience	"… I felt nervous because my colleagues in the staff room were unfriendly as I expected. I love my students, but the politics in the office always make me feel suffocated. The other senior year schoolmates suggested I behave and not cause any trouble. So, I dare not to talk with my mentor about my emotions because I think it will affect my grade… …" (P3)
P4	19	Student (University Undergrad)	(a) Negative social self-efficacy perception	negative self-image due to trauma	"… My father is an agreeable person at the workplace. When he is at home, I think he gets too close to me. He molested me when I was a child. I remember he watched pornography in front of me and once touched me. I was shocked that he did this to me … . mother doesn't believe that her husband sexually abused me and said that it was only my delusion. My sisters just ignored me. They thought I was a troublemaker. I always feel that I am not their daughter and I was not loved. I should have called the police, but I feel bad to ruin this "normal" family. It was difficult to share my feelings with others as well. (P4)
			(d) Participants' self-wounding habits met some addictive criteria mentioned in DSM-V		"… Frequently, I feel empty and leave this world. I went to the drugstore and looked for drugs. I cut myself. I took more medicine than I should. And I tried to get hit by cars. Most of the time I drew back because I thought I should give myself a chance. These thoughts worsened during examination time …" (P4)

(Continued)

Table 10.1 (Continued)

Participant	Age	Occupation	Theme	Subtheme	Opinion of NSSI
P5	17	Student (Secondary School)	(a) Negative social self-efficacy perception	negative self-image due to trauma	"… Every night I could not sleep at night. When I think about the school time and the fierce teachers at school, I would feel miserable. It is so painful. I would use a paper cutter to cut my wrist until I bleed or maybe take my mom's sleeping pills or drink my mom's wine, or burn myself with a lighter or cigarette … Bleeding is the best revenge for my parents. Also, I will make myself feel more relieved and I can sense I'm existing so I could go to bed easily until the next day and skip school …"(P5)
P6	23	Student (University Master,)	(c) NSSI as an emotion regulation strategy		"… I usually cut it at night. That is the time I feel lonely and sad. Cutting made me feel and sleep better at night …"(P6)
			(b) Alexithymia is a trait of Chinese females	Negative help seeking experience	"… My psychiatric doctor knows my self-harm behaviour, but he doesn't think it is a serious issue unless I faint on the street and I was sent to the Emergency department, and I dislike seeing psychologists. I am a very determined person, and I hate talking about my problems with them repeatedly … The psychiatrists have no time to talk about your feelings and self-harm at all. How can a doctor take care of you when they meet you within five minutes? They need to see a lot of patients. The queue for the public psychiatric service is super long. They won't bother a lot and ask you to be hospitalised because of your minor cuts as it is not life-threatening! They will just give you medicine and send you away …" (P6)
			e) The comorbidity of NSSI and other psychiatric disorders		"… I skipped school, went drinking, and took different drugs. I once had an illusion and walked on the rooftop of my house. My boyfriend was scared and brought me to seek help from a social worker. Soon I was seen by a government psychiatrist. I was diagnosed with major depression disorder …" (P6)

	Age	Occupation	Code	Theme	Quote
			(d) Participants' self-wounding habits met some addictive criteria mentioned in DSM-V		"… I did not take all the drugs that the doctor gave me because of the side effects that will affect my performance in school and social life. As I know the drugs well, I told lies to the doctor and made them prescribe the drugs that I want. My mother is paranoid and sarcastic to me. My sister always argued with her as well when she was young. I hate getting others into trouble. I learned to cut my wrist after my first episode of mental illness …"(P6)
P7	19	Student I (Diploma)	(a) Negative social self-efficacy perception	negative self-image due to Trauma	"… My life is worthless because my parents didn't want me. In addition, I feel disappointed with my dad as well. How could a person whom I respected the most touch me? When I was ten, I learnt to use a paper cutter to cut my hands and thighs. It was no pain at all. Then, I frequently cut my hand …" (P7)
			e) The comorbidity of NSSI and other psychiatric disorders		"… I feel depressed when I celebrate festivals such as the Mid-Autumn Festival, New Year, and the days when relatives and friends have gatherings. My mood was extremely depressed, so I used alcohol and drugs to numb myself …" (P7)
			(b) Alexithymia is a trait of Chinese females	NSSI as a negative emotional regulation tools	"… These scars can only represent less than one percent of the pain in my heart. I love my family, but it contradicts that this family hurt me a lot. I feel it's difficult to tell people about how much I got hurt …" (P7)
			(d) Participants' self-wounding habits met some addictive criteria mentioned in DSM-V		"… When I was 10, I took the pills at home. I once unconsciously used a knife to cut my hands and thighs. It was no pain at all. Then, I frequently cut my hand …"(P7)
			(b) Alexithymia is a trait of Chinese females	NSSI as a subtle way to express emotion	"… You know, the Chinese parents enjoy comparing their kids, talking about their academics, their jobs, how much money they made. Criticisms are annoying, but you cannot avoid them …. So I wore my sunglasses. I avoid going to family gatherings, talking and sharing my feelings with family members …" (P7)

(Continued)

Table 10.1 (Continued)

Participant	Age	Occupation	Theme	Subtheme	Opinion of NSSI
			(f) Gaining new perspectives on emotional distress and developing emotional sobriety as core factors of recovery		"… The social worker referred me to a psychologist. She taught me to accept sadness and to help me express my indignation. I learn to get rid of the trauma of my family. I know that I should take a step forward,,start to balance my life and take responsibility as an adult. I learn to face the difficulties and not to escape. After ten months of treatment, my mood improved significantly. I did not blame myself for my parents' marriage unhappiness. I have less self-destructive behaviour …" (P7)
P8	17	Student (Secondary School)	(b) Alexithymia is a trait of Chinese females	NSSI as a subtle way to express emotion	"… my mother will be angry if I tell others about my family issue. I need to use a more instant method such as cutting my hand to relieve it. I think it is the best way to deal with painful emotions."(P8)
			(b) Alexithymia is a trait of Chinese females	NSSI as a negative emotional regulation tools	".… Since I was in Grade six, Every time when I encountered unhappy things or am angry with my parents I use a paper cutter to cut my arm. It is not that painful if the scars and wounds are small. I feel relaxed. Cutting is better than talking about my grief and unhappiness …"(P8)
P9	21	Unemployed	(b) Alexithymia is a trait of Chinese females	NSSI as a subtle way to express emotion	"When the social worker explained this to my mother. She said, "Let her do it (cutting hands)! She is not taking drugs, and no one will know about it! If she feels better and does not affect her academic result, why not? What is the big deal for cutting? What is the harm of doing this?…" (P9)
			e) The comorbidity of NSSI and other psychiatric disorders		"My boyfriends need to make me a priority. If they don't obey me and listen to me, I will harm myself or threaten them by committing suicide. When I was 17 years old, after a quarrel with my ex-boyfriend, I had my first episode of psychosis. I experienced psychotic symptoms on the street. Passers-by called the ambulance and sent

	Age	Occupation	Code	Theme	Quote
P10	18	Student (Secondary School)	(d) Participants' self-wounding habits met some addictive criteria mentioned in DSM-V		"me to the hospital. I was surprised that the situation was serious. I had a series of examinations. Clinical psychologists and psychiatrists confirmed it was panic disorder and bipolar disorder ..."(P9) "... every time I break up, I will have emotional breakdown and I would do some dangerous behaviour such as meeting strangers and having sex with them, drinking and taking drugs. I want to numb myself and find happiness in other ways ... ." (P9)
			(b) Alexithymia is a trait of Chinese females	NSSI as a negative emotional regulation tools	"... I knew that the most difficult thing was to keep suppressing my emotions. I told myself that I shouldn't lose my temper or cry when I got home. So, I took a lot of different medicines and suppressed myself with medicines and I overdosed on it sometime." (P10)
P11	20	Student (University Undergrad)	(b) Alexithymia is a trait of Chinese females	NSSI as a subtle way to express emotion	"... Sometimes I found that the more I cried, the sadder I was. There is some unspeakable pain in my heart ... sometimes I feel I am crying without tears. I feel very numb, empty and lonely ...". (P11)
			(b) Alexithymia is a trait of Chinese females		"... My professors told us that University is a place to pursue knowledge. No competition is required! However, I do not think so. I strive to be an excellent student and a dutiful daughter. I don't want to disappoint my parents! Whenever I was nervous and worried, my anxiety rises ... Sometimes there is an unspeakable pain in my heart, and sometimes I feel like crying without tears, very numb, empty and lonely... ... Every time when the blade cuts through the skin, the pain from the wound seem to help me forget the pain in my heart. (P11)
P12	23	Housewife	(a) Negative social self-efficacy perception	negative self-image due to Trauma	"... Even my ex-boyfriend entered my house, captured me and confined me again, my parents did not care about this because they were too busy with gambling. My sister was too small to do anything for me. I thought I was wrong to be with him. I once had a suicidal thought. But, I remember that the old Chinese says that the spirit of the one who committed

(Continued)

Table 10.1 (Continued)

Participant	Age	Occupation	Theme	Subtheme	Opinion of NSSI
					suicide in a house would be tied up and stay in the place they die, so I stopped thinking it again. Isn't it horrible that I still have to stay with him again in afterlife? I was scared and felt helpless that I could not seek any friends to help, so I continued to pinch myself since I hated myself a lot …" (P12)
P13	19	Student (Secondary School)	(b) Alexithymia is a trait of Chinese females	NSSI as a subtle way to express emotion	"… Knowing that my parents' income decreased because of the epidemic, I did not express my worries to them. I pretend to be a cheerful and active daughter in front of my parents, but every night after closing the door of my bedroom, I thought a lot and sob so much that I fell asleep with tears soaking my entire pillow." (P13)
			(c) NSSI as an emotion regulation strategy		"… When the fourth wave of the epidemic came, everyone around me dared not go out. My mental health became worse as it made it difficult to concentrate on studying, and the crowded environment at home made me feel stressed. To escape from the tense emotion, I found out that cutting my hands and my abdomen with scissors on my arms made me feel better. Although cutting my arms made me forget the suffering in my heart for a short time …" (P13)

Negative Social Self-Efficacy Perception

Social self-efficacy refers to an individual's collaborative competency in a group. Participants (N = 8) reflected that they have insufficient ability to engage in social interactional tasks, which would help them to begin and sustain a positive human relationship (P1; see Table 10.1). Due to traumatic experiences such as parental emotional and physical negligence, and sexual abuse, the participants have a negative self-image, a personalized belief of the cause of some negative external event, and exclude themselves socially (P4, P2, P5, P7, P12).

Alexithymia is a Trait of Chinese Females That May Contribute to Their Addictive Self-Injury Behaviour

Most participants (N = 10) shared the subjective experience of alexithymia, a personality trait that features the disinterest or inability of identifying and expressing emotions (Berthoz et al., 2011) (P11). The participants shared some similar backgrounds, such as growing up in Chinese families in which parents have authoritative or permissive parenting styles. Living in a collectivist and comparatively conservative and competitive society, individuals are preferred to talk about successful experiences rather than discussing failure or emotion in front of others as it is regarded as "losing face". Maladjustment behaviour such as drug-using or self-harming might be methods for them to handle the discrepancy between their ideal and actual selves (P7, P8, P9, P11, P13). The participants internalized negative stereotypes that include expectations that expressions of feelings and emotions are not to be encouraged. They felt challenged by limited options in managing emotional pain and had difficulties with low acceptance of negative life events and responses to trauma. Gradually, the participants became prone to experiencing difficulties in establishing connections and showing emotions and thus may use self-injuries as emotional regulation tools (P3, P7, P8, P10). Help-seeking behaviours had also been limited because of the unsuccessful emotional expression experiences, mistrust, and dissatisfactory involvement of helping professionals (P1, P3, P6).

NSSI as an Emotion Regulation Strategy

Most of the participants (N = 11) adapted self-harming as a form of instantaneous way and automatic emotional regulation tool to escape from suppressed psychological pain and mental suffering (P1, P2, P6, P13).

Participants' Self-Wounding Habits Met Some Addictive Criteria Mentioned in DSM-V

Researchers analyzed the interview transcripts according to the criteria of substance dependence in DSM-V. Some reported cases (N = 10) of NSSI behaviour met criteria for substance abuse mentioned in DSM-V, such as tolerance, loss of control, and relapse. Apart from NSSI, individuals (N = 5) who use a broad variety of self-harm methods often reported that they had multiple addictions, such as prescription drug abuse, illicit drug use, and sexual addiction, which attempted to escape from their traumas from negative childhood events and cope with life distress. (P4, P6, P 7, P 9).

The Comorbidity of NSSI and Other Psychiatric Disorders

Participants (N = 5) who showed self-mutilating behaviour reported that they are diagnosed with psychiatric disorders such as bipolar, anxiety, depression, and eating disorder. People with trouble managing emotions and a tendency for impulsive behaviour are at a higher risk for NSSI (P6, P7, P9).

Gaining New Perspectives on Emotional Distress and Developing Emotional Sobriety as Core Factors of Recovery

People who self-harm regularly have difficulty in managing their emotions. As a result, when facing emotionally challenging situations, they react in impulsive ways. In this research, individuals with previous experience of NSSI (N = 7) agreed that they recognized the stress, gained more understanding and acceptance of their own stress, and coped with trauma symptoms with more positive self-regulation methods such as finding alternatives instead of autonomic self-harming behaviour (P2, P 7).

Discussion

This study explored psychosocial reasons for NSSI and the cultural pull factors on their help-seeking attitude among young women in a semi-structured interview. The results indicate that the social environment and traditional gender role expectations play a significant role in Chinese women's self-mutilation behaviour. In humanistic psychology theory, it is suggested individuals may experience discomfort, anxiety, and irritation if there is a disconnection between how they see themselves and how they wish they were to fit society's expectations. The over-emphasis on academic achievement and the extremely competitive lifestyle in Hong Kong puts citizens, especially students, and education practitioners, under constant stress. Being members of a collectivist society, it is not uncommon for some individuals to perceive that they are discouraged from displaying disengaging social emotions, such as anxiety and anger (Kitayama et al., 2006), which is produced by unresolved traumas and unsuccessful experiences. Because of prolonged negative thinking patterns and suppression of feeling, these young women may have a tendency to have poor emotion-cognition ability and inability to reflect on their own mental states. This result confirms a previous study on the relevance of difficulty in identifying and expressing feelings in NSSI. A possible explanation for the female participants' self-harm behaviours might be that self-mutilation and other addictive behaviours could be regarded as a method for them to alter their mood instantly.

In line with a study that found that NSSI can be regarded as an addiction (Blasco-Fontecilla et al., 2016), women in the current study agreed that their self-harm behaviours met some common features of behavioural addiction such as failure to quit cutting hands, tolerance, withdrawal, and consistently lying to conceal failure to resist from self-harm despite understanding that it is harmful. They also mentioned their polysubstance use and comorbidity of other psychological disorders which are suggested to be strongly associated with NSSI. Participants reported frequently that the function of their NSSI was automatic negative reinforcement, as a means to remove unpleasant emotions. At the same time, when the participants face a stressful life event, a self-injurious urge is aroused intrusively and a broader range and more severe self-harm methods are applied for alleviating their psychological pain over time.

The participants' tolerance for self-harm is in the line with prior studies (Gordon et al., 2010; Joiner, 2005; Van Orden et al., 2010) which suggested that individuals with NSSI may have a tolerance for the negative aspects of suicide based on the recurrent exposure to sensory stimuli, such as NSSI. Gradually, the self-harm behaviours are learned. If an individual encounters a painful event, through the means of self-mutilation, the individual's experience of negative aspects such as fear and physical pain weakens, while their positive experiences such as relief strengthen.

Interestingly, several participants stated that social rejection and discrimination linked to repetitive self-harm behaviour are less harmful than substance abuse in society. There is a strong probability that young female self-harmers might underestimate the potential harms of NSSI and internalize that self-harm is a comparatively "mild" and "acceptable" emotional outlet to express their latent feelings. Surprisingly, when the subjects were asked about their pathways to recovery, similar to the result of research in other behavioural addictions such as problem gambling (Leung, 2017), the majority confirmed the effectiveness of counseling service and that positive experiences in the family and social supports may encourage them to maintain abstinence from NSSI. Participants' responses showed that positive family and social support play a core role in successful help-seeking behaviour. It would be helpful to not only offer unconditional emotional support and a more objective perspective on their behaviour but also information on seeking professional help. With counseling help and evidence-based interventions such as Cognitive Behavioural Therapy, individuals will be guided to manage their mental distress by changing their thinking patterns and behaviour. Participants stated the effectiveness of several emotional self-help programs, such as the Wellness Recovery Action Plan and Mental Health First Aid, where individuals who deliberately self-harm could also address their physical, mental health, and life issues by integrating core concepts of recovery (hope, personal responsibility, education, self-advocacy, and support) into daily life as they gain self-awareness on their wellbeing holistically. Meanwhile, these self-decided action plans could assist participants to explore appropriate emotion regulation tools, be aware of their mental states and create an emergency plan that specifies how members of the family or supporters should intervene if the individual cannot act on their own behalf. Participants could also customize post-crisis plans to use once the mental health issue has been resolved in order to encourage a return to wellness.

Limitation

Snowball sampling was adopted in this study, where participants help recruiting participants with NSSI experiences among their acquaintances. Although this sample provides some insight into the experiences of hard-to-reach, young Chinese participants who concealed their self-harm problems, the interviews with 13 young women may not provide a wide range of perspectives on self-mutilation. Further, the participants' social network might be limited to a single geographic area. Thus, it is difficult to interpret and generalize study results to the entire Asian Population. Subsequent, larger-scale studies could explore issues arising in this study in more detail; for example, comparing self-harm and help-seeking experiences among the Chinese population in urban, rural, and global settings and the potential factors for intervention and recovery.

Conclusion

This research may contribute to a better understanding of the socio-cultural elements that contribute to NSSI among young Asian women, as well as barriers may hinder their help-seeking behaviour. The current study indicated that NSSI behaviour, like other addictive behaviours, is characterized by emotional control and reinforcement. Behavioural therapy and self-help programs may be beneficial for this potential non-substance related addiction. Policymakers and other stakeholders are encouraged to learn more about the causes and functions of NSSI in Asian populations in order to build better preventive measures and psychoeducation strategies in the future.

References

Berthoz, S., Pouga, L., & Wessa, M. (2011). Alexithymia from the social neuroscience perspective. In: J. Decety & J. Cacciopo, editors. *The Oxford Handbook of Social Neuroscience*, (pp. 906–934). New York: Oxford University Press.

Blasco-Fontecilla, H., Fernández-Fernández, R., Colino, L., Fajardo, L., Perteguer-Barrio, R., & de Leon, J. (2016). The addictive model of self-harming (non-suicidal and suicidal) behavior. *Frontiers in Psychiatry, 7*, 8. 10.3389/fpsyt.2016.00008

Chang, W.C., Wong, C., Chen, E., Lam, L., Chan, W.C., Ng, R., Hung, S.F., Cheung, E., Sham, P.C., Chiu, H., Lam, M., Lee, E., Chiang, T.P., Chan, L.K., Lau, G., Lee, A., Leung, G., Leung, J., Lau, J., van Os, J., & Bebbington, P. (2017). Lifetime prevalence and correlates of schizophrenia-spectrum, affective, and other non-affective psychotic disorders in the Chinese Adult Population. *Schizophrenia Bulletin*, *43*(6), 1280–1290. 10.1093/schbul/sbx056

Cheung, Y.T.D., Wong, P., Lee, A., Lam, T., Fan, Y., & Yip, P. (2012). Non-suicidal self-injury and suicidal behavior: Prevalence, co-occurrence, and correlates of suicide among adolescents in Hong Kong. *Social Psychiatry and Psychiatric Epidemiology*. *48*. 10.1007/s00127-012-0640-4.

Forrester, R.L., Slater, H., Jomar, K., Mitzman, S., & Taylor, P.J. (2017). Self-esteem and non-suicidal self-injury in adulthood: A systematic review. *Journal of Affective Disorders*, *221*, 172–183. 10.1016/j.jad.2017.06.027

Gordon, K.H., Selby, E.A., Anestis, M.D., et al. (2010). The reinforcing properties of repeated deliberate self-harm. *Arch Suicide Res*, *14*(4), 329–341. 10.1080/13811118.2010.524059

Joiner, T.E. (2005). *Why people die by suicide*. Cambridge, MA: Harvard University Press.

Kitayama, S., Mesquita, B., & Karasawa, M. (2006). Cultural affordances and emotional experience: Socially engaging and disengaging emotions in Japan and the United States. *Journal of Personality and Social Psychology*, *91*(5), 890–903. 10.1037/0022-3514.91.5.890

Law, B.M., & Shek, D.T. (2013). Self-harm and suicide attempts among young Chinese adolescents in Hong Kong: Prevalence, correlates, and changes. *Journal of Pediatric and Adolescent Gynecology*, *26*(3 Suppl), S26–S32. 10.1016/j.jpag.2013.03.012

Leung, A. (2017). A review of literature: Gambling problems among the female populations in Hong Kong. In: H. Bowden-Jones & F. Prever (Eds.), *Gambling disorders in women: An international female perspective on treatment and research* (pp. 87–96). Routledge/Taylor & Francis Group. 10.4324/9781315627625-10

Ni, M.Y., Yao, X.I., Leung, K., Yau, C., Leung, C., Lun, P., Flores, F.P., Chang, W.C., Cowling, B.J., & Leung, G.M. (2020). Depression and post-traumatic stress during major social unrest in Hong Kong: a 10-year prospective cohort study. *Lancet (London, England)*, *395*(10220), 273–284.

Nixon, M.K., Cloutier, P.F., & Aggarwal, S. (2002). Affect regulation and addictive aspects of repetitive self-injury in hospitalized adolescents. *Journal of the American Academy of Child and Adolescent Psychiatry*, *41*(11), 1333–1341. 10.1097/00004583-200211000-00015

Nock, M.K., Joiner, T.E., Jr, Gordon, K.H., Lloyd-Richardson, E., & Prinstein, M.J. (2006). Non-suicidal self-injury among adolescents: diagnostic correlates and relation to suicide attempts. *Psychiatry Research*, *144*(1), 65–72. 10.1016/j.psychres.2006.05.010

Sifneos, P.E. (1973). The prevalence of 'alexithymic' characteristics in psychosomatic patients. *Psychotherapy & Psychosomatics*, *22*, 255–262. 10.1159/000286529

Van Orden, K.A., Witte T.K., Cukrowicz, K.C., Braithwaite, S.R., Selby, E.A., & Joiner, T.E., Jr (2010). The Interpersonal Theory of Suicide. *Psychological Review*, *117*, 575–600.

Yau, C. (2017). One in three primary school students in Hong Kong at risk of suicide. *South China Morning Post.* https://www.scmp.com/news/hong-kong/education-community/article/2094561/one-three-primary-school-students-hong-kong-risk

Zetterqvist, M. (2015). The DSM-5 diagnosis of non-suicidal self-injury disorder: A review of the empirical literature. *Child and Adolescent Psychiatry and Mental Health, 9,* 31. 10.1186/s13034-015-0062-7

Higher Burden of Withdrawal Symptoms, Depressive Mood, Loneliness, Anxiety and Agitation among Women with Internet Gaming Disorder in South Korea

Soo-Young Bhang

According to the 2020 survey on smartphone overdependence in South Korea, conducted by the "Ministry of Science and ICT" (MSIT), 3.7% of women were categorized as being at high risk and 18.4% at potential risk of smartphone addiction. There has been little literature on female behavioural addiction in the past. Therefore, data from the Nowon-gu Addiction Center project were analyzed in a secondary data analysis. This survey was conducted in 2017 and included 3,937 students. Of the total sample, 62 women (1.7%) showed high risk for Internet gaming disorder. Symptoms of depression, anxiety, and withdrawal were significantly higher among women than among men.

Introduction

This chapter describes the prevalence of behavioural addiction among women in Korea, using current National statistics. In addition, the results of a subgroup analysis by gender of Internet gaming disorder (IGD) among adolescents in the community is presented. These results are also included in a forthcoming article by Ji Ho et al, "Is I-PACE (Interaction of Person-Affect-Cognitive- Execution) model valid in South Korea? - Effects of Adverse Childhood Experiences (ACEs) on Internet Gaming Disorder and Mediating Effect of Stress in South Korean Adolescents." There has been little research specifically focusing on female behavioural addiction; therefore, this is considered a meaningful analysis. My guiding hypothesis was that women with IGD may (1) have different demographic variables than men, (2) experience key symptoms of addiction such as withdrawal and tolerance more frequently or more intensely than men, and (3) be more emotionally and socially vulnerable.

DOI: 10.4324/9781003203476-16

Current Internet Addiction Statistics for Women in South Korea

Korea has been conducting annual surveys to understand the status of information service dysfunction caused by problematic Internet use (since 2004), and problematic smartphone use (since 2013) evaluating the performance of smartphone dependence prevention and resolution policies, and creating effective policies and improvement measures. This survey is based on Article 12 of the Framework Act on Intelligent Informatization and National Approval Statistics (No. 120019). The smartphone overdependence scale used in the survey consists of questions about control failure, salience, and problematic results. "Overdependence risk" is defined as a state in which serious interpersonal conflict, daily role problems, and health problems occur while one loses control over the use of smartphones.

In the 2020 survey on smartphone overdependence in South Korea, conducted by the "Ministry of Science and ICT" (MSIT; ICT & Agency, 2020), participants were smartphone (Internet) users aged 3 to 69 years, using their smartphone at least once within the last month. A total of 10,000 households and 30,927 people within these households were surveyed: 2,701 infants (ages 3–9), 5,032 adolescents (ages 10–19), 20,304 adults (ages 20–59), and 2,890 people in their 60s. The reference point for the survey was August 1, 2020, and it consists of a one-year household visit interview survey. Almost one-fourth (23.3%) of smartphone users in Korea (total N = 43,828,000) were categorized as a risk group for smartphone dependence – the largest increase since the start of this survey in 2013. The proportion of people at risk of smartphone dependence increased by 2.0% in 2015, 1.6% in 2016, 0.8% in 2017, 0.5% in 2018, showing a slowing trend. It then gradually increased by 0.9% in 2019 and 3.3% in 2020. Among those at risk of dependence, 4.0% were categorized as the high-risk group, an increase of 1.1% from the previous year. Almost one-fifth (19.3%) were categorized as the potential-risk group, an increase of 2.2%. Adults (20–59 years old) were found to be more vulnerable compared to the low-age groups, and men were more vulnerable to the risk of overdependence than women.

Let's take a closer look at the trend of changes in risk over time with respect to gender. In 2020, 24.4% of men and 22.1% of women were at risk of dependence. Compared to the previous year, the proportion of men in the high-risk group increased by 1.5% (vs increases of 2.7% in 2019 and 4.2% in 2020), and in the potential risk group by 2.7% (vs increases of 17.5% in 2019 and 20.2% in 2020). For women, the proportion in the high-risk group increased by 0.7% (vs increases of 3.0% in 2019 and 3.7% in 2020), and in the potential risk group by 2.7% (vs increases of 16.6% in 2019 and 18.4% in 2020).

Looking at the status by year, gender, and subject, compared to the previous year, the male at-risk groups showed a large increase in infants (5.7%) and adolescents (5.8%), whereas female at-risk groups showed a decrease by 0.8% only among women in their 60s.

Comparison between Women and Men with Internet Gaming Disorder from a Korean Community Sample: Addiction Symptoms and Other Socio-Psychological Variables

While preparing this chapter, I found very limited data on behavioural addiction specifically focusing on women and I received similar feedback from experts in this field in South Korea. I am currently the director of the Nowon-gu Addiction Management Center and received permission to analyze community data collected by the Center in 2017 for this chapter. The Nowon Community Addiction Management Center is a community-centered addiction management agency that detects addicts early and offers support through counseling, treatment, and rehabilitation. It is in charge of 53,2905 people (population as of December 31, 2019) in Nowon-gu, Seoul, and is operated by the Ministry of Health and Welfare. My guiding hypothesis was that women with IGD may have different (1) demographic variables than men, (2) symptoms of addiction such as withdrawal and tolerance, and (3) characteristics from men in terms of socio-psychological variables.

Participants and Procedure

This survey was conducted from March to October 2017. The smart digital media survey project is conducted annually at local schools and local children's centers to identify Internet and smartphone addiction targets for individual intervention after identifying trends in Internet smartphone use necessary to prevent addiction. Participants included 3,937 students from 23 elementary, middle, and high schools and 11 local children's centers. Students were asked to respond to self-report questionnaires before the team conducted neuroscience-based education to prevent Internet addiction in all classes. Of the 3,937 respondents, 344 surveys with missing values were excluded. As a result, 3,593 final samples were analyzed.

Measures

Besides gender (male/female), the survey queried academic achievement (1 "high" - 5 "low"), parents' attitude toward Internet/smartphone use (1 "completely restricted" - 7 "indifference"), Internet/smartphone addiction prevention education experience, and cohabitation.

The severity of IGD was assessed with the Internet Game Use-Elicited Symptoms Screen (I-GUESS), a self-report screening measure based on the diagnostic criteria of DSM-5. In this measure, nine IGD diagnostic criteria are rated from 0 to 3 points depending on the frequency of past experience. A total score of 10 or more indicates high risk of IGD.

This study used the adverse experiences in children (ACE) scale of the CDC-Kaiser ACE study (Felitti et al., 1998). The ACE scale consists of 10 items assessing verbal/emotional abuse, physical abuse, verbal/emotional neglect, physical neglect, sexual violence, domestic violence, family mental health, family addiction, crime in the family, separation/divorce. The number of ACEs was calculated by summing the scores, where "yes" was measured as 1 point and "no" as 0 points. The higher the score, the more ACE experienced.

A stress scale developed by the Korea Youth Policy Institute was used for stress evaluation (Choi et al., 2011). This Likert scale measures the level of stress that participants feel about parental relationships, siblings, appearance, health, home environment, friendship, rational relationships, seniors, teacher relationships, job problems, and academic problems, ranging from 1–7 points. The sum of problem scores represents an individual's perceived level of stress.

Statistical Analysis

All statistical analyses were conducted using SPSS 25.0 (IBM Corp., Armonk, NY, USA). First, frequency statistics and Descriptive statistics were calculated to analyze the general characteristics of the sample. Second, Chi-square analysis was used for the differences of variables between genders. In this analysis, 95% confidence level was used.

Ethics

This study was approved by the Institutional Review Committee of Eulji University Eulji Hospital (IRB No. EMCS 2018-06-014). For the current analysis, data containing Non-Personal Identifiable Information (PII) were used with IRB approval.

Results

The sample included 1,533 male students (42.7%) and 2,027 female students (56.4%). Demographic and sociopsychological profiles of participants are shown in Table 11.1. Among the participating students (n = 3,593), 1,771 students (49.3%) were in elementary school (1st to 6th grades), 1,224 students (34.1%) in middle school (7th to 9th grades), and 598 (16.6%) in high school.

Of the total sample, 193 (5.3%) students were in the high-risk group for IGD; 125 (3.5%) were men, and 62 (1.7%) were women. In the high-risk group of IGD, the average age was significantly higher in women (Mean = 14.35, SD = 2.39) than in men (Mean = 13.21, SD = 1.48; p = 0.001) (Table 11.1).

In addition, among the symptoms of addiction, women reported experiences of withdrawal symptoms more frequently than men (38.7% vs 25.8%; p = 0.05). Depressive mood and loneliness while using the Internet were reported by 15.9% of women, but only by 3.9% of men (p = 0.006). Further, the percentage of women who experienced anxiety and agitation while using the Internet was significantly higher than the percentage of men (39.4% vs 10.2%; p = 0.041) (Table 11.1).

Table 11.1 Demographic and sociopsychological profiles of the total sample (N = 3,593), participants with internet gaming disorder (N = 193; measured by I-GUESS), and by gender

Category		Total Participants (n = 3593)		Internet gaming addiction (n = 193)		Boys (n = 125)		Girls (n = 62)		Statistics
		N/M	SD/%	N/M	SD/%	N/M	SD/%	N/M	SD/%	
Age		13.76	2.23	13.57	1.9	13.21	1.48	14.35	2.39	-3.462^{**}(p = 0.001)
Economic status	High	1287	35.8%	54	28.0%	38	28.4%	16	25.4%	4.703(p = 0.319)
	Middle	1892	52.7%	106	54.9%	68	50.7%	36	57.1%	
	Low	373	10.4%	29	15.0%	19	14.2%	10	15.9%	
	NA	41	1.1%	4	2.1%					
Parents' attitude toward Internet/ smartphone use	Completely prohibited	86	2.4%	10	5.2%	9	7.2%	1	1.5%	7.557(p = 0.272)
	Mostly prohibited	278	7.7%	9	4.7%	5	4.0%	4	6.1%	
	Mostly prohibited and Partially allowed	738	20.5%	44	22.8%	30	24.0%	14	21.2%	
	Partially prohibited and Mostly allowed	1183	32.9%	54	28.0%	34	27.2%	20	30.3%	
	Mostly allowed	937	26.1%	48	24.9%	28	22.4%	19	28.8%	
	Completely allowed	181	5.0%	16	8.3%	14	11.2%	2	3.0%	
	Indifference	155	4.3%	9	4.7%	5	4.0%	3	4.5%	
	NA	35	1.0%	3	1.6%					
Number of cohabitant(s)	1	131	3.6%	11	5.7%	6	4.8%	4	6.8%	5.279(p = 0.383)
	2	2406	67.0%	124	64.2%	87	69.6%	37	62.7%	
	3	595	16.6%	30	15.5%	15	12.0%	14	23.7%	
	4	297	8.3%	18	9.3%	11	8.8%	7	11.9%	
	5 or more	122	3.4%	6	3.1%	5	4.0%	1	1.7%	
	None	13	0.4%	1	0.5%	1	0.8%	0	0.0%	
	NA	29	0.8%	3	1.6%					
Stress scale score		20.30	6.74	25.83	7.39	25.19	7.7	27.12	6.7	-1.688(p = 0.93)

(Continued)

Table 11.1 (Continued)

Category		Total Participants (n = 3593)		Internet gaming addiction (n = 193)		Boys (n = 125)		Girls (n = 62)		Statistics
		N/M	SD/%	N/M	SD/%	N/M	SD/%	N/M	SD/%	
Number of Adverse childhood experiences		0.43	1.05	1.03	1.62	0.97	1.49	1.20	1.88	−0.945(p = 0.346)
Withdrawal symptom	Yes	272	7.6%	57	29.5%	33	25.8%	24	38.7%	3.324+(p = 0.05)
	No	3304	92.0%	135	69.9%	95	74.2%	38	61.3%	
	NA	17	0.5%	1	0.5%					
Tolerance symptom	Yes	1832	51.0%	165	85.5%	107	83.6%	56	88.9%	0.946(p = 0.228)
	No	1734	48.3%	28	14.5%	21	16.4%	7	11.1%	
	NA	27	0.8%	0	0.0%					
Depressive mood and loneliness	Yes	76	2.1%	15	7.8%	5	3.9%	10	15.9%	8.355**(P = 0.006)
	No	3517	97.9%	175	90.7%	123	96.1%	53	84.1%	
Anxiety and agitation	Yes	129	3.6%	26	13.5%	13	10.2%	13	39.4%	3.942(P = 0.041)
	No	3464	96.4%	164	85.0%	115	89.8%	20	60.6%	

Note
I-GUESS = the Internet Game Use-Elicited Symptoms Screen questionnaire, * p<0.05, ** p < 0.01, *** p < 0.001.

Discussion

According to DSM-5, the prevalence of IGD is unclear because of varying questionnaires, standards, and criteria for symptom evaluation. Nonetheless, it is presumed high in Asian countries and among male adolescents aged 12 to 20. Among Asian countries, there are many reports, especially in China and Korea, but fewer in Europe and North America, and estimates of prevalence have been reported with wide ranges. In an Asian study cited in DSM-5, five standard items were used as criteria to estimate the prevalence of IGD among adolescents (15–19 years old). In their study, the point prevalence of IGD was 8.4% for male adolescents and 4.5% for females (APA, 2013), whereas the prevalence of IGD in the community was reported as 3.5% for men and 1.7% for women in this study. This is similar to reports from Europe and North America, reflecting the characteristics of communities that are active in preventive education and have high parental interest in preventing IGD.

According to DSM-5 (APA, 2013), the risk and prognosis factors of IGD are largely environmental (e.g., access to Internet-connected computers and game types that are highly related to IGD), genetic and physiological. The age at which women access games is historically higher than the age at which men access Internet games; thus, Internet use problems may occur later in female than in male adolescents (Su et al., 2019). Research or interest in female IGD is still scarce since problematic Internet use among male adolescents is highlighted and it is easier to recruit subjects.

Withdrawal symptoms are a key symptom of substance use disorders, and several studies have reported that they can also accompany behavioural addiction. In the present study, women reported withdrawal symptoms more often than men. Women may be more vulnerable to withdrawal symptoms associated with IGD and this vulnerability may affect long-term prognosis. In a study conducted by Reed and colleagues (Reed et al., 2017), changes in heart rate, systolic blood pressure, state of anxiety, and mood were measured after an Internet session was stopped in a Problematic Internet Use (PIU) group. Changes after stopping the Internet session were similar to symptoms observed among people with substance use disorder after cutting off sedative or opiate drugs. This result supports PIU's classification as an addictive disorder. However, reports on differences between men and women in regard to withdrawal symptoms related to IGD are lacking. Long-term prospective research is needed to better understand the withdrawal system in IGD among women.

A report analyzing 73,238 Korean adolescents (male:38,391, female:34,847), using data from the Six Korea National Youth Risk Behaviour Web-based Survey 2010, showed gender differences in Internet addiction (Park & Jeon, 2013). There were significant differences between women and men in all variables of mental health and Internet addiction. For both male and female students, smoking experience, habitual drug use experience, subjective health status, stress, depression, suicidal thoughts, happiness, and sleep satisfaction had significant effects on the occurrence of Internet addiction. The authors showed that female students had higher mental health-related factors than male students. In Korea, suicide among female adolescents is not significantly different from that of male adolescents (Jung et al., 2019). This is very different from statistics for other countries where male adolescents' suicide rates are reported several times higher, which may reflect the serious mental health problems of female adolescents in Korea. In the study by Jung et al. (2019), depressive mood, loneliness, anxiety, and agitation while using the Internet were four times higher in women than in men. A person at high risk of IGD may use Internet games as a way to reduce previously existing anxiety or depression. Avoidance of anxiety may explain the relationship between trait anxiety and high PIU scores (Romano et al., 2013). Of course, there are numerous alternative possibilities. An important question is why addiction is maintained at the individual level and reinforced positively and negatively.

Limitations

The results presented in this chapter have several limitations. First, a secondary data analysis was carried out for this chapter and the data were not primarily collected for research purposes. Second, depressive mood, loneliness, anxiety, and agitation were assessed by asking simple questions without using standardized scales. Third, data were collected in schools that participated in the project, so randomization was not possible. Fourth, data were collected in a region with an addiction prevention center that actively conducts IGD prevention activities, and residents are very interested in it. Therefore, caution should be taken to generalize this data to Korea or other countries in Asia. However, despite the low prevalence of IGD, it may be valuable to observe the characteristics of subjects with IGD.

Conclusion

In this chapter, through a secondary analysis of data from a community sample, I report psychological symptom differences between men and women with regard to Internet addiction. In this study, although the prevalence of Internet addiction was less than that of other Asian countries, the symptoms of depression, anxiety, and withdrawal among female students were significantly higher than that of male students. For future research, I would like to emphasize that it may be helpful to plan research by comprehensively including aspects such as mood, anxiety, withdrawal, and resistance among men and women to adapt different approaches according to the differential characteristics of men and women with IGD.

References

APA. (2013). *Diagnostic and statistical manual of mental disorders (DSM-5)*. Arlington, VA: American Psychiatric Association Publishing.

Choi, I.J., Mo, S.H., Kang, J.H., Kim, Y.H., & Lee, J.Y. (2011). A study on mental health improvement policy for children and adolescents: National youth policy institute study report

Felitti, V.J. M. D., Facp, Anda, R.F. M. D., Ms, Nordenberg, D. M. D., Williamson, D.F. M. S., ... Mph. (1998). Relationship of childhood abuse and household dysfunction to many of the leading causes of death in adults: The adverse childhood experiences (ACE) study. *American Journal of Preventive Medicine, 14*(4), 245–258. 10.1016/S0749-3797(98)00017-8

ICT, M.o.S.a., & Agency, N.I.S. (2020). The survey on smartphone overdependence: Ministry of Science and ICT and National Information Society Agency.

Jung, S., Lee, D., Park, S., Lee, K., Kweon, Y.-S., Lee, E.-J., ...Hong, H.J. (2019). Gender differences in Korean adolescents who died by suicide based on teacher reports. *Child and Adolescent Psychiatry and Mental Health, 13*(1), 12. 10.1186/s13 034-019-0274-3

Park, M., & Jeon, H. (2013). Relationships between health behaviors, mental health and internet addiction by gender differences among Korean adolescents. *Journal of the Korea Academia-Industrial Cooperation Society, 14*(3), 1283–1293. 10.5762/ KAIS.2013.14.3.1283

Reed, P., Romano, M., Re, F., Roaro, A., Osborne, L.A., Viganò, C., & Truzoli, R. (2017). Differential physiological changes following Internet exposure in higher and lower problematic internet users. *PLOS ONE, 12*(5), e0178480. 10.1371/journal. pone.0178480

Romano, M., Osborne, L.A., Truzoli, R., & Reed, P. (2013). Differential psychological impact of internet exposure on internet addicts. *PLOS ONE, 8*(2), e55162. 10.1371/journal.pone.0055162

Su, W., Han, X., Jin, C., Yan, Y., & Potenza, M.N. (2019). Are males more likely to be addicted to the Internet than females? A meta-analysis involving 34 global jurisdictions. *Computers in Human Behavior, 99*, 86–100. 10.1016/j.chb.2019.04.021

Chapter 12

Problematic Internet Usage among Women in Malaysia

*Su Tein Sim, Melisa Abdul Aziz, Norharlina Bahar,
Nik Ruzyanei Nik Jaafar, Normala Ibrahim,
Wan Salwina Wan Ismail, Azlin Baharudin, Kit-Aun Tan,
and Ling Shiao Ling*

Recent studies suggest gender differences in problematic internet usage and such differences could be attributed to usage patterns and motivation and could result in different psychological impacts. This chapter reviews the risk factors, internet-related activities, access to the internet, and internet usage sequelae among women in Malaysia. We conclude the chapter by summarizing current treatment models which could be used in managing problematic internet usage among Malaysian women. It is hoped that this chapter could provide insight into future research areas as new studies in the field continue to emerge.

Introduction

Malaysia is a multi-ethnic country in South-East Asia with 32 million people (Ying et al., 2021). According to the Malaysian Communications and Multimedia Commission (2020), there are 26.7 million Malaysian internet users and nearly half are women. The internet penetration in Malaysia has risen from 87.4% in 2018 to 131% in 2020 due to the Covid-19 pandemic. During the COVID-19 pandemic, the internet plays a vital role in maintaining work productivity, education, and social connections.

Despite the equal distribution of gender among internet users, most existing studies reported that men are more likely to engage in problematic use of the internet than women (Jaafar et al., 2017). However, the impact of problematic internet usage among women should not be neglected. As reported by some studies, men and women are equally at risk (Soh et al., 2013). Perhaps, women are more vulnerable to internet use related psychological distress than men (Mooi, 2019). Hence, this chapter highlights the internet usage pattern, motivation, and problematic internet usage sequelae among women in Malaysia.

DOI: 10.4324/9781003203476-17

Internet Usage Patterns among Women

Malaysian urban teenage girls spend as much as 8–10 hours a week on the internet (Soh et al., 2013). However, their internet usage is about 50% less than boys. Women tend to use more portable devices like smartphones, and tablets, whereas men prefer using laptops, game consoles, and personal computers (Jaafar et al., 2017). One possible explanation is that the functionality of these devices is customized for distinct types of internet-related activities. In contrast to the findings from past research, results from a local study reported no differences in devices used to access the internet between genders in Malaysia (Akin & Iskender, 2011).

Motivation in Problematic Internet Usage among Women

Only a few studies from other countries reported gender differences in internet motives. These studies reported that women use the internet to allow anonymous social interaction, information/surveillance, and online shopping (Jaafar et al., 2017). In other words, women prefer internet activities that involve social media and messaging applications. On the other hand, men use the internet to seek out dominance through either online games or online sexual fantasies (Jaafar et al., 2017). However, it was also reported that women increasingly access online gaming, which was previously considered a predominantly male activity (Shashaani, 1997).

Myriad motivational factors for women from different age groups to engage in internet usage exist. The young age group (14–18 years) usually uses the internet for social interaction, shopping and surveillance, and information searching (Soh et al., 2013). They are also keen to expand their social networks to gain peer interaction and acceptance (Jaafar et al., 2017). Women from other age groups (>18 years old) use the internet for information-searching and online shopping. However, they are more concerned with product quality and avoiding scammers and poor customer service (Majid & Firend, 2017).

Impacts of Problematic Internet Usage among Women

Problematic internet usage affects women in at least three aspects: biological, psychological, and social. As far as the biological aspect is concerned, the majority of devices used to access the internet involve screens that emit blue light. The harmful effects of bedtime blue light-emitting-device use on sleep have been reported previously (Jniene et al., 2019). In addition, there is cognitive stimulation and related sleep disturbances due to the brightness of the short blue wavelengths of light emitted by smartphone devices that disrupt the circadian rhythm. It has been shown that women become sedentary when their internet usage increased, resulting in higher risks of obesity, unhealthy eating habits, cigarette, and alcohol use (Jaafar et al., 2017). Lack of physical activities and long hours using devices in poor posture could lead to stiff necks along with other musculoskeletal problems (Jniene et al., 2019).

Regarding psychological impacts, women with problematic internet usage are vulnerable to developing depression and anxiety issues even though such a developmental pathway could not be causally determined (Mooi, 2019). The Internet provides escapism for people with psychological problems to positively reinforce their avoidant behaviour (Akin & Iskender, 2011). The associations between internet use, particularly online gaming, with emotional and behavioural issues (e.g., aggressive behaviour, cyberbullying, and dating violence) are more pronounced in young women than in young men (Jaafar et al., 2017).

Concerning social consequences, excessive internet use could result in high parental distraction and neglect of child safety, and low parental engagement (Aziz et al., 2016). However, no significant impacts of problematic internet usage on marital satisfaction were shown in the local population. In general, women are often considered to have lower digital literacy, digital self-efficacy, and higher technology anxiety than men (Shashaani, 1997). This was found to be pronounced in the middle and older age women groups, subjecting them to internet security issues and making them vulnerable to scams and cybercrime (e.g., fraud and love scams; Zulkipli, 2021).

Treatment Models for Internet-Related Problem

Treatment and preventive measures for problematic internet use are available, but such measures targeting young internet users are not gender-specific. Therefore, a bio-psycho-social model has been developed to address internet-related problems. Individuals who suffer from internet-related problems were found to have psychological comorbidities such as anxiety and depression (Mooi, 2019). Hence, biological treatment mainly consists of pharmacological medications to target such comorbidity or underlying mental illness. The most common pharmacological treatment options for internet-related issues among women are antidepressants and benzodiazepines (Jaafar et al., 2017).

As for psychotherapy options, cognitive-behavioural therapy (CBT) trials have shown promising outcomes to address problematic internet usage in a local study (Ke & Wong, 2018). In this study, a one-month intervention program known as Psychological Intervention Program-Internet Use for Youth, incorporating CBT and positive psychology theory, was delivered. This was found to reduce social anxiety, strengthen coping skills, and improve insights. The effectiveness of reality group therapy on problematic internet use was documented in another local study (Shafie et al., 2019). By addressing five basic needs (i.e., power, love and belonging, freedom, fun, and survival), this therapy approach may help individuals achieve self-actualization and enhance their interpersonal skills and inhibit problematic internet use behaviour.

More than two-thirds (68.6%) of participants had low to middle monthly income, earning 500,000 to 7,000,000 Rupiah (€29,20 to €408,74). Around one-third (30.9%) of participants reported liking high-fat foods, 33.0% flour-containing foods, 20.1% sweet foods, 14.4% salty snacks, and 1.5% sugary drinks. Women tended to cook at home (67.5%) rather than eating fast food (32.5%).

Measures

BMI. Participants self-reported their height and weight to calculate BMI (kg/m^2), which was then categorized according to the WHO Asia-Pacific BMI Classification as underweight (<18.5), normal (18.5–22.9), overweight (23–24.9), and obese (≥25).

YFAS 2.0. The Yale Food Addiction Scale (YFAS) was developed as a scale for measuring addictive-like-eating behaviour and was revised to the YFAS version 2.0 in 2016 (Gearhardt et al., 2016). The scale is based on the 11 criteria for the diagnosis of Substance-Related and Addictive Disorders in the Diagnostic and Statistical Manual of Mental Disorders, 5th edition (DSM-5) (American Psychiatric Association, 2013) to measure the presence or absence of FA. In addition, FA severity can be classified as mild (two to three symptoms), moderate (four to five symptoms), and severe (six or more symptoms). The 11 symptoms included in the YFAS 2.0 are as follows: 1) Substances that are consumed in greater quantities and for a longer period of time than intended; 2) Persistent desire or repeated unsuccessful attempts to quit; 3) Lots of time/activity to acquire, use, and recover from eating; 4) Important social, occupational, or recreational activities are stopped or reduced; 5) Continue to use despite knowing the adverse consequences; 6) Tolerance (significant increase in amount, marked decrease in effect); 7) Characteristics of withdrawal symptoms, eating to relieve withdrawal; 8) Continue to use despite social or interpersonal problems; 9) Failure to fulfill lead role obligations; 10) Use in physically hazardous situations; 11) Craving, or a strong desire or urge to use. These symptoms were summed into a continuous score. FA diagnosis also required the presence of clinically significant impairment or distress. The YFAS 2.0 has shown high internal reliability and a unidimensional structure in several studies, supporting its construct validity (Meule & Gearhardt, 2019). In the current study, a reliability analysis with the alpha coefficients of the Indonesian YFAS 2.0 adaptation resulted in $\alpha = .87$. The items showed item-rest correlations between .45 and .65. Test validation results using Confirmatory Factor Analysis indicated that the one-factor model is adequate in our data ($x^2/df = 2.34$, RMSEA = .08, SRMR = .05, CFI = .92, GFI = .91). In summary, the psychometric properties of the Indonesian YFAS 2.0 adaptation indicated that the scale is reliable and valid.

Results

Participant characteristics are shown in Table 13.1. Around 3.6% of participants met FA criteria and 14.3% of those were classified as moderate and 85.7% as severe. Overall, the average number of symptoms met was 1.36 (range = 0–11). YFAS 2.0 symptom criteria met by participants from the total sample varied from 4.1% for "use causing significant impairment or distress" to 18.6% for "persistent desire or repeated unsuccessful attempts at quitting." The average score of those with FA was 8.14 (range = 5–11) and the most common symptom was the presence of characteristic withdrawal symptoms. Among participants who met the diagnosis of FA, 57.1% lived in Java (an urban area), 85.7% lived with other people, all were highly educated, and all worked as professionals or employees. More than one-fourth (28.6%) of participants with FA had low income and 71.4% had a medium income. Participants with FA preferred high-sugar foods (42.9%), flour-containing food (42.9%), and fatty foods (14.3%). About 71.4% had a weight above average, but 28.6% had normal BMI.

Bivariate comparisons showed that the prevalence of FA did not differ by age group, domicile, with whom participants lived, educational level, occupation, income, BMI categories, favorite food, or eating habit (all $p>0.05$). However, there was a positive correlation between BMI score and the continuous YFAS 2.0 score ($r = .178, p = .013$). Positive correlations were also found between BMI score and some diagnostic indicators in the YFAS 2.0, such as substance taken in larger amount and for longer period than intended ($r = .180, p = .012$), withdrawal ($r = .148, p = .040$), and continued use despite social or interpersonal problems ($r = .257, p = .000$).

Discussion

In this study, we aimed to determine how common FA is in the adult Indonesian female population, with a higher prevalence of obesity compared to the male population. Determining the prevalence of FA will enable us to learn more about the FA construct which is still a controversy. We also aimed to observe the relationship between sociodemographic factors with FA and the YFAS 2.0 score, respectively, to determine which factors may influence the occurrence of FA.

Our findings indicate that the prevalence of FA in Indonesian women is around 3.6%. A study from Brazil that also used a non-clinical sample found a similar prevalence in adult women of 5.3% (Nunes-Neto et al., 2018). Another study found that the prevalence varies from 3% to 20%, where the prevalence is higher in people with obesity, eating disorders, or bulimia nervosa (Meule & Gearhardt, 2019). In terms of severity, several studies showed that participants with FA tend to show severe expressions rather than moderate FA or mild FA (Gearhardt et al., 2016; Meule et al., 2017). This is

Table 13.1 Participant characteristics (N = 194)

Variable	Total	FA	No FA	P-value
	(N = 194)	(n = 7)	(n = 187)	
Age (Years)				0.090
Median (Minimum-Maximum)	28 (18–70)	25 (23–27)	29(18–70)	
Domicile (N, %)				0.054
Java	163 (84)	4 (57.1)	159 (85)	
Sumatera	7 (3.6)	1 (14.3)	6 (3.2)	
Sulawesi	7 (3.6)	1 (14.3)	6 (3.2)	
Kalimantan	4 (2.1)	0 (0)	4 (2.1)	
Nusa Tenggara	9 (4.6)	0 (0)	9 (4.8)	
Bali	1 (0.5)	0 (0)	1 (0.5)	
Bangka Belitung	1 (0.5)	0 (0)	1 (0.5)	
Maluku	1 (0.5)	1 (14.3)	0 (0)	
Papua	1 (0.5)	0 (0)	1 (0.5)	
Living with (N, %)				1,000
Alone	22 (11.3)	1 (14.3)	21 (11.2)	
Parents/Family/Friends	172 (88.7)	6 (85.7)	166 (88.8)	
Educational Level (N, %)				0.779
Basic Education	20 (10.3)	0 (0)	20 (10.7)	
Higher Education	174 (89.7)	7 (100)	167 (89.3)	
Occupation (N, %)				0.447
Student	38 (19.6)	0 (0)	38 (20.3)	
Employee	28 (14.4)	2 (28.6)	26 (13.9)	
Teacher/Lecturer	10 (5.2)	0 (0)	10 (5.3)	
Entrepreneur	11 (5.7)	0 (0)	11 (5.9)	
Civil Servant	5 (2.6)	0 (0)	5 (2.7)	
Professional	88 (45.4)	5 (71.4)	83 (44.4)	
Housewife	6 (3.1)	0 (0)	6 (3.2)	
Other	8 (4.1)	0 (0)	8 (4.3)	
Income (N, %)				0.558
<Rp. 500.000	21 (10.8)	0 (0)	21 (10.8)	
Rp. 500.000 - Rp. 3.500.000	55 (28.4)	2 (28.6)	53 (28.4)	
Rp. 3.600.000 - Rp. 7.000.000	57 (29.4)	2 (28.6)	55 (29.4)	
Rp. 7.100.000 - Rp. 14.000.000	38 (19.6)	3 (42.9)	35 (19.6)	
Rp. 14.100.000 - Rp. 30.000.000	10 (5.2)	0 (0)	10 (5.2)	
>Rp. 30.000.000	11 (5.7)	0 (0)	11 (5.7)	
No Answer	2 (1)	0 (0)	2 (1)	
BMI (N, %)				0.185
Median (Minimum-Maximum)	23.24 (16.22–44.08)	25.15 (19.29–28.40)	23.23 (16.22–44.08)	
Obese	63 (32.5)	4 (57.1)	59 (31.6)	
Overweight	43 (22.2)	1 (14.3)	42 (22.5)	
Normal	73 (37.6)	2 (28.6)	71 (38)	
Underweight	15 (7.7)	0 (0)	15 (8)	
Favorite Food (N, %)				0.079
Sweets	39 (20.1)	3 (42.9)	36 (19.3)	
Starches	64 (33)	3 (42.9)	61 (32.6)	
Salty Snacks	28 (14.4)	0 (0)	28 (15)	
Fatty Foods	60 (30.9)	1 (14.3)	59 (31.6)	
Sugary Drinks	3 (1.5)	0 (0)	3 (1.6)	

(Continued)

Table 13.1 (Continued)

Variable	Total	FA	No FA	P-value
	(N = 194)	*(n = 7)*	*(n = 187)*	
Eating Habit (N, %)				0.684
Home Cooking	63 (32.5)	3 (42.9)	60 (32.1)	
Eating out	131 (67.5)	4 (57.1)	127 (67.9)	
YFAS 2.0 Score				
Mean (Minimum-Maximum)	1.36 (0–11)	8.14 (5–11)	1.10 (0–11)	

Note

BMI: Body Mass Index; YFAS: Yale Food Addiction Scale.

possible because participants with lower symptom levels rarely meet the criterion of clinically significant impairment and distress.

More than half of participants (54.7%) in our study were overweight or obese, but not all participants who were overweight or obese have FA. Only 4.7% of overweight or obese participants had FA, and 28.6% of participants with FA had a normal BMI. Our results indicate that the BMI category is not significantly different in participants with FA compared to those without FA. Our findings were supported by 12/29 studies included in a systematic review and meta-analysis which found no difference between the BMI of individuals with or without FA (Fernandes et al., 2020). However, another nine studies observed that FA was more common in people with a higher BMI.

We also assessed types of food participants favored. Of participants who met the diagnosis of FA, 42.9% liked eating sweets, 42.9% starches, and 14.3% fatty food. Several studies have shown that men report more cravings for savory foods (e.g., meat, fish, eggs), whereas women report more cravings for sweet foods (e.g., chocolate, pastries, ice cream) (Halllam et al., 2016). The present study did not reveal any differences between participants with and without FA in eating habits (home-cooked food vs. fast food) or living situation (either alone or with others). Therefore, these recreational and socialization factors did not seem to affect the occurrence of FA in our sample.

Further, there was no significant difference between the FA and the non-FA group regarding age, domicile, occupation, monthly income, or education level. This is in line with previous research (Gearhardt et al., 2016) which did not find a relationship between age, ethnicity, and education level with the total score of FA symptoms or the likelihood of meeting the FA diagnostic threshold. However, this study found a relationship between gender and FA symptoms, where women had more symptoms than men.

Although the current study used a sample of women from a non-clinical population with a wide age range, participants were not representative of the general Indonesian population. Most participants lived in Java and centrally in the city, especially in Jakarta, one of the largest urban areas in Indonesia.

People who live in urban areas tend to have higher education compared to rural areas. The use of a nationally representative sample of Indonesian adult women in future studies would certainly help estimate the prevalence of FA more accurately. The prevalence of FA as assessed with YFAS 2.0 criteria was relatively low, which prevented us from carrying out more complex analyzes. Moreover, BMI was based on self-report. Second, because this study was only conducted with women, the results cannot be generalized to both sexes. Third, due to the cross-sectional design of our study, it is not possible to determine whether sociodemographic characteristics, eating habits, or BMI contribute to the development of FA among women over time.

In conclusion, we were able to show that a non-negligible proportion of Indonesian women are affected by FA. Further investigation is needed, particularly longitudinal studies, to determine the relationship between the phenomenon of FA and obesity.

References

American Psychiatric Association. (2013). *Diagnostic and statistical manual of mental disorders*. 5th ed. American Psychiatric Association.

Fernandes, M.S., Master, G.C., Master, R.M., Oliveira, T.L., Ribeiro, I.D., Silva, L.D., et al. (2020). Relation of food addiction in overweight/obesity, depression and impulsivity: A systematic review and meta-analysis. *Health Science Journal, 14*(5), 737.

García-García, I., Jurado, M.A., Garolera, M., Segura, B., Marqués-Iturria, I., Pueyo, R., et al. (2013). Functional connectivity in obesity during reward processing. *Neuroimage*, 232–239.

Gearhardt, A.N., Corbin, W.R., & Brownell, K.D. (2016). Development of the yale food addiction scale version 2.0. *Psychology of Addictive Behaviors, 30*(1), 113–121.

Halllam, J., Boswell, R.G., DeVito, E.E., & Kober, H. (2016). Gender-related differences in food craving and obesity. *Yale Journal of Biology and Medicine, 89*(2), 161–173.

Harbuwono, D.S., Pramono, L.A., Yunir, E., & Subekti, I. (2018). Obesity and central obesity in Indonesia: Evidence from a national health survey. *Medical Journal of Indonesia, 27*(2), 114–120.

Kenny, P.J. (2011). Reward mechanisms in obesity: New insights and future directions. *Neuron, 69*(4), 664–679.

Lutter, M., & Nestler, E.J. (2009). Homeostatic and hedonic signals interact in the regulation of food intake. *The Journal of Nutrition, 139*(3), 629–632.

Meule, A., & Gearhardt, A.N. (2019). Ten years of the yale food addiction scale: A review of version 2.0. *Current Addiction Reports, 6*, 218–228.

Meule, A., Müller, A., Gearhardt, A.N., & Blechert, J. (2017). German version of the yale food addiction scale 2.0: Prevalence and correlates of 'food addiction' in students and obese individuals. *Appetite, 115*, 54–61.

Nunes-Neto, P.R., Köhler, C.A., Schuch, F.B., Solmi, M., Quevedo, J., Maes, M., et al. (2018). Food addiction: Prevalence, psychopathological correlates and associations with quality of life in a large sample. *Journal of Psychiatric Research*, 145–152.

Rachmi, C.N., Li, M., & Baur, L.A. (2017). Overweight and obesity in Indonesia: Prevalence and risk factors-a literature review. *Public Health*, 20–29.

Randolph, T.G. (1956). The descriptive features of food addiction; addictive eating and drinking. *Quarterly Journal of Studies on Alcohol*, *17*(2), 199–224.

Stice, E., Yokum, S., Blum, K., & Bohon, C. (2010). Weight gain is associated with reduced striatal response to palatable food. *The Journal of Neuroscience*, *30*(39), 13105–13109.

The GBD 2015 Obesity Collaborators. (2017). Health effects of overweight and obesity in 195 countries over 25 years. *New England Journal of Medicine*, *377*(1), 13–27.

Volkow, N.D., Wang, G.-J., Telang, F., Fowler, J.S., Thanos, P.K., Logan, J., et al. (2008). Low dopamine striatal D2 receptors are associated with prefrontal metabolism in obese subjects: Possible contributing factors. *Neuroimage*, *42*(4), 1537–1543.

Volkow, N.D., Wise, R.A., & Baler, R. (2017). The dopamine motive system: Implications for drug and food addiction. *Nature Reviews Neuroscience*, (18), 741–752.

Wang, G.-J., Tomasi, D., Convit, A., Logan, J., Wong, C.T., Shumay, E., et al. (2014). BMI modulates calorie-dependent dopamine changes in accumbens from glucose intake. *PloS One*, *9*(7), 1–4.

Yu, Y.-H., Vasselli, J.R., Zhang, Y., Mechanick, J.I., Korner, J., & Peterli, R. (2015). Metabolic vs. hedonic obesity: A conceptual distinction and its clinical implications. *Obesity Reviews*, *16*(3), 234–247.

Part V

Europe

Chapter 14

Shielded from View? Gender Bias in Gambling Research, Prevention, and Treatment

Heather Wardle and Fay Laidler

Like other health-related issues, our understanding of gambling harms has a gender bias. By tracing how knowledge about gambling harms has developed, we see research systematically focusing on the experiences of men and translating what works for men to women. Women with lived experience of harm appear less likely than men to advocate for themselves, a situation exacerbated by the shame and stigma attached to gambling. Stereotypes of gambling as male-dominated arguably reinforce these norms, which then may become self-perpetuating. It is essential to critically examine our corpus of knowledge and to assess if and how gender biases have influenced, and continue to influence, our understanding of gambling harms.

Gender Bias in Gambling Research, Prevention, and Treatment

For good reason, gambling is known as the "hidden" addiction (Ladouceur, 2004). Those experiencing harm from behavioural addictions can be adept at hiding difficulties and behaviours from their loved ones and, arguably, from themselves. With few visible symptoms, all too often, family, friends, or employers of those affected by gambling harms say they were unaware of the full extent of problems experienced until it was too late. For some, this awareness only begins with the emergence of a legal or financial crisis, with attendant emotional impacts on all involved at the point of "discovery" (Holdsworth et al., 2013). Furthermore, those experiencing harm often don't speak out because of feelings of shame and stigma surrounding gambling, something that Livingstone and Rintoul (2021) have argued is exacerbated by policy focus on "responsible gambling." According to Livingstone and Rintoul (2021), this decades-old focus on "responsible gambling" extends notions of shame and self-stigmatization among those experiencing harm because "it carries with it a message of irresponsibility and shame for those who supposedly cannot control their gambling." This shame and stigmatization have very real consequences. In Britain, we see a large disconnect between the number of people likely to be in need for treatment and support from gambling harms and those actually accessing these services. Subsequent studies examining this identify shame and stigma as major barriers to accessing help and support

DOI: 10.4324/9781003203476-20

(NatCen, 2020). This is further underpinned by societal-level negative perceptions of those experiencing gambling difficulties even though gambling is something that is normalized by many governments and industry alike (Carroll et al., 2013). Extending this, Baxter et al. (2015) looked at experiences and perceptions of gambling-related shame and stigma through a gendered lens, concluding that "efforts to engage people who face gambling problems need to consider gendered perceptions of what is viewed as stigmatizing." In short, men and women may have very different perspectives of gambling-related stigma which is likely bound with a whole range of other normative perceptions and experiences relating to roles, expectations, and responsibilities.

At a societal level, gambling tends not to attract the same kind of policy attention or resources of other similar public health issues; the impact of this being to effectively minimize gambling as public health concern. Alongside this is a growing network of increasingly global corporations who are adept at lobbying governments, and the wider public, promoting their views of gambling as "leisure" with harms affecting only a "tiny" minority and extending notions of "responsible gambling" among individuals as the solution to managing harms. Advocates for policy and regulatory change work within an exceptionally difficult political landscape and whilst excellent advocacy networks (in Britain, at least) have developed, the broader environment in which gambling is situated, also arguably, conspires to shield the full nature and extent of gambling harms from view.

Within this environment, our understanding of women's experiences of gambling, their gambling careers, and their pathways to harm are even less well understood. Lack of understanding about the gendered nature of harm and its impact on health is not a phenomenon unique to gambling, but something that pervades health research more generally. However, until recently, there have been few steps within gambling research, prevention, and treatment to understand or correct this bias. This has potentially profound implications for how women are supported in their recovery and how we design and implement female-centered policies to prevent harm from occurring in the first place. In this chapter, we explore some potential reasons this situation has occurred and situate this within broader trends evident within the health field.

In 2010, Richard Horton (editor-in-chief of The Lancet) wrote an editorial arguing that despite international and concerted action to focus on the health of women and children, they continued to be invisible, outlining ten reasons why he believed this to be the case. Whilst further exemplifying how issues of gender bias are far from unique to gambling, this provides a useful framework around which to assess why women (and to some extent children also) may continue to be invisible within gambling policy and practice.

First and foremost for Horton (2010) was "The Mission." For him, focus on women's health was originally conceived as an issue of social justice, a focus which has gradually been eroded by agencies concentrating increasingly on technical solutions than broader issues of social and political equity.

Within the gambling policy environment, there is clear reticence to engage with or explore how gambling fits within broader social and political theories and movements. Whilst some argue that gambling policy should be considered an issue of social justice and highlight how gambling contributes towards and reinforces inequities (Reith, 2018; Wardle et al., 2019), there is limited adoption of these perspectives among policy makers. Instead, there is disproportionate focus on technical solutions – such as self-exclusion, pre-commitment, deposit limits, and enforcement of responsible gambling tools. Few of these technical solutions have been examined through a gendered lens.

For Horton, "evaluation" was another critical element contributing to the invisibility of women within health research and practice. He argued we have spent far too little time monitoring the effects of policies on maternal health, and that with no data, women and children struggle to be seen. The same is true for women within gambling. There is and continues to be a systematic bias towards understanding male experiences. In 2021 alone, hundreds of new empirical research studies on gambling behaviours, prevention, and treatment were published. Whilst many included both men and women in their samples, results were not generally presented separately by sex. Closer examination of these studies reveals a bias towards male participants, whereby men out-number women in the sample or where the population of focus (i.e., sports bettors, online bettors, or treatment populations) naturally favors the over-inclusion of men. Results reported for all are naturally skewed towards male behaviours and experiences, with female behaviours seen as an extension of this (Mark & Lesieur, 1992). Even in gender-specific studies focus on men outweighs focus on women by a factor of nearly 2:1.[1] Our knowledge about gambling continues to be dominated by the male experience.

Relatedly, Horton noted how women's health and death were not valued in the same way as others. Here we are forced to confront a series of un-settling questions: is the systematic gender bias in gambling knowledge part of this broader trend whereby women's experiences are simply not valued in the same way as those for men? As researchers, if we adhere to the idea of gambling being a "male" dominated pursuit, does this naturally reinforce the male subtype as the primary object of inquiry?

This is also likely compounded by another of Horton's explanations – that of "translation." Here he argued that failure to account for differences between groups of people compounds one invisibility with another. Given the bias towards male experience, gambling research, policy, and practice almost certainly suffers from issues of translation in that what is assumed to hold true for men will also hold true for women. This has implications for the type and nature of prevention strategies implemented. The antecedents of this can be traced back to the seminal research of Robert Custer, whose work in-formed how gambling came to be understood as a medical issue (Rosenthal, 2020). Custer's early work on gambling was based on either studies of male veterans or overwhelmingly on male samples from those attending GA.

Subsequent studies replicated and extended this, with an over-representation of men or, where women were included, a lack of clarity regarding gender-specific analyzes. This generates some uncertainty around the extent to which understanding of gambling as mental health disorder and the criterion used to diagnose it have taken female experiences into account.

Extending this, Horton highlighted "prevention" as a critical issue, drawing attention to the lack of strategic action to tackle the determinants of child and maternal ill-health. Again, too often there is an assumption of what works for men will also work for women (Mark & Lesieur, 1992) and little strategic action aimed at preventing gambling harms among women, though arguably there is little strategic action or consensus around prevention of gambling harms more generally.

Horton also argued that a lack of integration within the health community, especially between science, practice, and advocacy, continued to reinforce existing biases and further exacerbate the exclusion of women and children from health. Gambling policy and practice also suffer from a lack of integration between communities of researchers, practitioners, and policy makers. Despite the growth of gambling as a multi-national industry, where corporations transcend national boundaries through a complex web of mergers, acquisitions, and partnerships, there is little integrated or international collaboration focusing on gambling as a global health issue. Positive steps have been taken, with the World Health Organization showing interest in gambling policy and reform, but there is arguably a lack of leadership (another of Horton's factors) to drive the kind of integration needed. This is arguably amplified for women. Organizations focusing on female gambling are even more dispersed and, in some jurisdictions, do not exist. In the UK, a lack of integrated understanding between treatment needs and support provision means that, in some areas, women have a greater reliance on joining Gamblers Anonymous (GA) for support, where they are welcome. However, GA may not cater to their specific needs and groups may often be dominated by men. Some women report finding them intimidating and unhelpful. A similar situation is reported in Italy and other countries alike.

Expanding on these structural themes, Horton also identified empowerment, organization, and advocacy as key contributors to the continuing invisibility of women's health. These certainly have resonance when applied to gambling specifically. Empowerment and advocacy are needed to support women to drive policy and deliver improvements in health outcomes. Within gambling, we see (certainly in the UK at least) increasing empowerment among those with lived experience of harm, be it those who themselves have struggled with gambling or those who have been affected by the gambling of someone else. This has given rise to an increasing number of advocacy groups and movements. And they have been successful, one charity which focuses on providing peer-to-peer support for gambling harms recently won the Royal Society for Public Health's Health on the High Street award for their work providing rapid support to people gambling in betting shops.

Yet, many of these support organizations and networks have been founded by men whose own experience of and recovery from gambling harms provided a catalyst for them to help others. Interestingly, we have not seen women organizing and advocating on the same scale, or a focus on female-centered advocacy – rather they are subsumed within existing networks and structures. Where women have provided powerful advocacy, it is commonly through their role as an individual affected by the gambling of others – too often women are bereaved by death from gambling-related suicide of a child or partner. Grief and anger have been powerful catalysts for their empowerment and advocacy. Arguably, the same barriers of shame and stigma surrounding treatment seeking and support may be applied to women's willingness to engage, organize, and advocate for themselves. In the UK, an increasing number of high-profile sports men are speaking out about their experiences with gambling, with media interviews and television documentaries showcasing their journeys. Yet, there is a lack of well-known females providing similar representation, arguably reinforcing the perception of gambling harms as a male-centric experience.

All these factors may serve to further obscure women's experiences of gambling from view and serve to reinforce the invisibility of women from gambling research, policy, and practice. Gambling behaviour is gendered, yet work exploring this is relatively cursory focusing on women's stated preference for chance-based games (without exploring why) or simply mapping basic descriptive differences between men and women – potentially doing a disservice to both.

We are not the first to call attention to this. Mark and Lesieur highlighted the same in 1992 when reviewing gambling studies published to date. They noted that most research about gambling was male orientated and asserted that gender was rarely considered in the literature because gambling is seen as a male-dominated pursuit. Female gamblers are viewed by many researchers as the exception rather than the rule, or as a group to which male-orientated theories can be applied with similar results. Mark and Lesieur (1992) encouraged researchers to pay close attention to these processes, especially when developing diagnostic screening instruments.

Unfortunately, these warnings have not always been heeded. Numerous screening tools and standardized instruments continue to be developed with limited attention to gendered behaviours, attitudes, or experiences. As previously, these studies still often include systematic biases in their samples towards men and rarely conduct or adequately detail differences by gender. Many instruments aimed at measuring problem gambling or gambling harm regularly show large differences between men and women. Yet, the lack of attention to gender-specific development raises questions about where some of this may, in part, be a legacy of their development.

In other public health and mental health areas, there is increasing recognition that their diagnosis and measurement may require more consideration of gendered behaviours and experiences than previously acknowledged. For example, researchers examining autism are increasingly recognizing gender-specific behaviours (such as imitation of social interactions) that may mask autism among women, with researchers concluding that existing autism measures may under-represent women with autism (Brugha et al., 2016). Similar arguments have been levied at the measurement and diagnosis of non-suicidal self-harm, with researchers this time highlighting the female bias in research and evidence, stemming from the early assumption that this behaviour was more apparent in females than males (Victor et al., 2018).

These brief examples show how our gendered norms and biases can be easily absorbed, wittingly or otherwise, into our understanding of behaviours. These then may become self-perpetuating as the evidence base generated reflects and reinforces these norms. Now is the time to critically reflect upon our corpus of knowledge and to assess if and how similar issues may have influenced our conceptualization of gambling disorders and harms. Put simply, one reason we know little about how gambling harms affect women is that we haven't adequately asked them, or we haven't asked them in enough depth or in the right environments. This relates to both women who gamble and women who experience harm as an affected other. Neither have we created the conditions to support women with lived experience to join the debate and contribute to setting policy and research agendas. This focus has simply not been a policy or research priority and thus has not been explored in detail. Acknowledging this is the first step. Researchers, policy makers, and clinicians should critically reflect on how our knowledge about gambling has been generated, the processes involved, and the ongoing impact of this, especially upon women, and question whether now is the time for change.

Note

1   This is based on screening all articles published in 2021 (up to September 2021) on the PubMed database with gambling either as a keyword, in abstract, or title.

References

Baxter, A., Salmon, C., Dufresne, K., Carasco-Lee, A., & Matheson, F.I. (2015). Gender differences in felt stigma and barriers to help-seeking for problem gambling. *Addictive Behaviors Reports*, *3*(3), 1–8. 10.1016/j.abrep.2015.10.001. PMID: 29531995; PMCID: PMC5845950.

Brugha, T., Spiers, N., Bankart, J., Cooper, S., McManus, S., et al. (2016). Epidemiology of autism in adults across age groups and ability levels. *British Journal of Psychiatry*, *209*(6), 498–503. 10.1192/bjp.bp.115.174649

Carroll, A. et al. (2013). Stigma and help seeking for gambling problems. *Gambling and Racing Commission*. Available at: https://www.gamblingandracing.act.gov.au/__data/assets/pdf_file/0005/745034/Stigma-and-help-seeking-for-gambling-problems-Report-November-2013.pdf

Holdsworth, L., Nuske, E., Tiyce, M., *et al.* (2013). Impacts of gambling problems on partners: Partners' interpretations. *Asian Journal of Gambling Issues and Public Health, 3*, 11. 10.1186/2195-3007-3-11

Horton, R. (2010). The continuing invisibility of women and children. *Lancet, 375*(9730), 1941–1943. 10.1016/S0140-6736(10)60902-6. PMID: 20569823.

Ladouceur, R. (2004). Gambling: The hidden addiction. *The Canadian Journal of Psychiatry, 49*(8), 501–503. 10.1177/070674370404900801

Livingstone, C., & Rintoul, A. (2021). Gambling-related suicidality: Stigma, shame, and neglect. *Lancet Public Health, 6*(1), e4–e5. 10.1016/S2468-2667(20)30257-7.

Mark, M.E., & Lesieur, H.R. (1992). A feminist critique of problem gambling research. *British Journal of Addiction, 87*(4), 549–565. 10.1111/j.1360-0443.1992.tb01957.x

NatCen. (2020). A needs assessment for treatment and support services. Available at: https://www.begambleaware.org/sites/default/files/2020-12/a-needs-assessment-for-treatment-and-support-services.pdf

Reith, G. (2018). *Addictive consumption: Modernity, capitalism and excess.* London: Routledge.

Rosenthal, R.J. (2020). Inclusion of pathological gambling in DSM-III, its classification as a disorder of impulse control, and the role of Robert Custer. *International Gambling Studies, 20*(1), 151–170, 10.1080/14459795.2019.1638432

Victor, S.E., Muehlenkamp, J.J., Hayes, N.A., Lengel, G.J., Styer, D.M., & Washburn, J.J. (2018). Characterizing gender differences in nonsuicidal self-injury: Evidence from a large clinical sample of adolescents and adults. *Comprehensive Psychiatry, 82*, 53–60. 10.1016/j.comppsych.2018.01.009

Wardle, H., Reith, G., Langham, E., & Rogers, R.D. (2019). Gambling and public health: We need policy action to prevent harm. *BMJ, 365*, l1807. 10.1136/bmj.l1807

Chapter 15

Gender-Specific Personalized Care Delivery for Problematic Use of Internet in Switzerland

Sophia Achab

The proportion of women treated for problematic internet use (PIU) is growing. In addition, women play a major role in facilitating treatment seeking for their partners and children. PIU in women has specific motives and determinants that must be assessed and acknowledged to adjust the care response. Treating women for addictive behaviours is a human endeavor, which would benefit from a female care providers' lens for in-depth and comprehensive assessment and treatment. I capitalized on 15 years of experience to shed light on clinical and public health issues related with PIU in Swiss women and the fit-for-purpose care response I fine-tuned including gender considerations.

Introduction

In Switzerland, Internet addiction has been considered a public health issue since mid-2000. This has led to the progressive implementation of public health actions. Its inclusion in the National Addictions Strategic Plan 2017–2024 has been a major step for the policy response to health harms related to Internet use (Achab, 2021). In 2013, the Federal Office of Public Health commissioned an advisory board on cyber addiction in Switzerland for scientific follow-up and for informing national policy making. I have been part of this gender-balanced (50% of women) taskforce since then. As a woman scientist and clinician, I have a particular focus on gender issues related to prevention needs and care response to Internet addiction in my country.

Problematic internet use (PIU) affects 3.8% of the Swiss population over 15 years old, with men (4.3%) slightly more affected than women (3.3%) (Hermann et al., 2020). However, in a national survey, we conducted on specialized facilities in addiction medicine in 2017, assistance for PIU was reported to be primarily sought for men, whereas women were reported to be the major facilitators of counseling and treatment seeking for their relatives (Hermann et al., 2020). We recommended further investigating this potential gender bias and the reasons behind women being underrepresented in assistance seeking for themselves (Hermann et al., 2020).

DOI: 10.4324/9781003203476-21

I have been conducting research in Swiss samples since 2009, to understand driving forces of problematic patterns of engagement in several online activities. In this chapter, I will present and discuss some of those findings in women.

During the same period, I have been leading the national pioneering outpatient facility specialized in addictive behaviours including PIU. To date, we treated more than 800 patients and relatives. I continuously adapted the care offered to meet emerging and changing needs. In this chapter, I will share the concept and strategies I designed for meeting the female clients' needs. I will also discuss the driving forces of my actions and those of my female multicultural and multidisciplinary team members.

Understanding Driving Forces of PIU in Women in Switzerland

Moving towards a personalized response to public health issues related with PIU in women in Switzerland and understanding female PIU profiles and their underlying psychosocial characteristics is a crucial preliminary step. I am drawing upon the evidence we collected during the last decade from different Swiss samples.

Problematic Mobile Phone Use in Young Adult Women

A recent European study conducted in university students aged 18–29 years, included a Swiss sample (n = 142; 65% female respondents) (Lopez-Fernandez et al., 2017). It showed that mobile PIU is most likely overrepresented in women, associated with patterns of heavy use, and particularly with some specific online activities including communication, buying, video gaming, and video watching. These findings can serve to orient national prevention measures against PIU, tailored to women. They can also guide clinical assessment for PIU in women, which should cover the amount of time devoted to mobile phone use and the types of online activities they engage in.

PIU in Senior Women

In 2016–2017, we conducted another study in a Swiss general population sample aged 60+ years. We investigated PIU and underlying psychological factors (Rochat et al., 2021). PIU was found to be associated with reduced psychological well-being and life satisfaction in 15% of seniors screening positive for PIU (Rochat et al., 2021). Some impulsivity dimensions (i.e., negative urgency, lack of premeditation, and perseverance) and low life satisfaction were found to be predictors of PIU in Swiss seniors (Rochat et al., 2021). Regardless of gender, problematic engagement in online activities was associated with maladaptive strategies to cope with life dissatisfaction and negative emotions (Rochat et al., 2021).

As caregivers, it is important to have these data in mind when screening for PIU in seniors of both genders and to design treatment plans accordingly, including strategies against life dissatisfaction, dysfunctional emotional coping, and impulsivity.

PIU in Treatment-Seeking Women

Analyzing clinical data (institutional electronic records) of individuals seeking treatment at the Swiss pioneering outpatient clinic for addictive behaviours (ReConnecte), having answered over a thousand treatment requests over more than a decade, is very informative regarding the treatment-seeking motives of women.

Of 557 treatment requests between 2007 and 2016, 90.5% were for psychotherapy for the person affected (the women's rate evolved from 2% to 27% during the period) and 9.5% for support and counseling of relatives (mainly requested by women).

Female patients' age ranged from 12 to 73 years and women sought treatment for themselves (31%) or were referred by a healthcare professional (46%) or by relatives (17%). Over 40% sought treatment for PIU: social networks (38%), sex addiction (33%), video games (28%), video watching (9%), shopping and gambling (4%), and non-specific PIU (19%). Interestingly, women present a broad range of motives for PIU beyond social networking. In some cases, the treatment-seeking motive hides another diagnosis. This was the case for 24% of those suffering from sex addiction, referred for social networking, and 9% of those presenting problematic video gaming, initially referred for video watching.

In most female patients, PIU was the primary disorder, with up to 8% presenting comorbid conditions such as depression, anxiety, borderline personality, or alcohol use disorder. This has important implications for the design of specific psychotherapeutic approaches for women and for the addiction medicine field in general – PIU should not merely be considered as a symptom of mood or anxiety disorders.

Taken together, these data highlight the need for a careful and comprehensive assessment of patients seeking treatment for PIU. Personalized assessment is even more crucial for women to avoid gender bias in referrals. Comprehensive assessment should include comorbid conditions along with underlying psychosocial drivers (e.g., low life satisfaction, high impulsivity, and self-esteem impairment).

In our specialized clinic, the majority of relatives (75%) seeking help are women – mothers (91.4%), spouses (6%), or daughters (3%). Support and information for relatives make up nearly 10% of our activity, and the work with them has been useful since it allows direct access to the patient – mainly men (89%) – for specialized psychotherapy. The period between the first meeting with the female relative initiating the treatment process and the first meeting with the patient with a PIU (80% of these cases are sons with gaming disorder) ranged from 1 week to 2 years. It seems that the alliance we developed with relatives, and the support we provided to them, was able to trigger, sooner or later, a treatment demand from the patient himself. Thus, a crucial need we identified during our experience in the last decade is including relatives, mostly women, in the treatment process – be it in the presence and absence of the patient.

Adapting to Women's Care and Counseling Needs

In response to the lack of a blueprint for treatment in this emerging field of medicine, I developed a treatment concept which was based on helping patients to reconnect to themselves, to their life goals, and to their loved ones. My conceptual approach was opposite to the few existing care offers a decade ago, which were based on the implicit or explicit goal of referees or patients, that of "disconnecting" individuals from an addictive product. The underlying concept for our work in Geneva is shared by each of the new collaborators I hired over time. It constitutes our core "WHY" and it led me to relabel the clinic "ReConnecte" in 2017, at its tenth anniversary (Pozniak, 2021).

During the 15 years of experience in leading ReConnecte, one of the first lessons learned was that assessing treatment expectancies, representations of the problem and habits of "limit-setting" for media use is a crucial prelimi-nary element to purposefully answer mothers' counseling demands (Achab, 2019; Achab et al., 2020; Achab & Zullino, 2017). Indeed, nearly one-third of clients presenting for treatment do not meet diagnostic criteria for PIU. In those cases, problems arise from intra-family conflicts about divergence in adopting technology or from different limits set by the two parents for their child's screen use. Our mission in responding to these issues is mainly counseling parents, mainly mothers, on setting limits and addressing potential prejudices about their children's media use. We also provide psychoeducation on media content, its benefits, and on the richness of interpersonal bonds which can develop in digital platforms. This requires good digital skills by the clinician (i.e., knowledge of categories of online activities and their features in terms of interactions, motivational components, perceived benefits from users, and associated risks for addictive patterns of use). It also requires specific therapeutic skills in the child psychiatry field (i.e., psychology of children and adolescents and purposeful work with parents in clinical set-tings) (Achab, 2019; Achab & Zullino, 2017).

A second lesson learned was that there can be many motives for seeking treatment for PIU, with three main categories: (a) intra-family conflicts crystallized around Internet use, (b) expression of a mild to severe primary acute psychiatric disorder (i.e., depression, anxiety, or ADHD), and (c) pri-mary PIU with/or without a comorbid psychosocial or somatic condition.

From the beginning of my clinical and research involvement in this specific field in 2006, I have gotten used to this type of clinical practice, and I have been creative in adapting to the demands of female relatives and of patients, including women. These skills still have to be developed in new health professionals entering the field, even if they are specialized in mental health and addictive disorders. I first noticed this need in 2013, when the treatment and counseling demands had grown in a magnitude that I had to hire a psychiatric nurse to cope with them. I had to train her and supervise her closely to develop the required skills mentioned above, capitalizing on her natural compassion and therapeutic skills.

This was the opportunity that led me to design a standardized decision-making diagram for the evaluation of treatment demands for PIU. In addition, I set up a comprehensive care process model (see Figure 15.1) based on the profiles of patients with PIU (Achab, 2016, 2018; Achab et al., 2015). Some recurrent clinical profiles were specific to women, such as emotion dysregulation as the main driving force of gaming disorder in girls, as well as affective dependence or addiction to social networks in women seeking treatment for sex addiction.

This decisional flowchart has now been implemented since 8 years, and has been considered very useful, satisfying, simple to use, and beneficial in

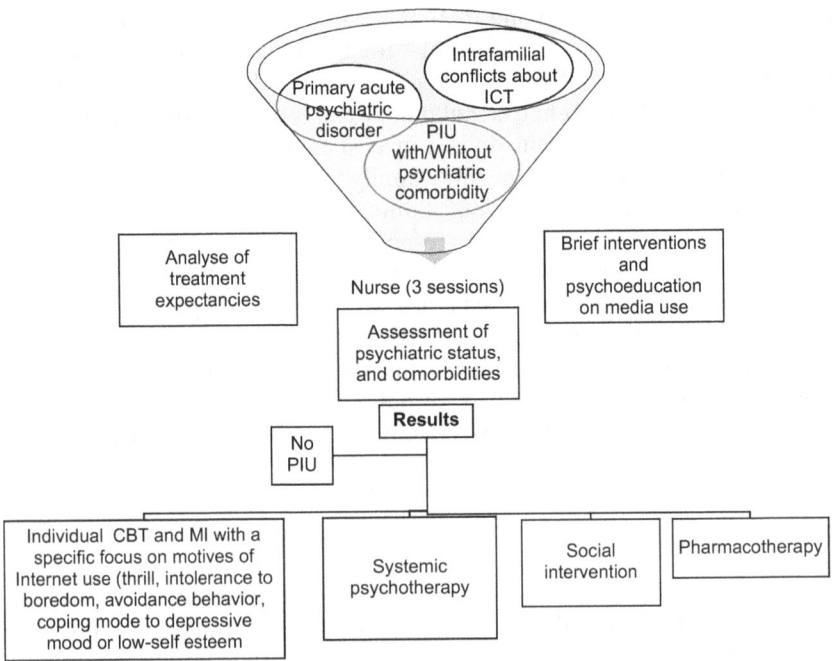

Figure 15.1 Care process model: decision-making diagram for evaluation of problematic internet use and suitable treatment options and approaches. *CBT = Cognitive and Behavioural Therapy; ICT = Information and Communication Tools; MI = Motivational Interview; PIU = Problematic Internet Use.*

offering a landmark for clinical practice by five of the six respondents to an evaluation survey I ran in May 2021, targeting all collaborators that have worked at the clinic since 2014. Only one of the six respondents found it useless, fearing duplication between the nurse's and the therapist's assessment, and a potentially increased risk of embarrassment and shame in patients assessed for sexual disorders.

For me, the care process model has been very useful for team management purposes, in terms of standardization, to achieve cohesion between assessors and therapists, and to plan the treatment trajectory for patients in the care system. Indeed, eight more colleagues (70% women) have progressively joined the clinic since 2014 – a multicultural and multidisciplinary taskforce consisting of nurses, medical trainees, psychiatrists specialized in addiction medicine or sexology, psychologists, and a social worker.

Conclusion

PIU is an increasing driver of treatment and counseling demands, with a broad range of psychosocial determinants, individual representations, and care driving forces. To meet the needs of female patients and female relatives, we need to view these topics from a female perspective.

Running a specialized clinic and conducting psychotherapy with people with PIU and other addictive behaviours and with their relatives has led me to design a fit-for-purpose care response, including gender-specific needs.

Acknowledgments

Many thanks to my team for the amazing work achieved all these years for patients and families trusting us.

References

Achab, S. (2016). *Features of gambling disorder and internet gaming disorder in the spectrum of addictive disorders*. University of Geneva.

Achab, S. (2018). Clinical practice in behavioural addictions, heterogeneous realities under homogeneous complaints in Switzerland. [Meeting abstract oral communication]. *Journal of Behavioral Addictions, 7*(Suppl. 1), 38.

Achab, S. (2019). Repères pour les praticiens concernant les troubles d'addiction aux jeux vidéo en ligne. *Le Courrier des Addictions, 4*, 9–11.

Achab, S. (2021). Internet patterns of use and which health promotion in Switzerland? *Revue medicale suisse, 17*(742), 1118–1121.

Achab, S., & Zullino, D. (2017). The digital age: A time of change for the medicine of addiction. *Psychotropes, 23*(3), 184.

Achab, S., Soulignac, R., Zullino, D., & Khazaal, Y. (2015). Addict sex-types, overview of clinical data of treatment seekers for problematic sexual behaviors. [Meeting abstract oral communication]. *Journal of Behavioral Addictions, 4*(Suppl. 1), 6.

Achab, S., Weber, N., Willemse, I., & Perissinotto, C. (2020). *Intervention guide for professionals regarding screens' use.* Retrieved from https://www.bag.admin.ch/dam/bag/fr/dokumente/npp/kinder-und-jugend/mediennutzung_model_zur_zusammenarbeit_mit_eltern.pdf.download.pdf/GREA_ecrans_FR_web_OK_FINAL.pdf.

Hermann, M., Stortz, C., & Perissinotto, C. (2020). *Problematic use of internet in Switzerland: Conclusions and recommendations from national expert group 2018-2020.* Bern: Swiss Federal Office of Public Health.

Lopez-Fernandez, O., Kuss, D.J., Romo, L., Morvan, Y., Kern, L., Graziani, P., et al. (2017). Self-reported dependence on mobile phones in young adults: A European cross-cultural empirical survey. *Journal of Behavioral Addictions, 6*(2), 168–177.

Pozniak, H. (2021, July). A very modern addiction. *Tech for good,* pp. 42–51. Retrieved from https://issuu.com/digitalbulletin/docs/tfg_issue13new?e=33076197/86387587

Rochat, L., Wilkosc-Debczynska, M., Zajac-Lamparska, L., Rothen, S., Andryszak, P., Gaspoz, J., et al. (2021). Internet use and problematic use in seniors: A comparative study in Switzerland and Poland. *Front Psychiatry, 12,* 609190.

Chapter 16

Gambling Disorders among Women with Suicidality

Guidance and Specificities

Mélina Andronicos and Monique Séguin

Gambling is strongly associated with male gender; therefore, pathological gambling (or gambling disorder) is predominantly considered a problem in men although 20% to 40% of pathological gamblers are women. While pathological gambling is a risk factor for suicide, it has been demonstrated that women have difficulties consulting specific services for their addiction due to social stigma, isolation, fear of being judged, or being threatened by their partners. Moreover, often obscured by a multitude of risk factors, gambling problems as well as suicidal behaviour can remain undetected in women. An empathetic and non-judgmental attitude is necessary for screening suicidal thoughts in women with problematic gambling.

Gambling Disorders among Women with Suicidality

Globally, more than 703,000 people die by suicide every year and at least ten times as many attempt suicide. Statistically, more than one in every hundred deaths (1.3%) is the result of suicide (WHO, 2021). Sociodemographic factors such as age and gender have been shown to be linked to the risk of death by suicide (Beck et al., 2011). Men tend to be more likely to complete suicide, whereas women are more likely to engage in a suicide attempt that does not lead to their death. Overall, the rates of completed suicide in women are substantially lower than in men, this being explained by men's tendency to choose more violent methods, but recently, in some countries, the rate of completion among women has been increasing (WHO, 2021). Research on suicide among women is still underdeveloped, particularly amongst gamblers.

A psychiatric disorder is the most robust risk factor for suicide. More specifically, suffering from a mood disorder—especially depression—substance abuse or a substance use disorder, a personality disorder, an impulsive control disorder, or an anxiety disorder is associated with higher suicide rates. Some environmental factors are linked to higher suicide risk, such as social isolation, loneliness, trouble with the law, or suicidal behaviours in the family. Some life trajectories are also associated with higher risk of suicide, and these are characterized by a heavy burden of adversity across several life domains, including mental health disorders,

DOI: 10.4324/9781003203476-22

social life and family ties, professional issues, etc. Indeed, most victims of suicide have been confronted with multiple adverse life events, such as divorce, a period of unemployment, the death of a loved one (possibly also due to suicide), or abusive or violent experiences throughout their life course (Séguin et al., 2014).

Suicide generally happens in the wake of a suicidal crisis, with varying evolution and variable psychological factors, including cognitive constriction over time. Everyday life requires dealing with good and bad moments, and people generally maintain a balance in their life by using various coping strategies to deal with negative events. These strategies can be emotional (e.g., crying), cognitive (e.g., rationalizing), or behavioural (e.g., seeing friends or practicing physical activities). Because gambling addiction can involve many kinds of adversity, such as financial stress, complications in one's professional life, lack of self-esteem, loss of a beloved person's trust, or feelings of shame or guilt, it is considered a risk factor for suicide. Indeed, up to 80% of individuals with a problematic gambling disorder express suicidal thoughts (Ledgerwood & Petry, 2004; Ledgerwood et al., 2005; Potenza et al., 2001). In the general population, this rate is estimated to be much lower, at 10–18% (Weissman et al., 1999). Some negative events can be particularly hard to cope with, to the point that some individuals may feel powerless and very vulnerable over a certain period of time and they might engage in inefficient coping strategies such as gambling. Researchers have found that 18% of problem gamblers reported having considered suicide, which is six times more often than non-problem gamblers (Zangeneh & Hason, 2006). An Austrian study observed that one in ten pathological gamblers had a history of suicide attempts (Thon et al., 2014). Gambling problems evolve over time. Ensuing issues such as social isolation and financial problems may lead to a suicidal crisis.

Regardless of gender, some pathological gamblers do not seek treatment due to feeling ashamed and embarrassed about their situation (Suurvali et al., 2012). Only 5–7% of gamblers seek treatment or join support groups to treat their gambling problems. When gambling becomes a problem, women wait on average 11 years before seeking help, whereas for men, this delay averages 4–5 years (Andronicos et al., 2015; Haw & Holdsworth, 2016). Gamblers who die by suicide are less likely to have a history of visits to mental health professionals or their general practitioner (Séguin et al., 2005).

Gamblers who have considered or attempted suicide have a greater number of psychiatric complications than non-suicidal gamblers, especially depression and substance abuse disorders (Komoto, 2014). Compared to the general population, gamblers in treatment reported more suicidal ideation, had more psychiatric symptoms, were less satisfied with their life situation, and had to deal with more difficulties in everyday life (Petry & Kiluk, 2002). Studies on suicidal ideation and suicide attempts in treatment-seeking pathological gamblers report that gamblers who had experienced suicidal behaviour were more likely to be unmarried, to have an early onset of problem gambling, to have been diagnosed with depressive or substance abuse disorders, and to have an immediate relative or family member with an alcohol use disorder. Impulsivity is a core characteristic of pathological gambling. Childhood adversity, such as exposure to parental violence, family tension, negligence, lack of or too much discipline, and physical or sexual abuse, is another clinical risk factor associated with pathological gambling (Andronicos et al., 2015).

Since gambling is strongly associated with male activity and therefore with men's care services, prevention programs, and research are designed to reach men (Andronicos et al., 2015; Merkouris et al., 2016). Yet 20–40% of pathological gamblers are women (Grant et al., 2012). It is important to highlight that women gamble for different reasons and in distinctive ways from men. Therefore, it is important that women be screened and treated differently for gambling addiction, as well as for other addictions and mental health disorders (Sanchis-Segura & Becker, 2016).

Most investigations suggest that, compared to male gamblers, female gamblers have lower self-esteem and suffer more frequently from mood and anxiety disorders, including major depression, dysthymia, panic disorder, social phobia, and generalized anxiety disorder (Desai & Potenza, 2008; Echeburúa et al., 2011; Grant et al., 2012). During adulthood, male pathological gamblers frequently live alone (widowed, separated, or divorced) and face professional difficulties, while female pathological gamblers are often victims of intimate partner violence (Andronicos et al., 2015). Women also show a higher vulnerability to suicidal behaviour than men (Fröberg et al., 2013). Furthermore, men and women may experience different emotions towards their gambling behaviours; women are more likely to feel guilt and shame about their gambling problems, while men are more likely to detach themselves from their gambling behaviours by attributing them to external causes (Suurvali et al., 2012). Women with gambling addiction particularly seek help for feelings of anguish, emptiness, loneliness, and fear of death (Domic, 2013). For gambling-related difficulties, women are more likely than men to admit their addiction problem and seek counseling; however, they are also less likely to experience remissions without intervention (Slutske et al., 2009).

Regrettably, female gamblers are often identified with the representation of vice, a stigma that causes deep suffering and fear of exclusion and leads women to hide their gambling activity. Researchers have underlined that it is difficult for women to consult addiction services, in particular for gambling problems, due to social stigma, social isolation or the fear of being judged, and sometimes due to being victims of partner violence (Andronicos et al., 2015; Domic, 2013). It has also been shown that women tend to seek consultation at a more advanced stage in their gambling pathology than men; they prioritize consultations in psychiatric services, psychotherapy, and medical advice from their general practitioner. In general, when women seek medical advice, they ask more questions during consultations than men (Beaulac et al., 2017). However, since a gambling problem can be obscured by a multitude of other risk factors, it may remain undetected (Andronicos et al., 2015).

Shame seems to be strongly associated with reluctance to enter treatment, particularly among women. Indeed, studies have shown that perceptions of normativity can influence seeking help, the impact on self-esteem being greater when a problem is perceived as non-normative. Accordingly, in order to support women seeking help, there is still much work to be done. Simplifying women's access to treatment or group support by destigmatizing female gambling, reducing waiting lists, or offering free treatment could be effective strategies. Post-mortem studies of women who were victims of suicide observed disadvantages regarding work, income, living alone, parental responsibilities, and education, highlighting that access to well paid jobs and access to daycare for children are important determinants of health for women (Séguin et al., 2021). Most importantly, it is well established that a prior history of attempting suicide is one of the strongest predictors of completed suicide. A Canadian study of women who had died by suicide found that 28% of the women in the sample had previously attempted suicide at least once in their life (Séguin et al., 2021).

From a public health perspective, suicidality in women may be detectable at several points during their life trajectories: when they face adversity during key developmental periods, in childhood (e.g., being a victim of violence or negligence), adolescence (e.g., academic difficulties, social isolation, mental health problems) and adulthood (e.g., abuse/misuse of alcohol or drugs, mental health problems, being a victim of violence, facing interpersonal difficulties) (Séguin et al., 2021), and even more so if they use gambling as a coping strategy. In addition, when women face contextual problems, such as loneliness or marital difficulties, gambling disorder strongly accelerates (González-Ortega et al., 2013). Women with gambling addiction tend to lose their money slowly and discreetly and find hidden sources of income, such as spending their savings, getting money in exchange for sex, or borrowing from their loved ones under the pretext of asking for help with their daily expenses (Tschibelu & Elman, 2010). Furthermore, being threatened by a lender or a loan shark, particularly when in personal bankruptcy, can have a strong influence on suicidal behaviour (Park et al., 2010; Wong et al., 2010). The context and social pressures related to gambling activity in women must be further investigated.

By way of illustration, a mother may be afraid that she could lose custody of her children due to her gambling problem and therefore hide it and not seek specific help. For that reason, social and mental health services should learn to systematically detect compulsive disorders such as gambling addiction. Primary care services workers should pay particular attention to exploring gambling problems once it has been observed that a woman is experiencing anxiety and difficulties in her relationships or finances. When we treat a woman with gambling problems, it is essential to spontaneously and frequently ask questions about suicidal behaviour and thoughts: for example, has she ever had suicidal thoughts or a suicide plan, is she currently having suicidal thoughts or planning suicide, and if so, the temporality of her plan, and the method and means being considered. Once she has revealed the temporality, method, and means of a plan to attempt suicide, counselors should protect her by calling on trusted relatives' support, by prescribing treatment or hospitalization and by removing the means. The evaluation of suicidal behaviour must be multi-faceted: the entire socio-health situation must be carefully assessed. The substance misuse or problematic activity must not be the only concern for the clinician: clinicians should examine their patient beyond problematic behaviours or behavioural addiction.

From the perspective of an early prevention approach, including relatives in therapeutic and social work can significantly promote recovery by providing relevant clues regarding the patient's everyday situation. This also provides a valuable opportunity to care for any relatives in distress.

In conclusion, among people with gambling problems, clinicians should be particularly attentive during a sudden increase in symptoms of mental health disorders, such as mood, substance use, and anxiety disorders, as these are all warning signs of risk of suicide. Monitoring such signs should be a routine part of screening for suicidality, particularly in the case of co-morbid disorders in patients and especially when a person is reporting debt. We must keep in mind that people with mental health problems are on average 17 times more likely to develop a gambling problem than the general population (Kessler et al., 2008). Moreover, the COVID-19 pandemic has triggered a 25% increase in the prevalence of anxiety and depression worldwide.

The issue of suicide is essential; any suicidal behaviour should be directly addressed. Suicide plans must be investigated in detail (where, when, how, and the means). Clinicians, social workers, and any person in contact with problem gamblers should be trained to investigate suicidal behaviour with a non-judgmental approach and should be able to call upon co-workers or supervisors when needed. Working to demystify mental health disorders, especially addictions such as pathological gambling, contributes to supporting women in need of help and thereby to preventing suicide in this population. Improving women's autonomy and social role (housing, work, leisure, etc.) and developing their social bonds is greatly helpful in that regard. Indeed, social support plays a key role in providing a sense of security for people with addictions and suicidal behaviours. The loss of relationships, separations, and criminal offenses may have a strong impact on suicidal behaviour: maintaining intensive contact with the patient is essential during such adversity. Overall, a multifactorial preventive approach, including universal, selective, and indicated interventions, is key to reducing suicide rates.

References

Andronicos, M., Beauchamp, G., DiMambro, M., Robert, M., Besson, J., & Séguin, M. (2015). Do male and female gamblers have the same burden of adversity over their life course? *International Gambling Studies*, *15*(2), 224–238. DOI 10.1080/14459795.2015.1024706

Beaulac, É., Andronicos, M., Lesage, A., Robert, M., Larochelle, S., & Séguin, M. (2017). Quelle est l'influence du genre dans la recherche de soins chez les joueurs? *Journal of Gambling Issues, 35.* DOI 10.4309/jgi.2017.35.5

Beck, F., Guignard, R., Du Roscoät, E., & Saïas, T. (2011). Tentatives de suicide et pensées suicidaires en France en 2010. *Bull Epidémiol Hebd, 47,* 488–492.

Desai, R.A., & Potenza, M.N. (2008). Gender differences in the associations between past-year gambling problems and psychiatric disorders. *Social Psychiatry and Psychiatric Epidemiology, 43*(3), 173–183. DOI 10.1007/s00127-007-0283-z

Domic, Z. (2013). L'addiction aux jeux d'argent chez la femme. *Psychotropes, 19*(3), 75–93. DOI 10.3917/psyt.193.0075

Echeburúa, E., González-Ortega, I., De Corral, P., & Polo-López, R. (2011). Clinical gender differences among adult pathological gamblers seeking treatment. *Journal of Gambling Studies, 27*(2), 215–227. DOI 10.1007/s10899-010-9205-1

Fröberg, F., Hallqvist, J., & Tengström, A.J.T.E.J.O.P.H. (2013). Psychosocial health and gambling problems among men and women aged 16–24 years in the Swedish. *National Public Health Survey, 23*(3), 427–433. DOI 10.1093/eurpub/cks129

González-Ortega, I., Echeburúa, E., Corral, P., Polo-López, R., & Alberich, S. (2012). Predictors of pathological gambling severity taking gender differences into account. *European Addiction Research, 19*(3), 146–154.

Grant, J.E., Chamberlain, S.R., Schreiber, L.R., & Odlaug, B.L. (2012). Gender-related clinical and neurocognitive differences in individuals seeking treatment for pathological gambling. *Journal of Psychiatric Research, 46*(9), 1206–1211. DOI 10.1016/j.jpsychires.2012.05.013

Haw, J., & Holdsworth, L. (2016). Gender differences in the temporal sequencing of problem gambling with other disorders. *International Journal of Mental Health and Addiction, 14*(5), 687–699. DOI 10.1007/s11469-015-9601-y

Kessler, R.C., Hwang, I., LaBrie, R., Petukhova, M., Sampson, N.A., Winters, K.C., & Shaffer, H.J. (2008). DSM-IV pathological gambling in the National Comorbidity Survey Replication. *Psychological Medicine, 38*(9), 1351–1360. DOI 10.1017/S0033291708002900

Komoto, Y. (2014). Factors associated with suicide and bankruptcy in Japanese pathological gamblers. *International Journal of Mental Health and Addiction, 12*(5), 600–606. DOI 10.1007/s11469-014-9492-3

Ledgerwood, D.M., & Petry, N.M. (2004). Gambling and suicidality in treatment-seeking pathological gamblers. *The Journal of Nervous and Mental Disease, 192*(10), 711–714. DOI 10.1097/01.nmd.0000142021.71880.ce

Ledgerwood, D.M., Steinberg, M.A., Wu, R., & Potenza, M.N. (2005). Self-reported gambling-related suicidality among gambling helpline callers. *Psychology of Addictive Behaviors, 19*(2), 175. DOI 10.1037/0893-164X.19.2.175

Merkouris, S.S., Thomas, A.C., Shandley, K.A., Rodda, S.N., Oldenhof, E., & Dowling, N.A. (2016). An update on gender differences in the characteristics associated with problem gambling: A systematic review. *Current Addiction Reports, 3*(3), 254–267. DOI 10.1007/s40429-016-0106-y

Park, S., Cho, M.J., Jeon, H.J., Lee, H.W., Bae, J.N., Park, J.I., ... Epidemiology, P. (2010). Prevalence, clinical correlations, comorbidities, and suicidal tendencies in pathological Korean gamblers: Results from the Korean. *Epidemiologic Catchment Area Study, 45*(6), 621–629. DOI 10.1007/s00127-009-0102-9

Petry, N.M., & Kiluk, B.D. (2002). Suicidal ideation and suicide attempts in treatment-seeking pathological gamblers. *The Journal of Nervous and Mental Disease, 190*(7), 462. DOI 10.1097/01.NMD.0000022447.27689.96

Potenza, M.N., Steinberg, M.A., McLaughlin, S.D., Wu, R., Rounsaville, B.J., & O'Malley, S.S. (2001). Gender-related differences in the characteristics of problem gamblers using a gambling helpline. *American Journal of Psychiatry, 158*(9), 1500–1505. DOI 10.1176/appi.ajp.158.9.1500

Sanchis-Segura, C., & Becker, J.B. (2016). Why we should consider sex (and study sex differences) in addiction research. *Addiction Biology, 21*(5), 995–1006. DOI 10.1111/adb.12382

Séguin, M., Beauchamp, G., & Notredame, C.-É. (2021). Adversity over the life course: A comparison between women and men who died by suicide. *Frontiers in Psychiatry, 1249.* DOI 10.3389/fpsyt.2021.682637

Séguin, M., Beauchamp, G., Robert, M., DiMambro, M., & Turecki, G. (2014). Developmental model of suicide trajectories. *The British Journal of Psychiatry, 205*(2), 120–126. DOI 10.1192/bjp.bp.113.139949

Séguin, M., Lesage, A., & Tousignant, M. (2005). Comparaison des trajectoires de vie chez des personnes ayant un problème de jeu excessif: Conséquences et difficultés de vie: Rapport de recherche dans le cadre du programme thématique Jeux de hasard et d'argent, *FQRSC.*

Slutske, W.S., Blaszczynski, A., & Martin, N.G. (2009). Sex differences in the rates of recovery, treatment-seeking, and natural recovery in pathological gambling: Results from an Australian community-based twin survey. *Twin Research and Human Genetics, 12*(5), 425–432. DOI 10.1375/twin.12.5.425

Suurvali, H., Hodgins, D.C., Toneatto, T., & Cunningham, J.A. (2012). Hesitation to seek gambling-related treatment among Ontario problem gamblers. *Journal of addiction medicine, 6*(1), 39–49. DOI 10.1097/ADM.0b013e3182307dbb

Thon, N., Preuss, U.W., Pölzleitner, A., Quantschnig, B., Scholz, H., Kühberger, A., ... & Wurst, F.M. (2014). Prevalence of suicide attempts in pathological gamblers in a nationwide Austrian treatment sample. *General Hospital Psychiatry, 36*(3), 342–346. DOI 10.1016/j.genhosppsych.2014.01.012

Tschibelu, E., & Elman, I. (2010). Gender differences in psychosocial stress and in its relationship to gambling urges in individuals with pathological gambling. *Journal of Addictive Diseases, 30*(1), 81–87. DOI 10.1080/10550887.2010.531671

Weissman, M.M., Bland, R.C., Canino, G.J., Greenwald, S., Hwu, H.-G., Joyce, P.R., ... Lepine, J.-P. (1999). Prevalence of suicide ideation and suicide attempts in nine countries. *Psychological Medicine, 29*(1), 9–17. DOI 10.1017/S0033291798007867

Wong, P.W., Chan, W.S., Conwell, Y., Conner, K.R., & Yip, P.S. (2010). A psychological autopsy study of pathological gamblers who died by suicide. *Journal of Affective Disorders, 120*(1–3), 213–216. DOI 10.1016/j.jad.2009.04.001

World Health Organization. (17 June 2021). One in 100 deaths is by suicide. WHO guidance to help the world reach the target of reducing suicide rate by 1/3 by 2030. https://movendi.ngo/news/2021/07/27/new-who-guidance-to-reduce-global-suicide-rate-by-1-3/

Zangeneh, M., & Hason, T. (2006). Suicide and gambling. *International Journal of Mental Health and Addiction, 4*(3), 191–193. DOI 10.1007/s11469-006-9030-z

Chapter 17

Online Gambling in France

Comparison of Women and Men

*Anaïs Saillard, Marie Grall-Bronnec, Morgane Rousselet,
Elsa Thiabaud, Juliette Leboucher, Julie Caillon, and
Gaëlle Challet-Bouju*

Background. In France, the prevalence of online gambling has largely increased over the last decade, and women represent a third of problem gamblers. **Objective.** Our study aimed to compare gambling habits between women and men among 450 non-problematic and at-risk online gamblers. **Method.** Participants completed a structured interview exploring their gambling habits, gambling-related motives, and negative consequences. **Results.** Women were more likely than men to report spending money as the main negative consequence, although they had a lower self-imposed budget per week dedicated to gambling. **Discussion.** Our results raise the question of control and guilt over money that women may experience regarding online gambling.

Introduction

In France, online gambling has constantly increased since its legalization in 2010. In 2019, 7.1% of the French population aged 18–75 declared having gambled on the internet, which represents a 70% increase compared to 2014 (4.2%) (Costes et al., 2020). Although gambling has predominantly involved men, the proportion of women has consistently increased and reached one-third of French online gamblers in 2017 (Costes et al., 2020).

The feminization of gambling has not only been observed in France; the international literature also reported an increasing number of female gamblers, their growing interest in online gambling (Gainsbury et al., 2013), and an increase in problem gambling and recourse to care among women (Castrén et al., 2018). Indeed, women's perception of gambling has evolved in recent decades in response to the modernization of certain gambling venues, allowing destigmatization of their practice (Holdsworth et al., 2012). Moreover, the spread of online gambling has accentuated this phenomenon, affording greater anonymity and privacy (McCormack et al., 2012).

Several studies have reported that men and women differ regarding their favorite gambling activity and their gambling motives. Women seem to have

DOI: 10.4324/9781003203476-23

a predilection for pure chance games, such as lotteries, scratch cards, or slots, whereas men seem to prefer skill and chance games, such as sports and horse race betting or poker (Holdsworth et al., 2012; LaPlante et al., 2006). Moreover, women tend to gamble to escape negative emotional states or to avoid boredom (Holdsworth et al., 2012; McCormack et al., 2012), whereas men gamble more for excitement, to demonstrate their skills, or for money (Holdsworth et al., 2012).

Despite evidence supporting gender-related differences, the majority of studies on gambling do not take gender into account and/or often pay little attention to this characteristic (Holdsworth et al., 2012; Svensson et al., 2011), especially since the expansion of online gambling (Piquette-Tomei et al., 2008). It is, however, of high importance to integrate gender differences in research on gambling, particularly online gambling, where the gambling landscape has dramatically changed over the past two decades.

The present chapter aims to investigate gender differences in socio-demographic and gambling-related characteristics in a sample of French recreational and at-risk online gamblers.

Methods

Procedure

This work is part of the MOD&JEU research program conducted at the Hospital of Nantes in France between 2013 and 2018 (ClinicalTrials.gov identifier NCT01789580). The objective of this program was to determine the effectiveness of online gambling moderators with an experimental design (Caillon et al., 2015). All participants underwent several interviews, and a baseline interview collected sociodemographic and gambling-related characteristics, independent of the research intervention. The present chapter focuses on baseline data only.

Participants

Participants were recruited through media announcements. They were aged between 18 and 65, screened as recreational (score 0–2) or at-risk (score 3–7) gamblers based on the Problem Gambling Severity Index (PGSI) (Ferris & Wynne, 2001), and had a current online gambling practice (past month) on a licensed French gambling website.

Excessive gamblers (PGSI ≥8), those in treatment for a gambling problem or having a history of cognitive impairment or psychosis, pregnant women, and gamblers under curatorship or guardianship or indebted were excluded.

Measures

The following information was collected during the baseline interview.

- **Sociodemographic data:** gender, age, education level, marital status, employment status, and monthly income.
- **Gambling habits:**
  - Gambling problems: the severity of gambling problems was assessed with the PGSI. A PGSI score of 0 indicates the absence of gambling problems, a score of 1–2 indicates a low risk of gambling problems, a score of 3–7 indicates a moderate risk of gambling problems, and a score of 8 or more indicates excessive gambling (Ferris & Wynne, 2001). Excessive gamblers were not included in the present study due to ethical constraints. Non-problem and low-risk gamblers were defined as recreational gamblers, whereas moderate-risk gamblers were defined as at-risk gamblers.
  - Gambling habits: age of regular gambling, gambling practice duration, and type and frequency of online gambling.
  - Gambling account information: money wagered and time spent per gambling session, number of sessions per day during the last 7 active days (active day meaning a day in which the participant gambled at least once).
  - Gambling budget: self-imposed budget dedicated to gambling, amount in euros per week, and whether the participant finds this amount reasonable given his or her income.
  - Gambling time limit: self-imposed time limit for gambling, duration in minutes per day, and whether the participant finds this duration reasonable.
- **Gambling-related motives:** main motives for gambling (pleasure, money, strategy, worry, loneliness, social aspects, to create an online life, other).
- **Gambling-related negative consequences:** main negative consequences of gambling, perception of the gambler on his or her financial situation regarding gambling since the creation of his or her online gambling account (has won money, has lost money, has neither won nor lost).

Data Analysis

A descriptive statistical analysis was conducted for the total sample. Continuous variables were described by the mean and standard deviation, while categorical variables were presented as numbers and percentages. Subsequently, we compared women and men using Student's or Mann-Whitney tests for continuous variables and chi-square or Fisher's exact tests for categorical variables. Since we made multiple comparisons, the risk of error was multiplied (alpha risk inflation). We used an adjustment method (Benjamini and Hochberg procedure) to correct the p-values (Benjamini & Hochberg, 1995). For both types of variables (categorical and continuous), a p-value below 0.05 was considered statistically significant. All statistical analyzes were conducted with TIBCO Statistica® 13.3.0 (Software, Inc., 2300 East 14th Street. Tulsa, OK, USA 74104).

Ethics

Participants were informed about the research and gave their written informed consent prior to inclusion in the study. This study was approved by the French Research Ethics Committee (CPP) on January 8, 2013.

Results

The description of the sample and the comparison of women and men regarding sociodemographic characteristics, gambling habits, gambling-related motives, and negative consequences are shown in Table 17.1.

Description of the Sample

Sociodemographic Characteristics

Among the 450 participants recruited, approximately one-quarter were women (23.8%). The participants' average age was 36.9 years. Most gamblers had an education level higher than or equal to a high school diploma. They mainly lived with other people (58.7% with a partner and 7.1% with their parents). Two-thirds of the sample were working, whereas 20.0% were not working and 12.9% were students, retired, or other. The average monthly income was 1652.9 euros.

Gambling Habits

As required by the study design, approximately half of the sample were at-risk gamblers (52.4%). The average age of regular online gambling was 31.9 years, and the average gambling duration was 5.0 years. The main types of online gambling were poker (43.1%), sports betting (39.8%), lotteries (34.2%), horse betting (21.6%), and scratch cards (20.0%). The participants gambled on average once or more per week (53.8%) or every day or almost every day (25.8%). The participants wagered, on average, 5.3 euros and gambling sessions during the last 7 active days lasted 67.8 minutes, with an average of 1.2 sessions per day. Less than half of the participants (42.0%) reported having a self-imposed budget for gambling, with an average amount of 18.9 euros per week, and 90.9% of participants thought that this amount was reasonable regarding

Table 17.1 Sociodemographic characteristics, gambling habits, gambling-related motives, and negative consequences reported by the sample (N = 450) and compared between women and men

n (%) or M (SD)	Entire Sample (N = 450)	Women (n = 107)	Men (n = 343)	p-value	Adjusted p-value	Statistical Test
Sociodemographic characteristics						
Age (years)	36.9 (11.1)	39.6 (11.0)	36.0 (11.0)	**0.004**	**0.012**	Student's t
Education level (yes)				0.474	0.596	Chi²
≤ high school diploma	82 (18.2)	17 (15.9)	65 (19.0)			
> high school diploma	368 (81.8)	90 (84.1)	278 (81.1)			
Marital status (yes)				0.440	0.569	Chi²
Alone	126 (28.0)	30 (28.0)	96 (28.0)			
With a partner	264 (58.7)	65 (60.8)	199 (58.0)			
With parents	32 (7.1)	4 (3.7)	28 (8.2)			
Other	28 (6.2)	8 (7.5)	20 (5.8)			
Employment status (yes)				0.900	0.985	Chi²
Active	302 (67.1)	70 (65.4)	232 (67.6)			
Inactive	90 (20.0)	23 (21.5)	67 (19.5)			
Other (student, retired, and other)	58 (12.9)	14 (13.1)	44 (12.8)			
Monthly income (euros) (N = 447)	1652.9 (884.0)	1483.2 (573.9)	1706.4 (955.6)	**0.010**	**0.022**	Mann Whitney
Gambling habits						
Severity of gambling problem (PGSI score)						
Recreational gambling (0–2)	214 (47.6)	61 (57.0)	153 (44.6)	**0.025**	0.055	Chi²
At-risk gambling (3–7)	236 (52.4)	46 (43.0)	190 (55.4)			
Age of regular online gambling (years)	31.9 (10.5)	35.2 (10.3)	30.8 (10.3)	**<0.001**	**<0.001**	Student's t
Gambling practice duration (years)	5.0 (4.2)	4.4 (3.4)	5.2 (4.4)	0.207	0.314	Mann Whitney
Type of online gambling (yes)						
Scratch cards	90 (20.0)	50 (46.7)	40 (11.7)	**<0.001**	**<0.001**	Chi²
Slot machine	4 (0.9)	1 (0.9)	3 (0.9)	1.000	1.000	Fisher two tailed
Roulette	5 (1.1)	1 (0.9)	4 (1.2)	1.000	1.000	Fisher two tailed
Poker	194 (43.1)	26 (24.3)	168 (49.0)	**<0.001**	**<0.001**	Chi²
Horse betting	97 (21.6)	18 (16.8)	79 (23.0)	0.173	0.271	Chi²
Lotteries	154 (34.2)	67 (62.6)	87 (25.4)	**<0.001**	**<0.001**	Chi²

Videopoker	2 (0.4)	0 (0)	2 (0.6)	1.000	1.000	Fisher two tailed
Blackjack	7 (1.6)	2 (1.9)	5 (1.5)	0.673	0.759	Fisher two tailed
Sports betting	179 (39.8)	7 (6.6)	172 (50.2)	**<0.001**	**<0.001**	Chi²
Others	3 (0.7)	2 (1.9)	1 (0.3)	0.142	0.232	Fisher two tailed
Frequency (yes)				**<0.001**	**<0.001**	Chi²
Less than once a month/once or more per month	92 (20.4)	38 (36.5)	54 (15.7)			
Once or more per week	242 (53.8)	54 (51.9)	186 (54.2)			
Every day or almost every day	116 (25.8)	12 (11.5)	103 (30.0)			
Gambling account information during the last 7 active days						
Money wagered per session (euros) (N = 448)	5.3 (26.1)	5.2 (9.0)	5.3 (29.5)	**0.036**	0.072	Chi²
Time spent per session (minutes)	67.8 (85.6)	43.8 (66.3)	75.3 (89.5)	**<0.001**	**<0.001**	Mann Whitney
Number of sessions per day (N = 449)	1.2 (0.6)	1.1 (0.2)	1.3 (0.7)	**<0.001**	**0.001**	Chi²
Budget						
Self-imposed budget (yes)	189 (42.0)	61 (57.0)	128 (37.3)	**<0.001**	**0.001**	Chi²
Amount of the budget (euros/week) (N = 188)	18.9 (26.4)	10.7 (9.4)	22.8 (30.8)	**<0.001**	**0.001**	Mann Whitney
Money spent reasonable (yes)	409 (90.9)	97 (90.7)	312 (91.0)	0.923	0.991	Chi²
Time limit						
Self-imposed time limit (yes)	25 (5.6)	4 (3.7)	21 (6.1)	0.347	0.474	Chi²
Amount of time (minutes/day) (N = 23)	82.6 (80.4)	15.0 (11.5)	96.8 (81.5)	0.054	0.096	Mann Whitney
Time spent reasonable (yes)	408 (90.7)	102 (95.3)	306 (89.2)	0.057	0.098	Chi²
Gambling-related motives						
Pleasure (yes)	258 (57.3)	45 (42.1)	213 (62.1)	**<0.001**	**0.001**	Chi²
Money (yes)	276 (61.3)	71 (66.4)	205 (59.8)	0.222	0.325	Chi²
Strategy (yes)	70 (15.6)	10 (9.4)	60 (17.5)	**0.042**	0.081	Chi²
Worry (yes)	6 (1.3)	4 (3.7)	2 (0.6)	**0.031**	0.064	Fisher two tailed
Loneliness (yes)	25 (5.6)	5 (4.7)	20 (5.8)	0.648	0.750	Chi²
Social Aspects (yes)	28 (6.2)	1 (0.9)	27 (7.9)	**0.010**	**0.022**	Chi²
To create an online life (yes)	1 (0.2)	0 (0)	1 (0.3)	**0.006**	**0.015**	Fisher two tailed
Other (yes)	100 (22.2)	26 (24.3)	74 (21.6)	0.554	0.677	Chi²

(Continued)

Table 17.1 (Continued)

	Entire Sample (N = 450)	Women (n = 107)	Men (n = 343)	p-value	Adjusted p-value	Statistical Test
Negative consequences						
Negative consequences of gambling (yes)						
None	328 (72.9)	89 (83.2)	239 (69.7)	**0.006**	**0.016**	Chi²
One or more	122 (27.1)	18 (16.8)	104 (30.3)			
Which ones? (yes) (N = 122)						
Too much money wagered	44 (36.1)	12 (66.7)	32 (30.8)	**0.003**	**0.011**	Chi²
Too much time spent	53 (27.1)	4 (22.2)	49 (47.1)	**0.050**	0.090	Chi²
Being anxious, stressed, depressed	53 (11.8)	6 (33.3)	47 (45.2)	0.349	0.474	Chi²
Disrupted work or school life	10 (2.2)	0 (0)	10 (9.6)	0.355	0.474	Fisher two tailed
Perceived financial situation regarding gambling (yes)						
Having lost money	308 (68.4)	87 (81.3)	221 (64.4)	**0.001**	**0.004**	Chi²
Having won money	82 (18.2)	4 (3.7)	78 (22.7)	**<0.001**	**<0.001**	Chi²
Having neither lost nor won money	60 (13.3)	16 (15.0)	44 (12.8)	0.573	0.681	Chi²

N, n: number; **%:** percentage; **M:** mean; **SD:** standard deviation.

their financial situation. Having a self-imposed time limit was much rarer (only 5.6% of the sample), with an average of 82.6 minutes per day, and similar to the self-imposed budget, 90.7% of the participants thought that this duration was reasonable regarding their own situation.

Gambling-Related Motives

Most gamblers reported that they gambled to earn money (61.3%) or for fun and excitement (57.3%).

Negative Consequences

Of the 122 participants who reported having experienced gambling-related negative consequences, 36.1% mentioned the excess money wagered, 27.1% the excess time spent, and 11.8% reported being anxious, stressed, and/or depressed because of gambling.

Comparison of Women and Men Gamblers

Results of our comparison between women and men are shown in Table 17.1.

Sociodemographic Characteristics

Women were significantly older than men and had significantly lower monthly incomes. However, no significant differences were found in education level, marital status, or employment status between women and men.

Gambling Habits

There was no significant difference in problem gambling status (recreational or at-risk) between women and men. Women started to gamble significantly later than men (35.2 vs. 30.8 years), although there was no significant difference regarding gambling practice duration. Women were significantly more likely to gamble at scratch cards and lotteries than men, who were more likely to gamble at poker and sports betting. Regarding gambling frequency, men gambled significantly more often than women. Based on the gambling account information from the last 7 active days, men spent significantly more time per session and gambled more times a day than women. Women and men did not differ in the amount of money they wagered per session. Regarding budgets, women were significantly more likely to have a self-imposed budget, which was also more restricted than that of men (10.7 vs. 22.8 euros). In contrast, no significant difference between women and men regarding a gambling time limit was found.

Gambling-Related Motives

Compared to men, women tended to gamble more "to forget about worries," although the difference did not reach significance. In contrast, men gambled more for "pleasure," "social aspects," and "to create an online life."

Negative Consequences

Men were significantly more likely to report one or more negative consequences of gambling than women. Women reported spending too much money at gambling more often than men and were significantly more likely to think that they had lost money since the creation of their online gambling account. In contrast, men were more likely to report that they had won money.

Discussion

Main Results

This study aimed to observe gender differences in sociodemographic and gambling-related characteristics in a sample of recreational and at-risk online French gamblers.

While women and men were similar regarding their educational level, marital status, and employment status, they differed based on their age, gambling habits, gambling-related motives, and gambling-related negative consequences they experienced. Indeed, women were older and preferred playing pure chance games, with a lower gambling frequency. These results are in line with the extant literature, especially the strong preference of women for pure chance games (Holdsworth et al., 2012).

One interesting finding of this study was the differential money and time management regarding involvement in gambling of men and women. Women tended to spend less money, spent less time gambling, and have fewer gambling sessions per day than men. In contrast, women were paradoxically more likely to have a self-imposed gambling budget, which was half that of men, and to report negative financial consequences of gambling. This paradox between, on the one hand, lower monetary involvement in gambling and, on the other hand, a higher tendency to report negative financial consequences may be due to gender differences in monthly income. Consequently, as women earned less money than men, financial damage may be more visible to women. This may also explain why women were more likely to admit they lost money in gambling compared to men.

One important framework of gender differences relates to gender role theory (Money et al., 1957). This theory includes standards, values, and expectations assigned to women or men in a society (Phillips, 2005). Therefore, socialization is defined as the process by which an individual learns to act like a woman or a man to meet the rules and expectations of a society or culture (Browne, 2005). Traditional gender role theory (women at home, men at work) was used to explain the "telescoping effect," which relates to the observation that women tend to start gambling later in life but progress to gambling-related problems more quickly than men (McMillen et al., 2004; Nelson et al., 2006). This theory postulates that women's social isolation accelerates their progression towards gambling addiction (McMillen et al., 2004) and that women tend to experience feelings of shame, guilt, and stigmatization when they fail to achieve the expectations of their assigned role in society (Piquette-Tomei et al., 2008). As a correlate of the gender role assigned to women, mental load is described as the managerial dimension of family and domestic work that generally falls to women. It involves physical, mental, and emotional overload that prompts women to take charge of the needs of others to the detriment of their own needs (Gagnon, 2019).

Although gender role theory and the related socialization and mental load may partially explain the observed differences, we should admit that the norms, values, and expectations of society are evolving and tend to progressively diminish the influence of these assigned outdated social roles. From another perspective, one could assume that women opt for gambling activities that do not mobilize too much financial resources or too much time, which may allow them to maintain control of their practice, compared to men who prefer more addictive games which require more financial resources and more daily time (Afifi et al., 2010). They tend to maintain financial independence and time management and make their gambling session a time that remains recreational. We could therefore perceive women gamblers in our study as less predisposed to gambling for long periods of time and spending much money but also as being more independent from gambling. This could explain why the prevalence of gambling problems is generally lower in women than in men (Costes et al., 2020) because their daily life does not allow gambling to take a predominant role in a way that protects them from addiction. They may also be more lucid in the face of the dangers of gambling because they are more sensitive to the value of time and money.

Strengths and Limitations

We had a large sample size, which provided good statistical power. Our group of women was comparable to men in terms of education, marital status, and professional status. The study took place between 2013 and 2018, a long time period that allowed us to observe overall gambling patterns. However, it would have been interesting to compare the groups of recreational and at-risk gamblers of each gender. Moreover, the fact that we excluded excessive gamblers may have impacted the results because excessive gamblers are those who experience more serious gambling-related harm.

Conclusion

Women and men have distinctly different behaviours and sensitivities to gambling. As a result, the susceptibility to addiction is unique to each group and must be considered in prevention and care strategies directed at gambling problems.

References

Afifi, T.O., Cox, B.J., Martens, P.J., Sareen, J., & Enns, M.W. (2010). The relation between types and frequency of gambling activities and problem gambling among women in Canada. *Canadian Journal of Psychiatry. Revue canadienne de psychiatrie*, *55*(1), 21–28.

Benjamini, Y., & Hochberg, Y. (1995). Controlling the false discovery rate: A practical and powerful approach to multiple testing. *Journal of the Royal Statistical Society, Series B (Methodological)*, *57*(1), 289–300.

Browne, K. (2005). An introduction to sociology, Third edition. https://books.google.fr/books?hl=fr&lr=&id=YN2JqlLg0UsC&oi=fnd&pg=PR4&dq=browne+introduction+&ots=tbrDQBaU8S&sig=tFOaGxR4yZ3LCuggqmYh-xl4V2c&redir_esc=y#v=onepage&q=browne%20introduction&f=false

Caillon, J., Grall-Bronnec, M., Hardouin, J.-B., Venisse, J.-L., & Challet-Bouju, G. (2015). Online gambling's moderators: How effective? Study protocol for a randomized controlled trial. *BMC Public Health*, *15*, 519. 10.1186/s12889-015-1846-7

Castrén, S., Heiskanen, M., & Salonen, A.H. (2018). Trends in gambling participation and gambling severity among Finnish men and women: Cross-sectional population surveys in 2007, 2010 and 2015. *BMJ Open*, *8*(8), e022129. 10.1136/bmjopen-2018-022129

Costes, J.-M., Richard, J.-B., Eroukmanoff, V., Le Nézet, O., & Philippon, A. (2020). Les Francais et les jeux d'argent et de hasard—Résultats du Baromètre de Santé publique France 2019. *Tendances*, *138*, 1–6.

Ferris, J., & Wynne, H. (2001). L'indice canadien du jeu excessif: Rapport final (pp. 1–72). *Centre canadien de lutte contre l'alcoolisme et les toxicomanie*s. http://www.jogoremoto.pt/docs/extra/Jbsm2N.pdf

Gagnon, C. (2019). Charge mentale et éthique critique du care: La division du travail dans la sphère domestique comme enjeu de justice sociale. *Ithaque*, *25*, 23–44.

Gainsbury, S., Parke, J., & Suhonen, N. (2013). Consumer attitudes towards internet gambling: Perceptions of responsible gambling policies, consumer protection, and regulation of online gambling sites. *Computers in Human Behavior*, *29*(1), 235–245. 10.1016/j.chb.2012.08.010

Holdsworth, L., Hing, N., & Breen, H. (2012). Exploring women's problem gambling: A review of the literature. *International Gambling Studies*, *12*(2), 199–213. 10.1080/14459795.2012.656317

LaPlante, D.A., Nelson, S.E., LaBrie, R.A., & Shaffer, H.J. (2006). Men & women playing games: Gender and the gambling preferences of Iowa gambling treatment program participants. *Journal of Gambling Studies*, *22*(1), 65–80. 10.1007/s10899-005-9003-3

McCormack, A., Shorter, G.W., & Griffiths, M.D. (2012). An empirical study of gender differences in online gambling. *Journal of Gambling Studies*, 1–18. 10.1007/s10899-012-9341-x

McMillen, J., McMillen, J., Australian Capital Territory Gambling and Racing Commission, Australian National University, & Centre for Gambling Research. (2004). *Help-seeking by problem gamblers, friends and families: A focus on gender and cultural groups.* ANU Centre for Gambling Research. http://www.gamblingandracing. act.gov.au/Documents/pdf/Help-seeking-FINAL.pdf

Money, J., Hampson, J.G., & Hampson, J.L. (1957). Imprinting and the establishment of gender role. *AMA Archives of Neurology & Psychiatry, 3*(77), 333–336. 10. 1001/archneurpsyc.1957.02330330119019

Nelson, S.E., Laplante, D.A., Labrie, R.A., & Shaffer, H.J. (2006). The proxy effect: Gender and gambling problem trajectories of Iowa gambling treatment program participants. *Journal of Gambling Studies, 22*(2), 221–240. 10.1007/s10899-006-9012-x

Phillips, S.P. (2005). Defining and measuring gender: A social determinant of health whose time has come. *International Journal for Equity in Health, 4*(1), 11. 10.1186/14 75-9276-4-11

Piquette-Tomei, N., Norman, E., Dwyer, S.C., & McCaslin, E. (2008). Group therapy for women problem gamblers: A space of their own. *Journal of Gambling Issues, 22,* 275–296.

Svensson, J., Romild, U., Nordenmark, M., & Mansdotter, A. (2011). Gendered gambling domains and changes in Sweden. *International Gambling Studies, 11,* 193–211. 10.1080/14459795.2011.581676

Buying-Shopping Disorder in German Women – When Everyday Actions Become an Addiction

Nora M. Laskowski, Maithilee Joshi, and Astrid Müller

Introduction: Excessive shopping can become a "buying-shopping disorder" (BSD) if it is characterized by impaired control over purchasing, mainly used to regulate emotions and driven by a compelling desire to instantly own a specific product. In the long run, BSD is associated with adverse consequences such as significant clinical distress and impairment in important areas of functioning. Questionnaire-based estimates indicate that about 5% of adults are at-risk for BSD within different cultural settings. Women seem to be more often affected than men, apparently due to social and cultural differences between the genders, especially in western cultures. This chapter discusses the phenomenology of BSD, buying preferences, and comorbidities of BSD using independently collected data of treatment-seeking women with BSD. **Methods:** A sample of 90 female patients was analyzed. Data were collected routinely at the Department of Psychosomatic Medicine and Psychotherapy of the Hannover Medical School. **Results:** The "mixed" form of buying/shopping, which includes offline and online buying/shopping, is the most common BSD subtype in our female sample. Clothing and cosmetics are reported as the preferred product categories. More than half of the women with BSD met the thresholds for hoarding disorder, somatoform disorder, or generalized anxiety disorder. **Conclusion:** The preferred product categories are in line with other studies as is the prevalence of comorbidities. These results illustrate the high level of distress associated with BSD in women. Given the negative consequences and the presumably high prevalence, it is concerning that BSD has not been included as a distinct psychiatric disorder in any classification systems of mental disorders.

Introduction

Buying is unavoidable in our modern society. For some people, however, excessive buying can become an addiction. The main characteristics of the resulting "buying-shopping disorder" (BSD) are preoccupations with buying/shopping, uncontrollable and irresistible urges to buy/shop, cravings, reduced control or

DOI: 10.4324/9781003203476-24

loss of control when it comes to buying/shopping, and continuation of buying/ shopping despite negative consequences such as social, emotional, financial, occupational, and even legal problems (Müller & Laskowski et al., 2021; McElroy et al., 1994).

Individuals with BSD often report positive feelings while buying/shopping in the earlier stages of the disorder (Müller et al., 2019). However, in the later stages, buying/shopping activities are rather used to escape from identity confusion and negative mood states such as loneliness, nervousness, and boredom (so-called "relief craving"; Claes et al., 2018; Müller & Laskowski et al., 2021). The purchased articles are rarely or never used, and more often either given away, forgotten, hidden, or discarded (Christenson et al., 1994).

Since the currently available prevalence estimate of BSD is based on questionnaire surveys and not on structured interviews, only a risk for this disorder can be reported. About 5% of the general population across different cultures seem to be affected (Maraz et al., 2016) and it can be assumed that there is an increase in the prevalence of BSD due to the development of the online market (Rose & Dhandayudham, 2014). In Germany, 4.8% of the population appears to be affected (Müller et al., 2015a). BSD often co-occurs with other mental disorders such as social anxiety, depressive disorder, binge-eating disorder, hoarding disorder, gambling disorder as well as substance use disorders (Laskowski et al., 2018; Mestre-Bach et al., 2017).

There is still little and inconsistent research regarding sociodemographic features such as partnership status, education, employment, or income, but it is unlikely that these variables are specific risk factors for BSD (Harvanko et al., 2013; Otero-López & Villardefrancos, 2014). Concerning individuals with BSD in general, younger groups and women are more likely to be affected as compared to older age groups and men (Müller et al., 2015a; Otero-López & Villardefrancos, 2014), even if the data is not always unambiguous (Müller et al., 2010; Neuner et al., 2005; Roberts & Tanner, 2002). One of the discussed possible reasons why women are more affected by BSD is social and cultural differences between the genders, especially in western cultures (Reisch, 2001). For example, women tend to do most of the buying/shopping activities in families as compared to men. Some authors suggest that this particular exposure to the activity may leave women more vulnerable to BSD (Reisch, 2001). Another possible explanation is that women tend to have more positive attitudes when it comes to buying/shopping and social interaction and may view it within a "leisure frame," while men may view it within a "work frame" and as something they want to do with minimum effort (Dittmar, 2005). With respect to younger age groups having a higher risk for developing BSD, many authors agree that young consumers tend to embrace more materialistic values than older age groups and possibly make more unplanned purchases that reach pathological levels (Dittmar, 2005; Duh & Thorsten, 2019; Unger & Raab, 2015).

Although there is a growing discussion about the recognition of BSD as a distinct mental disorder, it is still not mentioned as such in the 5th edition of the Diagnostic and Statistical Manual of Mental Disorders (DSM-5; APA, 2013) or in the 11th revision of the International Classification of Diseases (ICD-11; WHO, 2019). It is, however, considered in the ICD-11 as an example of "other specified impulse control disorders" (category 6C7Y) under the term "compulsive buying shopping-disorder" (WHO, 2019). Currently, however, due to considerable phenomenological and neurobiological similarities (e.g., craving, cue-reactivity) with other disorders in this group, it has been suggested that BSD should be classified as a behavioural addiction (Brand et al., 2020; Mestre-Bach et al., 2017; Müller et al., 2019). Considering the ongoing uncertainty about the classification of BSD, here we use the broader term "buying-shopping disorder" (BSD).

Since BSD has not yet been included in the current classification systems and is therefore not recognized as a distinct mental disorder, there are no official diagnostic criteria. This has significant implications not only for the patients (regarding therapy offers and funding), but also for research and consumer policy (Müller & Laskowski et al., 2021). Therefore, probable diagnostic criteria for BSD based on a Delphi study were recently published (Müller & Laskowski et al., 2021). These proposed criteria contain: 1) persistent/recurrent and dysfunctional buying/shopping behaviours/thoughts/ related phenomena, 2) diminished control over buying/shopping, 3) purchasing of items without utilizing them, 4) use of buying/shopping to regulate internal states, 5) negative consequences of the behaviour and impairment in important areas of functioning, 6) negative symptoms after reducing or quitting excessive buying/shopping.

This chapter will discuss the phenomenology of BSD, buying preferences, and comorbidities using independently collected data of treatment-seeking women with BSD in the Department of Psychosomatic Medicine and Psychotherapy of the Hannover Medical School (MHH).

Description of the Disorder

Case Vignette and Characteristics

Since longitudinal studies that systematically examine the course of the disorder are not yet available, the description of the development of BSD is based on the patients' own account. Case vignettes can serve to exemplify the phenomenology of a disorder. The woman whose case vignette is presented below attended the behavioural addiction consultation at the Department of Psychosomatic Medicine and Psychotherapy of the MHH and participated in group therapy for BSD.

For five years Ms. A.'s consumer behaviour has been out of control. She constantly has the urge to buy "something nice" and rarely ends up using it. Instead, she gives many things away. At least once a week she goes on a buying/shopping trip, and usually prefers shopping malls where she can remain "anonymous." Constant preoccupations about buying/shopping are making her feel very distressed. Buying/shopping episodes usually occur when she is annoyed, sad, or bored. Ms. A. has noticed that she avoids unpleasant emotions by engaging in buying/shopping behaviour. She hides the purchases from her partner, as she fears his critical comments. Although Ms. A. has identified the futility and negative consequences of her consumer behaviour for a substantial period, she is not able to stop it.

The main features of BSD as illustrated by the case vignette above are preoccupations with buying/shopping aspects (Müller & Laskowski et al., 2021) and a perceived irresistible urge to buy/shop (also called "craving" in addiction research; Sayette al., 2000). It is also characterized by frequently occurring buying/shopping episodes associated with reduced control or even a loss of control (McElroy et al., 1994).

Because people affected with BSD never or rarely use the purchased goods, it seems that they are more attracted to the activity of browsing, choosing, and shopping than to the actual purchase (Christenson et al., 1994; Müller et al., 2015b). In the early stages of the disorder, patients often describe positive feelings such as joy, excitement, or arousal. These feelings positively reinforce the buying/shopping behaviour, but after the purchase, many patients also describe feelings of shame, guilt and/or regret (Müller et al., 2015b, 2019). As the disorder progresses, positive feelings diminish more and more until they hardly seem perceptible anymore. Then the focus seems to be increasingly on avoiding negative feelings such as anger, sadness, and loneliness, so called "relief craving." Many individuals with BSD, therefore, try to manage their negative internal states through buying/shopping (Müller & Laskowski et al., 2021).

This irresistible, maladaptive, and excessive behaviour leads to massive problems and high distress for the affected people. The negative consequences are considerable: financial, social, relationship, family, and work problems are very commonly reported (McElroy et al., 1994); in severe situations, BSD can also lead to unlawful and/or antisocial behaviour (Mitchell et al., 2006).

Although BSD has psychological and socio-economic implications for the affected women and their significant others, it is difficult to observe since it is masked by other comorbid mental disorders and has popular misconceptions. In contrast to substance use, there are no visible signs of consumption or intoxication. There are no known differences in the symptoms or in the course of BSD between men and women. However, studies concluded that the preferred product categories differ.

Sample Characteristics and Buying Preferences

Sample Description

The data presented here were collected routinely in the Department of Psychosomatic Medicine and Psychotherapy of the MHH. Since this chapter

Table 18.1 Sample characteristics

Variable	n	%
Setting		
Stationary or day clinic of the Department of Psychosomatic Medicine and Psychotherapy of the MHH	20	22.2
Consulting hours for behavioural addictions in the Department of Psychosomatic Medicine and Psychotherapy of the MHH	70	77.8
School Years		
<12 years	51	58.6
≤12 years	51	41.4
Partnership Status		
With partner	41	46.6
Without partner	47	53.4

focuses on BSD in women, only female patients are considered below. At present, the number of men with BSD who attended the outpatient clinic is too low to enable comparisons between women and men with BSD. The sample consists of 90 females, aged between 19 and 69 years (median 37.5; Table 18.1).

The Pathological Buying Screener (PBS; Müller et al., 2015a) was used to measure symptom severity of BSD, and the Internet Addiction Test (Pawlikowski et al., 2013) modified for shopping (sIAT-shopping; Trotzke et al., 2015) to assess online BSD. The PBS, which was developed and validated in Germany, assesses the symptoms of BSD in 13 items. These 13 items are rated on a 5-point scale (Müller et al., 2015a). A total score of ≥29 indicates the prevalence of probable pathological buying (Müller et al., 2015a, 2021). The sIAT-shopping has 12 items, rated on a 5-point scale (Trotzke et al., 2015). A total score between >30 and 37 represents probable problematic online buying/shopping and a score of >37 reflects probable BSD (predominantly online; Trotzke et al., 2015).

The sum scores of these questionnaires in our sample were 46.75 (SD = 9.84, N = 89) for the PBS and 30.24 (SD = 12.93, N = 83) for the sIAT-shopping. The categorical analysis of the questionnaires showed that 81 patients (91.0%) were at risk for BSD according to the PBS. Eight patients (9.6%) seem to have problematic online buying/shopping, and 71 were above the cut-off for online-BSD (85.5%) according to the sIAT-shopping.

Preferred Medium and Product Categories

Data regarding buying and category preferences were available from a small subsample of patients. The category "online" includes purchase portals on the internet, apps, etc. The category "offline" includes stores, shopping malls, etc. The "mixed" form, which is the preferred medium in our sample, includes offline and online buying/shopping with equal frequency (Figure 18.1).

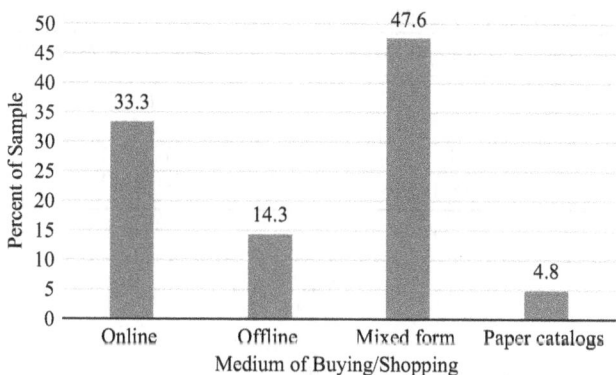

Figure 18.1 Preferred medium of buying/shopping in percent (N = 21).

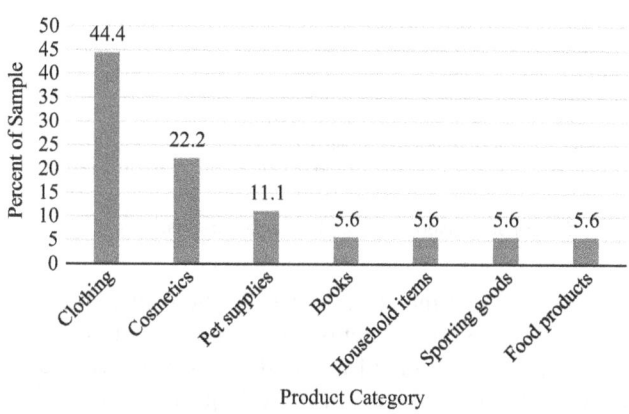

Figure 18.2 Preferred product category in percent (N = 17).

Also, regarding the preferred product category only a small sample can be reported (N = 17). As shown in Figure 18.2, by far the most frequently mentioned category was clothing, followed by cosmetics (multiple answers possible).

Psychiatric Comorbidities

To assess possible comorbid mental disorders in the same female sample, the German Compulsive Hoarding Inventory (FZH; Müller et al., 2009a), the Generalized Anxiety Disorder 7-Item Scale (GAD-7; Löwe et al., 2008), the Patient Health Questionnaire Somatic Symptom Severity (PHQ-15; Löwe et al., 2002) and the Patient Health Questionnaire for Depression (PHQ-9; Löwe et al., 2002) were used. Briefly described, the FZH has 19 items rated on

Table 18.2 Total scores of the questionnaires used assessing possible comorbidities

Questionnaire (Cut-off Score)	Sample Size n	Total Scores MW (SD)
FZH (≥29)	20	34.9 (16.60)
PHQ-15 (≥10)	70	15.5 (6.11)
PHQ-9 (≥20)	78	15.11 (6.13)
GAD-7 (≥11)	80	13.99 (4.69)

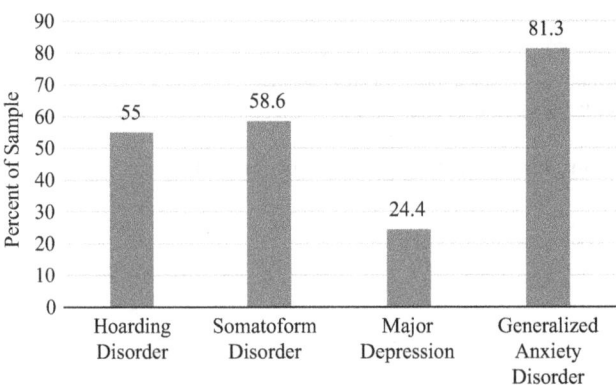

Figure 18.3 Probable comorbid disorder based on questionnaire cut-offs.

a 4-point scale. A sum score of ≥29 indicates a risk for hoarding disorder (Müller et al., 2009a). The PHQ-15 has 15 items rated on a 3-point scale. A sum score of ≥10 suggests high symptoms of a somatoform disorder (Löwe et al., 2008). Out of these 15 items, two questions (feeling tired and having little energy and trouble sleeping) are associated with depression and are a part of the PHQ-9 questionnaire (Kroenke et al., 2002). The PHQ-9 has nine items rated on a 4-point scale. Sum scores ≥20 reflect severe depression symptoms (major depression; Kroenke et al., 2001). Lastly, the GAD-7 has seven items rated on a 3-point scale. Sum scores ≥11 reflect severe GAD symptoms (Spitzer et al., 2006). Sum scores of these questionnaires in the current sample (N = 89) are shown in Table 18.2.

As shown in Figure 18.3, more than half of the sample scored above the questionnaire cutoffs for hoarding, somatoform and/or generalized anxiety disorder. About one-fourth met the questionnaire threshold for major depression.

Conclusion and Future Directions

In the current sample, most patients had schooling under 12 years and no partner. Nevertheless, the literature shows that sociodemographic variables probably have little influence on the development of BSD (Harvanko et al.,

2013; Otero-López & Villardefrancos, 2014). One study showed that partnership status is not associated with symptom severity of BSD (clinical sample, N = 157 women; Müller et al., 2016). In addition, partner satisfaction does not seem to be related to the presence of BSD (Schäfer et al., 2019). Future studies should examine whether the duration of BSD is associated with partnership quality or if education or other sociodemographic variables are specific risk factors for BSD.

The preferred way of buying-shopping in the current female sample was a mix of online and offline. This is in line with previous studies carried out at Hannover Medical School (Laskowski et al., 2018). Also, the preferred product categories (clothing and cosmetics) are in line with case reports and other studies on women with BSD (Dittmar et al., 1994; Georgiadou et al., 2021; Maccaronne-Eaglen & Schofield, 2020). Dittmar et al. (1994) described that many products are impulsively bought to reflect self-identity. Furthermore, women tend to buy more symbolic goods along with the goal of self-expression as compared to men (Dittmar et al., 1994). For this reason, maladaptive, excessive purchasing of clothing may play a significant role in BSD among women.

The categorical analysis of questionnaires assessing symptoms of comorbid mental disorders revealed that more than half of the women with BSD met the thresholds for a hoarding disorder, somatoform disorder, or generalized anxiety disorder. The prevalence estimates in the current female sample were considerably higher than those reported from population-based German samples: around 5% for pathological hoarding (N = 2307; Müller et al., 2009b), 10% for functional somatic symptoms (meta-analysis; Roenneberg et al., 2019) and 6% for generalized anxiety disorder (N = 9721; Hinz et al., 2016). Since the current sample was a clinical sample of treatment-seeking women, higher prevalence estimates are not surprising. Moreover, with respect to previous literature, these are the most common comorbidities in BSD. Other studies have found similarly high prevalence rates in clinical samples with BSD (Laskowski et al., 2021; Müller et al., 2007, 2009b). For example, in a previous German study, 41 out of 66 patients (55 women and 11 men) with BSD suffered from pathological hoarding (Müller et al., 2007). In another German study, the current estimated prevalence of any anxiety disorder was 3% in patients with BSD (Müller et al., 2009c). In contrast, symptoms of somatoform disorders seem to be more prevalent in the current sample as compared to other data. The point prevalence of somatoform disorder in an earlier German study was 17% (clinical female sample with BSD; Müller et al., 2009c). It is important to note that somatoform disorders (Bandelow & Michaelis, 2015) and anxiety disorders (Hinz et al., 2017) are generally more common in women. Taken together, the results of the current study illustrate the high level of distress associated with BSD.

Given this high distress and the presumably high prevalence of BSD (Maraz et al., 2016), it is questionable why BSD has not yet been included as a distinct psychiatric disorder in any classification systems of mental disorders. The recognition as a separate mental disorder is long overdue and could form the basis for the development of prevention approaches as well as for the (further) development of specific treatment services.

There are some limitations to mention regarding our data. One limitation is the small sample size for some variables (e.g., buying preferences). Moreover, it should be kept in mind that the present results cannot be generalized, especially since only women from Germany were considered here. Unfortunately, the number of men with BSD attending the outpatient clinic was very low. Therefore, we were not able to present findings concerning the comparison between women and men with BSD.

The enormous suffering and significant negative consequences for women and their families, as well as the increase in BSD and a shift to the online market, highlight the public health relevance of this problem. Although this article focuses on BSD in women, it is important to emphasize that men with BSD should not be ignored. Future studies should investigate, in a sufficiently large sample, whether there are gender differences in prevalence, comorbidity, and/or buying/shopping preferences regarding the medium and/or the product categories.

References

APA (American Psychiatric Press). (2013). *Diagnostic and statistical manual of mental disorders* (5th ed.). Washington, DC: American Psychiatric Press.

Bandelow, B., & Michaelis, S. (2015). Epidemiology of anxiety disorders in the 21st century. *Dialogues in Clinical Neuroscience, 17*(3), 327–335. doi: 10.31887/dcns.2015. 17.3/bbandelow

Christenson, G.A., Faber, R.J., de Zwaan, M., Raymond, N.C., Specker, S.M., Ekern, M.D., Mackenzie, T.B., Crosby, R.D., Crow, S.J., & Eckert, E.D. (1994). Compulsive buying: Descriptive characteristics and psychiatric comorbidity. *The Journal of Clinical Psychiatry, 55*(1).

Dittmar, H. (2005). Compulsive buying – a growing concern? An examination of gender, age, and endorsement of materialistic values as predictors. *British Journal of Psychology, 96*(4), 467–491. doi: 10.1348/000712605x53533

Dittmar, H., Beattie, J., & Friese, S. (1994). Gender identity and material symbols: Objects and decision considerations in impulse purchases. *Journal of Economic Psychology, 16*, 491–511.

Duh, H., & Thorsten, T. (2019). Preventing compulsive shopping among young South-Africans and Germans. *Young Consumers, 20*(1), 29–43. doi: 10.1108/yc-08-2 018-0842

Frost, R., Steketee, G., & Williams, L. (2002). Compulsive buying, compulsive hoarding, and obsessive-compulsive disorder. *Behavior Therapy, 33*(2), 201–214. doi: 10.1016/s0005-7894(02)80025-9

Georgiadou, E., Koopmann, A., Müller, A., Leménager, T., Hillemacher, T., & Kiefer, F. (2021). Who was shopping more during the spring lockdown 2020 in Germany? *Frontiers in Psychiatry.* doi: 10.3389/fpsyt.2021.650989

Harvanko, A., Lust, K., Odlaug, B., Schreiber, L., Derbyshire, K., Christenson, G., & Grant, J. (2013). Prevalence and characteristics of compulsive buying in college students. *Psychiatry Research*, *210*(3), 1079–1085. doi: 10.1016/j.psychres.2013.08.048

Hinz, A., Klein, A.M., Brähler, E., Glaesmer, H., Luck, T., Riedel-Heller, S., Wirkner, K., & Hilbert, A. (2017). Psychometric evaluation of the Generalized Anxiety Disorder Screener GAD-7, based on a large German general population sample. *Journal of Affective Disorders*, *210*, 338–344. doi: 10.1016/j.jad.2016.12.012

Kroenke, K., Spitzer, R.L., & Williams, J.B. (2001). The PHQ-9: Validity of a brief depression severity measure. *Journal of General Internal Medicine*, *16*(9), 606–613. doi: 10.1046/j.1525-1497.2001.016009606.x

Kroenke, K., Spitzer, R.L., & Williams, J.B. (2002). The PHQ-15: Validity of a new measure for evaluating the severity of somatic symptoms. *Psychosomatic Medicine*, *64*(2), 258–266. doi: 10.1097/00006842-200203000-00008

Laskowski, N.M., Georgiadou, E., Tahmassebi, N., de Zwaan, M., & Müller, A. (2021). Mental comorbidities in buying-shopping disorder compared to other mental disorders. Anxiety, depressive and somatoform symptoms as well as traumatic childhood experiences. *Psychotherapeut*, *66*(2), 113–118. doi: 10.1007/s00278-020-00487-x

Laskowski, N.M., Trotzke, P., & Müller, A. (2018). Needing versus buying: When excessive consumption of goods becomes an addiction. *Verhaltenstherapie*, *28*(4), 247–255. doi: 10.1159/000493888

Löwe, B., Decker, O., Müller, S., Brähler, E., Schellberg, D., Herzog, W., & Herzberg, P. (2008). Validation and standardization of the generalized anxiety disorder screener (GAD-7) in the general population. *Medical Care*, *46*(3), 266–274. doi: 10.1097/mlr.0b013e318160d093

Löwe, B., Zipfel, S., Herzog, W. (2002). *Gesundheitsfragebogen für Patienten (PHQ-D)*. Komplettversion und Kurzform. Testmappe mit Manual, Fragebögen, Schablonen. Karlsruhe: Pfizer.

Maraz, A., Griffiths, M.D., & Demetrovics, Z. (2016). The prevalence of compulsive buying: A meta-analysis. *Addiction*, *111*(3), 408–419. doi: 10.1111/add.13223

McElroy, S.L., Keck, P.E., Pope, H.G., Smith, J.M., & Strakowski, S.M. (1994). Compulsive buying: A report of 20 cases. *The Journal of Clinical Psychiatry*, *55*, 242–248.

Mestre-Bach, G., Steward, T., Jiménez-Murcia, S., & Fernández-Aranda, F. (2017). Differences and similarities between compulsive buying and other addictive behaviors. *Current Addiction Reports*, *4*(3), 228–236. doi: 10.1007/s40429-017-0153-z

Mitchell, J., Burgard, M., Faber, R., Crosby, R., & de Zwaan, M. (2006). Cognitive behavioral therapy for compulsive buying disorder. *Behaviour Research and Therapy*, *44*(12), 1859–1865. doi: 10.1016/j.brat.2005.12.009

Müller, A., Laskowski, N.M., Trotzke, P., Ali, K., Fassnacht, D.B., de Zwaan, M., Brand, M., Häder, M. & Kyrios, M. (2021). Proposed diagnostic criteria for compulsive buying-shopping disorder: A Delphi expert consensus study. *Journal of Behavioral Addictions*. doi: 10.1556/2006.2021.00013

Müller, A., Brand, M., Claes, L., Demetrovics, Z., De Zwaan, M., Fernández-Aranda, F., Frost, R.O., Jimenez-Murcia, S., Lejoyeux, M., Steins-Loeber, S., Mitchell, J.E., Moulding, R., Nedeljkovic, M., Trotzke, P., Weinstein, A., & Kyrios, M. (2019). Buying-shopping disorder – is there enough evidence to support its inclusion in ICD-11? *CNS Spectrums*, *24*(4), 374–379. doi: 10.1017/s1092852918001323

Müller, A., Crosby, R.D., Frost, R.O., Leidel, B., Bleich, S., Glaesmer, H., Osen, B., & de Zwaan, M. (2009a). German compulsive hoarding inventory (FZH) – Evaluation of the German version of the saving inventory-revised. *Verhaltenstherapie*, *19*(4), 243–250. doi: 10.1159/000253877

Müller, A., de Zwaan, M., Mitchell, J., & Zimmermann, T. (2016). Pathological buying and partnership status. *Psychiatry Research*, *239*, 122–123. doi: 10.1016/j.psychres.2016.03.013

Müller, A., Mitchell, J., & de Zwaan, M. (2015b). Compulsive buying. *The American Journal on Addictions*, *24*(2), 132–137. doi: 10.1111/ajad.12111

Müller, A., Mitchell, J.E., Crosby, R.D., Gefeller, O., Faber, R.J., Martin, A., Bleich, S., Glaesmer, H., Exner, C., & de Zwaan, M. (2010). Estimated prevalence of compulsive buying in Germany and its association with sociodemographic characteristics and depressive symptoms. *Psychiatry Research*, *180*(2–3), 137–142. doi: 10.1016/j.psychres.2009.12.001

Müller, A., Mitchell, J.E., Crosby, R.D., Glaesmer, H., & de Zwaan, M. (2009b). The prevalence of compulsive hoarding and its association with compulsive buying in a German population-based sample. *Behaviour Research and Therapy*, *47*, 705–709. doi: 10.1016/j.brat.2009.04.005

Müller, A., Mühlhans, B., Silbermann A., Müller, U., Mertens, C., Hornbach, T., Mitchell, J.E., & de Zwaan, M. (2009c). Compulsive buying and psychiatric comorbidity. *Psychotherapie Psychosomatik Medizinische Psychologie*, *59*(8), 291–299. doi: 10.1055/s-2008-1067438

Müller, A., Müller, U., Albert, P., Mertens, C., Silbermann, A., Mitchell, J.E., & de Zwaan, M. (2007). Hoarding in a compulsive buying sample. *Behaviour Research and Therapy*, *45*, 2754–2763. doi: 10.1016/j.brat.2007.07.012

Müller, A., Trotzke, P., Mitchell, J., de Zwaan, M., & Brand, M. (2015a). The pathological buying screener: Development and psychometric properties of a new screening instrument for the assessment of pathological buying symptoms. *PLOS ONE*, *10*(10), e0141094. doi: 10.1371/journal.pone.0141094

Neuner, M., Raab, G., & Reisch, L.A. (2005). Compulsive buying in maturing consumer societies: An empirical re-inquiry. *Journal of Economic Psychology*, *26*(4), 509–522. doi: 10.1016/j.joep.2004.08.002

Otero-López, J.M., & Villardefrancos, E. (2014). Prevalence, sociodemographic factors, psychological distress, and coping strategies related to compulsive buying: A cross scctional study in Galicia, Spain. *BMC Psychiatry*, *14*(1), 1–12. doi: 10.1186/1471-244x-14-101

Pawlikowski, M., Altstötter-Gleich, C., & Brand, M. (2013). Validation and psychometric properties of a short version of Young's Internet addiction test. *Computers in Human Behavior*, *29*(3), 1212–1223. doi: 10.1016/j.chb.2012.10.014

Reisch, L.A. (2001). Women and addictive buying: The gender question revised. *El Consumo y la Adicción a las Compras: Diferentes Perspectivas*, 169–195.

Roberts, J.A., & Tanner, J.F. (2000). Compulsive buying and risky behavior among adolescents. *Psychological Reports*, *86*, 763–770. doi: 10.2466/pr0.2000.86.3.763

Roberts, J. A. & Tanner Jr, J. F. (2002). Compulsive buying and sexual attitudes, intentions, and activity among adolescents: an extension of Roberts and Tanner.*Psychological Reports*, *90*(3_part_2), 1258–1260.

Roenneberg, C., Sattel, H., Schaefert, R., Henningsen, P., Hausteiner-Wiehle, C. (2019). Clinical practice guideline: Functional somatic symptoms. *Deutsches Ärzteblatt International*, *116*, 553–560. doi: 10.3238/arztebl.2019.0553

Rose, S., & Dhandayudham, A. (2014). Towards an understanding of Internet-based problem shopping behaviour: The concept of online shopping addiction and its proposed predictors. *Journal of Behavioral Addictions*, *3*(2), 83–89. doi: 10.1556/jba.3.2014.003

Sayette, M.A., Shiffman, S., Tiffany, S.T., Niaura, R.S., Martin, C.S., & Schadel, W.G. (2000). The measurement of drug craving. *Addiction*, *95*(8s2), 189–210. doi: 10.1046/j.13600443.95.8s2.8.x

Schäfer, G., Vogel, B., Zimmermann, T., Trotzke, P., Stenger, J., Tahmassebi, N., de Zwaan, M., & Müller, A. (2019). Buying-shopping disorder and partnership satisfaction. *International Journal of Mental Health and Addiction*, *17*, 247–257. doi: 10.1007/s11469-018-0016-4

Soares, C., Fernandes, N., & Morgado, P. (2016). A review of pharmacologic treatment for compulsive buying disorder. *CNS Drugs*, *30*(4), 281–291. doi:10.1007/s40263-016-0324-9

Spitzer, R., Kroenke, K., Williams, J., & Löwe, B. (2006). A brief measure for assessing generalized anxiety disorder. *Archives of Internal Medicine*, *166*(10), 1092. doi: 10.1001/archinte.166.10.1092

Trotzke, P., Starcke, K., Müller, A., & Brand, M. (2015). Pathological buying online as a specific form of internet addiction: A model-based experimental investigation. *PLOS ONE*, *10*(10), e0140296. doi: 10.1371/journal.pone.0140296

Unger, A., & Raab, G. (2015). The dark side of globalization and consumption: How similar are Chinese and German consumers toward their proneness to compulsive buying? *Journal Of Asia-Pacific Business*, *16*(1), 4–20. doi: 10.1080/10599231.2015.997624

WHO (World Health Organization). (2019). International Classification of Diseases updated 09/2019 (11th revision). Retrieved from: https://icd.who.int/en/, January 15th, 2021.

Chapter 19

Female Gamers

Psychosocial and Clinical Perspectives

Olatz Lopez-Fernandez and Daria J. Kuss

Research investigating female gamers is scarce with regards to psychosocial profile and clinical implications concerning potential gaming disorder. However, the stereotype of the male gamer and consequently the male gaming addict persists in our culture. The present chapter aims to (i) present an international female gamer profile, and to (ii) determine the clinical implications of addictive gaming behaviour in females. This chapter covers the gap in knowledge on the female gaming phenomenon from a global perspective to shed light on and prevent gaming disorder in this hidden population group, illuminating this gendered behaviour and the risks associated with gaming disorder in women.

Introduction

Research investigating female gamers is relatively scarce (Lopez-Fernandez et al., 2019a), and the prevalence of problematic gaming or Gaming Disorder among women remains unknown (World Health Organization [WHO], 2018). The common gamer stereotype of the young male gamer overshadows the reality of the female gamer population, as their number is higher than what is usually recognized, and females are skilled gamers who compete at the same levels as their male counterparts. Indeed, there are a few studies which have investigated female gamers starting with the development of the video gaming industry in the last decades of the 20th century until the present day using psychosocial and clinical perspectives. Women have been engaged with videogames from their inception in the 1970s and 1980s (e.g., "the lady arcades"; Worley, 1982). However, for decades, videogame designers mainly targeted male gamers and consequently developed videogames targeting males. This tendency has recently changed in gaming culture. However, female gamers are still not sufficiently recognized by the videogame industry (Lopez-Fernandez et al., 2019b).

DOI: 10.4324/9781003203476-25

Psychosocial Perspective

At present, half of the European population between six- and 64-years old play videogames, with an average age of 31 years, according to the video game industry (Interactive Software Federation of Europe [ISFE], 2021). Of those, 47% are female gamers; i.e., 56 million women play videogames across European markets. Women represent 53% of all mobile and tablet game players, which means they usually play on the move (e.g., whilst commuting), playing short and small games on mobile devices (e.g., casual games). The average age of a female gamer is 32 years; they are middle-aged women who are likely to be employed and/or a mother. In fact, almost 85% of parents have an agreement with their children regarding videogames, which has increased compared to 2018, in which the ISFE reported this to be 79%.

Similarly, in the United States, the gaming industry has collected comparable findings (Entertainment Software Association [ESA], 2021). Here, there are 227 million gamers across all ages with an average age of 31 years. Of those, 45% identify as women, and 32% are parents. Regarding families, 74% of parents play videogames with their children, and 31% of spouses or partners usually play together.

Thus, both European and American videogame market statistics are comparable, which may be due to the standardization of the gaming industry (e.g., genres played and devices used). Over 46% of the American and European gamers are now estimated to be female, usually a middle-aged woman who plays mobile games alone, or with family and friends (ESA, 2021; ISFE, 2021). Despite this fact, scientific knowledge on female gaming is still scarce.

During the COVID-19 pandemic, although gaming time increased overall during lockdowns, it decreased after the discontinuation of the safety measures for both genders and all ages (ISFE, 2021). This is consistent with 70% of North American parents letting their children play more often during the pandemic waves in 2020 (ESA, 2021). Of the games, parents encouraged their children to play, 59% included education and learning games within the available game genres, and 63% of surveyed parents believed these games are effective in supporting academic skills (e.g., 62% in terms of maths skills). Thus, it seems this increase of video gaming during the lockdowns in Europe and the United States predominantly affected those who were already gamers, as the figures on gaming behaviour at present are relatively steady compared to data before the pandemic (ESA, 2018; ISFE, 2018).

Clinical Perspective

Similar to the psychosocial perspective, female gamers are an understudied population in the clinical setting. Reports suggest that males are significantly more likely to experience addiction-related symptoms as a consequence of excessive gaming (Kuss & Pontes, 2019). Based on the scarce literature in this field, women appear to be less impacted by addiction-related problems due to problematic gaming. However, recent research indicates that they are a population that may experience significant impairment as a result of excessive gaming (Lopez-Fernandez et al., 2019a,b). In an international sample of female gamers, it was shown that one percent experience symptoms of Internet Gaming Disorder as measured by the Internet Gaming Disorder Screener 9 – Short Form (IGDS9-SF, Pontes & Griffiths, 2015). The identified problematic female gamers were aged between 18 and 32 years, and very diverse with regards to their educational and professional status, as well as nationalities, and all were introduced to gaming by family members. On average, their gaming time was approximately seven hours per day, with Massively Multiplayer Online Role-Playing Games (MMORPGs), Role-Playing Games (RPGs), First Person Shooters (FPSs), and Multiplayer Online Battle Arena (MOBAs) ranked as their favorite games (Lopez-Fernandez et al., 2019a). This work highlights a possibly problematic female gaming population.

Qualitative research evidence adds to our increasing knowledge on this population. Gamers undergoing outpatient cognitive behavioural therapy for gaming disorder appear to have different experiences when gaming, as indicated in the below excerpt:

> The most important question when you're a girl is why you're playing. You almost feel like something special because there are rarely girls who play, and then you feel like somebody who's unique. If you can play the game you're playing, then it's a bit better because this enthrals the boys, too, that you've not only got boys, but also somebody else, who you can swap ideas with because I think that girls have a completely different point of view than boys when it comes to game playing. (...) For instance, regarding the reaction to losing. When you lose, you lose. I think that we girls are a bit more relaxed in dealing with that. Boys flip out completely and become all worked up. (Kuss, 2015, p. 87)

To a significantly higher extent than males, female gamers report experiencing harassment whilst playing RPGs, FPSs, or MOBAs, and usually apply coping strategies, such as playing alone, playing anonymously, or moving groups regularly and looking for social support (i.e., social integration and networks) to avoid anxiety and loneliness (McLean & Griffiths, 2019). These negative experiences are mainly attributed to some male gamers, and the structural characteristics of specific games. Therefore, it seems there are still some concerns regarding online gaming communities and game genres that can negatively impact female gamers and lead to potential clinical concern.

From a clinical perspective, the fact that female gamer experiences appear to differ from that of males indicates that treatment approaches may need adapting in order to address the individual problem constellations experienced by females.

Conclusion

The present chapter has introduced the so far understudied female gamer population. It has been shown that from a psychosocial perspective, female gamers are an important population given that they make up a considerable proportion of the overall gaming population. The female gamer profile is that of a middle-aged woman who plays games by herself, with her partner and family. Moreover, even with the pandemic having initially increased the use of videogames during the lockdowns, there is a steady pattern of female gaming. More importantly, considering the high number of female gamers in Western societies, and recent research having demonstrated a small percentage can develop Gaming Disorder, it is surprising there is not more research attending to this hidden population group. These are usually women with work- and/or family-related responsibilities, and problems as a consequence of excessive gaming may not only negatively affect themselves, but also to those who depend on them.

Finally, the clinical perspective highlights how some women are affected by excessive gaming, and the potential peril they can experience. Future research should address both psychosocial and clinical implications for female gamers to prevent risks and tailor future interventions specifically to this group. Additional research is required to assess the extent to which the relatively small group of female gamers who experience addiction-related problems may benefit from adapted psychological treatment approaches given that their gaming experiences, including motivation and their participation in games, appear to differ from that of male gamers. We encourage future research to continue investigating this population and for stakeholders in the field, i.e., the gaming industry, researchers, and clinicians, to develop games targeted to female motivations and preferences, and to support this population with their individual needs.

References

Entertainment Software Association [ESA] (2018). Essential facts about the computer and video game industry. Available at https://www.theesa.com/resource/2018-essential-facts-about-the-computer-and-video-game-industry/ (Accessed September 20, 2021).

ESA (2021). 2021 Essential facts about the video game industry. Available at https://www.theesa.com/resource/2021-essential-facts-about-the-video-game-industry/ (Accessed September 20, 2021).

Interactive Software Federation of Europe [ISFE] (2018). Videogames in Europe: Consumer study videogames in Europe: Consumer study. Available at https://www.isfe.eu/wp-content/uploads/2018/11/euro_summary_-_isfe_consumer_study.pdf (Accessed September 20, 2021).

ISFE (2021). Key facts 2020. The year we played together. Available at https://www. isfe.eu/wp-content/uploads/2021/08/2021-ISFE-EGDF-Key-Facts-European-video-games-sector-FINAL.pdf (Accessed September 20, 2021).

Kuss, D.J. (2015). 'I can't do it by myself' – An IPA of clients seeking treatment for their MMORPG addiction. In J. Bishop (ed.), *Psychological and social implications surrounding Internet and gaming addiction* (pp. 78–11). Hershey, PA: IGI Global.

Kuss, D.J., & Pontes, H.M. (2019). *Internet addiction. Evidence-based practice in psychotherapy*. Hogrefe.

Lopez-Fernandez, O., Williams, A.J., Griffiths, M.D., & Kuss, D.J. (2019b). Female gaming, gaming addiction, and the role of women within gaming culture: A narrative literature review. *Frontiers in Psychiatry, 10*, 454. doi: 10.3389/fpsyt.2019.00454

Lopez-Fernandez, O., Williams, A.J., & Kuss, D.J. (2019a). Measuring female gaming: Gamer profile, predictors, prevalence, and characteristics from psychological and gender perspectives. *Frontiers in Psychology, 10*, 898. doi: 10.3389/fpsyg.2019.00898

McLean, L., & Griffiths, M. D. (2019). Female gamers' experience of online harassment and social support in online gaming: A qualitative study. *International Journal of Mental Health and Addiction, 17*, 970–994.

Pontes, H.M., & Griffiths, M.D. (2015). Measuring DSM-5 Internet Gaming Disorder: Development and validation of a short psychometric scale. *Computers in Human Behavior, 45*, 137–143.

World Health Organization (WHO) (2018). *International Classification of Diseases (ICD-11)*. Geneva, Switzerland: WHO. Available at https://icd.who.int/browse11/l-m/en#/http://id.who.int/icd/entity/1448597234 (Accessed September 20, 2021).

Worley, J. (1982). Women join the arcade revolution. *Electronic games (may): 31-32*. Available at https://imgur.com/gallery/EZpQo (Accessed September 20, 2021).

Chapter 20

Food Addiction

Exploring Underlying Shared Factors in Obesity, Eating Disorders, and Behavioural Addictions in Women

Lucía Camacho-Barcia, Lucero Munguía, and Susana Jiménez-Murcia

In recent years, the food addiction (FA) construct has become a topic of increasing interest in the scientific community. Although basic research has shown similar biological substrates between excessive food intake and addictive behaviours, the literature has provided seemingly contradictory results, and there have been limited longitudinal data generated from clinical populations. In this chapter, the state of the art of FA will be discussed. Different clinical populations, ranging from patients with eating disorders (ED) and obesity to behavioural addictions and the potentially shared and differential vulnerabilities among them will be covered. The main aim of this chapter is to explore underlying socio-cultural and psychological factors related to FA in women. The issues considered include the following: a) the current state of the FA construct and controversies; b) patients characteristics in different clinical pictures (ED, obesity, behavioural addiction, bariatric surgery patients) and associated risk factors; and c) therapeutic implications and future research.

Introduction

The prevalence of obesity is increasing worldwide. According to the World Health Organization, the global burden of disease has reached epidemic proportions, it has been even referred as the *real* pandemic of the 21st century. Because of its significant comorbidities, such as diabetes and cardiovascular diseases, that decrease the population's quality of life and owing to the substantial mortality and public health costs, there is a strong consensus that this pathology needs to be profoundly understood in order to be efficiently treated and prevented. Obesity effects are greater for women due to several reasons, including their smaller size, higher propensity to store body fat, and extra weight associated with each pregnancy, which is reflected in the worldwide incidence that has been higher in women in the last decades.

DOI: 10.4324/9781003203476-26

Obesity is a multicausal disease. The rapid increase in the prevalence of obesity cannot be attributed only to genetic causes. Even though hereditary factors are important, environmental factors play a key role in the development of this global obesity epidemic, creating the so-called "*obesogenic environment,*" characterized by an abundance of food and sedentary lifestyle. Spain, similar to several other regions around the world, has undergone great changes in recent decades that have drastically affected the way our citizens eat and move. The term "*nutritional transition*" refers to a sequence of quantitative and qualitative modifications in nutrition related to economic, social, and demographic changes. Traditional diets, like the Mediterranean Diet, have been quickly replaced by others with a higher energy density, which means more fat, mainly of animal origin, less complex carbohydrates, and more added sugar. These dietary changes are combined with behavioural changes that entail a reduction in physical activity at work and during leisure time. However, these factors are not the only ones that could offer an explanation. Obesity is related with several types of Eating Disorder (ED), especially those that present with binge behaviours, implying overeating and weight gain.

Although several prevention approaches have been implemented, obesity rates in Spain continue to increase, especially in women who may be considered a population at risk. In addition, treatment responses to obesity are limited. Therefore, to offer better prevention and treatment approaches, other potential explanations for increasing obesity rates particularly in women may have to be considered.

The *Food Addition Model* has been proposed as an alternative model of the development and maintenance of obesity and other weight and eating-related problems.

Current State of Food Addiction Construct and Controversies

The term *Food Addiction* (FA) was first introduced in 1956 by Theron Randolph. In recent years, its study has been continuously increasing, including its role as an alternative model to the development and maintenance of obesity and ED related with overeating (Gearhardt et al., 2012; Granero et al., 2014; Pursey et al., 2014).

Even though the term FA has been around for more than 60 years, it has not been recognized yet in the Diagnostic and Statistical Manual of Mental Disorders 5 (DSM-5) of the American Psychiatric Association (APA) and remains a controversial construct. Basically, two streams of thought have been postulated. The first refers to the *FA Model*, which focused on the similarities between the consumption of certain types of foods and addictive mechanisms related to substance abuse disorders (Gearhardt et al., 2011). On the other hand, some authors acknowledge *the action of eating* as the addictive process over considering a particular type of food as an addictive substance (Hebebrand et al., 2014).

According to the *FA Model*, the consumption of highly palatable and ultra-processed foods (sugary, salty, rich in saturated and trans fats) with high caloric content has an addictive effect similar to drugs in substance use disorders. This includes the search and compulsive consumption of certain foods, despite harmful physical and psychological consequences, the activation of the same brain areas of the reward pathways, as well as the presence of tolerance, abstinence, and a persistent desire or inability to reduce this consumption (Gearhardt et al., 2011).

Regardless of study results, some authors continue to be cautious, proposing the study of *the action of eating* as an explanation of the development of an addictive process instead of the consumption of certain foods (Hebebrand et al., 2014). This position focuses on the parallels between FA with other behavioural addictions, where the central aspect of the addiction process is not based on the substance.

Despite these two points of view, it cannot be denied that FA implies an addictive process, whether substance related (high palatable food) or through the action of eating.

A Clinical Picture of Women with FA and Associated Risk Factors

The evaluation of FA has been established through the *FA Model*, considering the behaviour and symptom patterns observed in other addictions. The Yale Food Addiction Scale (YFAS), developed by Gearhardt and her team (2009), was the first instrument to measure FA. It was constructed based on the criteria used by the Diagnostic Manual and Statistical of Mental Disorders (DSM-IV) of the APA for substance use and adapted to the context of food consumption. The same research team has designed a new version (YFAS 2.0) based on DSM-5 diagnostic criteria that have been accepted within the scientific community and translated and validated in several countries.

Based on the use of both scales, the prevalence of FA in different populations has been reported. The lowest prevalence was observed in people with normal weight (2–13%) (Pursey et al., 2014), contrary to what was reported in people with obesity (18–24%) and with ED, particularly in Binge Eating Disorder (70%) and Bulimia Nervosa (95%) (Gearhardt et al., 2012; Granero et al., 2014; Hilker et al., 2016). In a non-clinical female population, 45–64 years old, the reported prevalence of FA was 8.4% and decreased in the age group of 65–88 years to 2.7% (Flint et al., 2014).

Considering sex differences, previous studies have reported that women are more likely to engage in FA behaviours, with a mean prevalence of FA diagnosis of 12.2% compared to 6.4% in men (Pursey et al., 2014). Likewise, among patients with obesity or with a diagnosis of other behavioural addictions, FA seems to be more frequent in women than in men (Jiménez-Murcia et al., 2017; Pursey et al., 2014). In women with obesity, the prevalence of FA was 24.2%

(Stewart et al., 2018), while the prevalence among women with Gambling Disorder (GD) was 30.5% (Jiménez-Murcia et al., 2017). Yet, in patients with ED, the prevalence appears to be the same in both sexes (Gearhardt et al., 2012; Granero et al., 2014). FA has also been found in patients with obesity awaiting bariatric surgery (Guerrero-Pérez et al., 2018).

In addition, FA is a common comorbid condition of behavioural addictions such as GD. The prevalence of FA has been estimated at 7.8% in individuals with GD, and an association between body mass index and FA symptomatology has been described for patients with GD (Jiménez-Murcia et al., 2017).

Considering the most common comorbid disorders associated with FA (ED and GD), it is possible to detect similar characteristics in these different clinical pictures. FA and GD are both associated with difficulties in controlling behaviour, with impulsivity being a common feature in both disorders (Jiménez-Murcia et al., 2017). As with GD, higher psychopathology has been associated with FA (Jiménez-Murcia et al., 2019). Further, GD and FA may involve maladaptive emotional regulation, engaging in gambling or eating for negative reinforcement motivations, i.e., to alleviate negative emotions (Innamorati et al., 2017). As mentioned previously, in a sample of GD patients, women have higher FA rates (Jiménez-Murcia et al., 2017). We could hypothesize that women who present an addictive profile with high impulsivity and use the behaviour as a coping strategy might try to find a more socially accepted behaviour such as eating, while men may prefer other behaviours more associated with a constant search for gratification and novel stimulus, such as gambling.

Women with FA showed similar depression symptom profiles as women with substance use disorders and exhibited more problems with emotional dysregulation than women with no addictions (Hardy et al., 2018). Further, similar characteristics to FA have been found in binge-related impulsive behaviours present in Binge Eating Disorder and Bulimia Nervosa. A recent study provided a phenotypic characterization of FA by conducting a cluster analysis of FA in ED and obesity. Three clusters were found. Cluster 1 (dysfunctional) was characterized by the highest prevalence of Other Specified Feeding and Eating Disorder and Bulimia Nervosa, the highest ED severity and psychopathology, and more dysfunctional personality traits (low self-directedness and high harm avoidance). Cluster 2 (moderate) showed a high prevalence of Binge Eating Disorder and Bulimia Nervosa and moderate levels of ED psychopathology. Finally, cluster 3 (adaptive) was characterized by a high prevalence of obesity and Binge Eating Disorder, low levels of ED psychopathology, and more functional personality traits (the lowest levels of harm avoidance and self-transcendence, and the highest in cooperativeness and self-directedness) (Jiménez-Murcia et al., 2019). In addition, similar characteristics could be found in patients with FA and obesity: emotional eating and other problematic eating behaviour as well as high harm avoidance, low self-directedness, and emotion dysregulation (Ouellette et al., 2017). High harm avoidance implies higher anxiety that may lead to behaviours to regulate emotions considered safer for the society, i.e., eating instead of be-haviours that could imply higher risks such as gambling.

Given the high prevalence of FA in the population with obesity, the question arises whether FA could be associated with obesity risk factors and obesity-related comorbidities. Overall, studies that have searched for these links have not found significant differences in various metabolic parameters and obesity-related complications among patients with and without FA. It has been proposed that the presence of FA could be considered a contributing factor leading to obesity, but not to the development of the associated complications that are driven by several other factors (Camacho-Barcia et al., 2021). However, FA may have implications for obesity treatments. For example, patients with FA seeking bariatric surgery showed less weight loss after dietetic intervention and regain weight during dietary interventions (Guerrero-Pérez et al., 2018).

Therapeutic Implications and Future Research

Very little is known about the implications for therapeutic approaches on FA. Results from an interventional study in a sample of female patients with Bulimia Nervosa showed that following a 6-week intervention with a psychoeducational program, the severity and diagnosis of FA were reduced in those women who completed the treatment. Further, FA severity was observed as a short-term predictor of binge/purge episodes (Hilker et al., 2016). Likewise, in patients with Binge Eating Disorder, FA was found to act as a mediator between the severity of the ED and the outcome of treatment (Romero et al., 2019).

Among patients with obesity, there is evidence that suggests that FA symptoms can diminish after a weight reduction (Sevinçer et al., 2016). However, the traditional and simplistic weight loss treatment approach that works with a prescribed low-calorie diet and physical exercise has shown low success rates and is often associated with poor adherence (Adams et al., 2019). Additionally, longitudinal results suggest that the presence of FA could be an indicator of bad prognosis on the search for a successful weight loss process, having a negative impact on the final outcome (Camacho-Barcia et al., 2021; Guerrero-Pérez, et al., 2018). Therefore, a better strategy to enhance positive results might be implementing additional and specialized support to patients during treatment. Given that the prevalence of FA seems to be higher in women than in men, the design and implementation of treatment approaches focusing on this at-risk population is important. Based on what has been already mentioned, dietary patterns should be considered but other female-specific aspects implicated in the development and mainte-nance of FA should be addressed as well. Sociocultural aspects such as life-style, work, and maternity as well as psychological aspects such as emotional regulation and impulsivity should be considered when looking into biological vulnerability and risk factors.

Finally, although the YFAS 2.0 is an evaluation questionnaire that is based on DSM-5 diagnosis criteria for addictions and could be applied indiscriminately for women and men, it could be useful to assess FA with a standardized method that includes sociocultural and psychological aspects that are specific to women. A refinement of evaluation and treatment approaches for FA are important future research lines.

Acknowledgment

We would like to sincerely thank Fernando Fernández-Aranda, PhD for his wonderful work and constant support of our focus on sex and gender aspects in research.

References

Adams, R.C., Sedgmond, J., Maizey, L., Chambers, C.D., & Lawrence, N.S. (2019). Food addiction: Implications for the diagnosis and treatment of overeating. *Nutrients*, *11*, 2086.

Camacho-Barcia, L., Munguía, L., Lucas, I., de la Torre, R., Salas-Salvadó, J., Pintó, X., Corella, D., Granero, R., Jiménez-Murcia, S., González-Monje, I., Esteve-Luque, V., Cuenca-Royo, A., Gómez-Martínez, C., Paz-Graniel, I., Forcano, L., & Fernández-Aranda, F. (2021). Metabolic, affective and neurocognitive characterization of metabolic syndrome patients with and without food addiction. Implications for weight progression. *Nutrients*, *13*(8), 2779.

Flint, A.J., Gearhardt, A.N., Corbin, W.R., Brownell, K.D., Field, A.E., & Rimm, E.B. (2014 Mar). Food-addiction scale measurement in 2 cohorts of middle-aged and older women. *American Journal of Clinical Nutrition*, *99*(3), 578–586. doi: 10.3945/ajcn.113.068965. Epub 2014 Jan 22. PMID: 24452236; PMCID: PMC3927691.

Gearhardt, A.N., Corbin, W.R., & Brownell, K.D. (2009). Preliminary validation of the Yale Food Addiction Scale. *Appetite*, *52*(2). 430–436. 10.1016/j.appet.2008.12.003.

Gearhardt, A.N., Davis, C., Kuschner, R., & Brownell, K.D. (2011). The addiction potential of hyperpalatable foods. *Current Drug Abuse Reviews*, *4*(3), 140–145. 10.2174/1874473711104030140.

Gearhardt, A.N., White, M.A., Masheb, R.M., Morgan, P.T., Crosby, R.D., & Grilo, C.M. (2012). An examination of the food addiction construct in obese patients with binge eating disorder. *International Journal of Eating Disorders*, *45*(5), 657–663. 10.1002/eat.20957.

Granero, R., Hilker, I., Agüera, Z., Jiménez-Murcia, S., Sauchelli, S., Islam, M.A., ... Fernández-Aranda, F. (2014). Food addiction in a Spanish sample of eating disorders: DSM-5 diagnostic subtype differentiation and validation data. *European Eating Disorders Review*, *22*(6), 389–396. 10.1002/erv.2311.

Guerrero-Pérez, F., Sánchez-González, J., Sánchez, I., Jiménez-Murcia, S., Granero, R., Simó-Servat, A., ... Fernández-Aranda, F. (2018). Food addiction and preoperative weight loss achievement in patients seeking bariatric surgery. *European Eating Disorders Review*, *26*(6), 645–656. 10.1002/erv.2649.

Hardy, R., Fani, N., Iovanovic, T., & Michopoulos, V. (2018 Jan). Food addiction and substance addiction in women: Common clinical characteristics. *Appetite*, *1*(120), 367–373. doi: 10.1016/j.appet.2017.09.026. Epub 2017 Sep 27. PMID: 28958901; PMCID: PMC5680129.

Hebebrand, J., Albayraka, Ö., Adanb, R., Antel, J., Diéguez, C., De Jongb, J., ... Dickson, S.L. (2014). «Eating addiction», rather than «food addiction», better captures addictive-like eating behavior. *Neuroscience and Biobehavioral Reviews*. 10.1016/j.neubiorev.2014.08.016.

Hilker, I., Sánchez, I., Steward, T., Jiménez-Murcia, S., Granero, R., Gearhardt, A.N., ...Fernández-Aranda, F. (2016). Food addiction in bulimia nervosa: Clinical correlates and association with response to a brief psychoeducational intervention. *European Eating Disorders Review*, *24*(6), 482–488. 10.1002/erv.2473.

Innamorati, M., Imperatori, C., Harnic, D., Erbuto, D., Patitucci, E., Janiri, L., Lamis, D.A., Pompili, M., Tamburello, S., & Fabbricatore, M. (2017). Emotion regulation and mentalization in people at risk for food addiction. *Behavioral Medicine*, *43*(1), 21–30. 10.1080/08964289.2015.1036831.

Jiménez-Murcia, S., Granero, R., Wolz, I., Baño, M., Mestre-Bach, G., Steward, T., ... Fernández-Aranda, F. (2017). Food addiction in gambling disorder: Frequency and clinical outcomes. *Frontiers in Psychology*, *8*, 473. 10.3389/fpsyg.2017.00473.

Jiménez-Murcia, S., Agüera, Z., Paslakis, G., Munguia, L., Granero, R., Sánchez-González, J., ...Fernández-Aranda, F. (2019). Food addiction in eating disorders and obesity: Analysis of clusters and implications for treatment. *Nutrients*, *11*(11). 10.3390/nu11112633.

Ouellette, A.S., Rodrigue, C., Lemieux, S., Tchernof, A., Biertho, L., & Bégin, C. (2017). An examination of the mechanisms and personality traits underlying food addiction among individuals with severe obesity awaiting bariatric surgery. *Eating and Weight Disorders Studies on Anorexia, Bulimia and Obesity*, *22*(4), 633–640. 10.1007/s40519-017-0440-7.

Pursey, K.M., Stanwell, P., Gearhardt, A.N., Collins, C.E., & Burrows, T.L. (2014). The prevalence of food addiction as assessed by the yale food addiction scale: A systematic review. *Nutrients*. 10.3390/nu6104552.

Romero, X., Agüera, Z., Granero, R., Sánchez, I., Riesco, N., Jiménez-Murcia, S., ... Fernández-Aranda, F. (2019). Is food addiction a predictor of treatment outcome among patients with eating disorder? *European Eating Disorders Review*, *27*(6), 700–711. 10.1002/erv.2705.

Sevinçer, G.M., Konuk, N., Bozkurt, S., & Coskun, H. (2016). Food addiction and the outcome of bariatric surgery at 1-year: Prospective observational study. *Psychiatry Research*, *244*, 159–164.

Steward, T., Mestre-Bach, G., Vintró-Alcaraz, C., Lozano-Madrid, M., Agüera, Z., Fernández-Formoso, J.A., Granero, R., Jiménez-Murcia, S., Vilarrasa, N., García-Ruiz-de-Gordejuela, A., Veciana de Las Heras, M., Custal, N., Virgili, N., López-Urdiales, R., Gearhardt, A.N., Menchón, J.M., Soriano-Mas, C., & Fernández-Aranda, F. (2018 Nov). Food addiction and impaired executive functions in women with obesity. *European Eating Disorders Review*, *26*(6), 574–584. 10.1002/erv.2636. Epub 2018 Aug 30. PMID: 30159982.

Chapter 21

Psychological, Family, and Behavioural Factors Associated with Emotional Dependence

Ana Estévez and Janire Momeñe

In this chapter, we present some of the studies we have conducted in recent years on emotional dependence on a partner, which reflect conclusions relevant to the clinical setting. The results obtained suggest that as emotional dependence on the partner increases, the insecure attachment style developed in childhood increases in parallel, especially based on affective deprivation, substance use, impulsivity, behavioural addictions, eating disorders (ED), difficulties in emotional regulation, early maladaptive schemas, and permanence in violent relationships, as well as a parallel decrease in self-esteem and resilience.

Introduction

Individuals with emotional dependence have a deep affective need for a partner. Through the partner, they maladaptively try to cover or compensate for unsatisfied emotional needs that often originate in childhood, although maladaptive schema can also develop later in life (Urbiola et al., 2017). They place their partner at the center of their existence, idealizing and prioritizing them above all else. In addition, they perform a wide range of retentive strategies and adopt a submissive role in the relationship with the sole purpose of avoiding a breakup. Furthermore, emotionally dependent individuals are highly vulnerable to rejection, to the fear of no longer being loved, and they do not consider themselves to be a priority (Castelló, 2019). They tend to experience strong negative feelings, such as emotional emptiness, which translates into not feeling complete without the partner (Moral et al., 2018). This, together with continuous demands for displays of love, affection, and continuous contact makes them vulnerable to establishing pathological, asphyxiating, and unbalanced couple relationships (Castelló, 2005).

Emotional dependence on a partner, although it has not yet been included in the main diagnostic manuals (DSM-5; ICD-11), has been considered a behavioural addiction (Gómez-Llano and López-Rodríguez, 2013). Some authors have called it "love addiction" because it shows great similarity with other substance-related and addictive disorders (Castelló, 2012). The addiction

DOI: 10.4324/9781003203476-27

becomes the center of a person's existence (Castelló, 2005); it produces craving or an irresistible desire and withdrawal symptoms, loss of control and compulsion, and the affected person perseveres despite family, social, and work-related difficulties caused by the addiction. Moreover, in emotional dependence, reward systems are activated and psychopathological symptoms appear that are similar to those occurring in other addictive disorders such as substance use disorders or gambling disorder (Gómez & López-Rodríguez, 2017).

There is no consensus about differences between women and men in regard to the prevalence of emotional dependence. Previous studies have reported a higher score of emotional dependence in men (Estévez et al., 2017; Laca & Mejía, 2017; Momeñe et al., 2017; Urbiola & Estévez, 2015), while other studies mention a higher prevalence in women (Castelló, 2005; Lemos et al., 2012; Pradas & Perles, 2012), and yet other studies do not show statistically significant differences (Moral & Sirvent, 2009).

In this chapter, studies developed by me and my colleagues at the Universidad de Deusto in Bilbao, Spain in recent years on emotional dependence are presented. It is important to note that emotional dependence and intimate partner violence occur together with high frequency (Moral et al., 2017; Urbiola et al., 2014). People with emotional dependence develop an increasingly strong emotional bond with the abusive partner over time, they report continuing to love their partner despite the severity of the violence suffered, and try to resume the relationship even after a breakup. Moreover, when the relationship ends, they successively establish similar partner relationships following the same patterns of violence. Because of this co-occurrence of emotional dependence and intimate partner violence, some of the studies below include the evaluation of intimate partner violence.

Emotional Dependency and Attachment

The first experiences with attachment figures or primary caregivers in childhood, generally the parents, influence the establishment of couple relationships in adulthood. Throughout the scientific literature, early affective deficiencies have been pointed out as one of the etiological factors of emotional dependence toward the partner (Cubas et al., 2004; Momeñe & Estévez, 2018). Through emotional dependence, an attempt is made to maladaptively compensate for these early affective deficiencies. Accordingly, attachment styles developed in childhood in part as a result of parental styles experienced may persist into adulthood. Attachment styles have been reported to influence the process of choosing a partner, as well as the way of interacting and behaving in the relationship (Barroso, 2014). People with emotional dependence tend to present an insecure-ambivalent attachment style (Alonso-Arbiol et al., 2002; Yárnoz-Yaben, 2010). However, affective deficiencies during childhood also generate dysfunctional schemas or beliefs about oneself and others that serve as a guide when interpreting later events or situations. Thus, dysfunctional schemas influence the way of feeling, thinking, and relating to oneself and others and play an important role in emotional dependence (Young et al., 2013).

Attachment and Parenting Styles

In a study conducted by Momeñe and Estévez (2018), 269 people participated, of whom 219 were women and 50 men, with ages ranging from 18 to 65 years ($M = 28.34$, $SD = 10.15$). The results obtained show how parenting styles, and especially emotional deprivation in childhood, were related to emotional dependence, permanence in abusive relationships, and the establishment of relationships where emotional dependence is present along with psychological abuse. Thus, the present study allowed us to explore how affective relationships established with parents in childhood may influence establishing couple relationships in adulthood. Despite its importance, the relationship between adult attachment style and permanence in violent relationships is an area yet to be explored in detail. This study provides novel results that relate adult attachment to people who suffer psychological abuse in relationships in the Spanish population and may be used to inform and develop specific therapeutic strategies. It also contributes results that relate emotional dependence to psychological abuse.

Early Maladaptive Schemes

A recent study (Urbiola et al., 2019), composed of 1,975 school and university students, of whom 1,093 were from Spain and 882 from Colombia, indicates that the Spanish sample scored higher on the need for exclusivity, whereas the Colombian sample scored higher on the need to please. No differences were found in emotional dependence between the two samples. The cognitive schemas most strongly correlated with emotional dependence were subjugation, attachment, and grandiosity. Finally, the most valued characteristics in a partner in both samples were respect, humor, and intelligence. The results obtained may be useful for intervention and prevention in a young population. Verifying the existence of cultural differences between different countries, especially among countries with no historical antecedents that unite them, is proposed as a future line of research. This is of great relevance because when preventing and intervening in various problems it is important to take the context into account.

Emotional Dependence and Cognitive Emotional Factors

People with emotional dependence have low self-esteem and strong feelings of inferiority, and recent studies indicate a relationship between emotional dependence and low resilience (Estévez et al., 2017). Resilience consists of a capacity for coping, adaptation, overcoming, and subsequent strengthening in response to experiencing adverse events (Henderson, 2009). Emotional dependence and low resilience share certain underlying characteristics, such as low self-esteem, low perception of social support, difficulties in emotion regulation, inability to break up a relationship, and fear of loneliness (Castelló, 2005; Momeñe et al., 2017; Urbiola Estévez et al., 2017). Emotion regulation refers to the ability to experience and differentiate a wide range of emotions, as well as to modify intense emotional states. Its deficiency has been linked to emotional dependence (Gross, 1998).

Emotion Regulation

Momeñe et al. (2017) found in a sample consisting of 303 people (232 women and 71 men), aged between 18 and 75 years ($M = 25.93$, $SD = 8.66$), positive relationships between emotional dependence, psychological abuse, and difficulties in emotion regulation and these three variables increased in parallel in couple relationships. Furthermore, the results indicated greater difficulties in emotion regulation in women compared to men, while no significant differences were found in psychological abuse or emotional dependence. This study is relevant because several studies have related emotional dependence with physical abuse but its relationship with psychological abuse has been relatively understudied (Porrúa et al., 2010). Likewise, the relationship between emotional dependence on the partner and difficulties in emotion regulation have not been addressed sufficiently. In addition, difficulties in emotion regulation have been attributed to aggressors but, in the present study, the results suggest that it is also present in people who suffer violence. These results strongly suggest including aspects such as emotion regulation and emotional dependence in the approach to the prevention of and intervention for psychological violence. Emotion regulation could also be an important factor to understand the relationship between emotional dependence and psychological abuse because it is one of the underlying mechanisms of this relationship.

Self-esteem

Urbiola et al. (2019) found no gender or sexual orientation differences in emotional dependence in a sample of 550 Spanish youth (462 females and 88 males; 498 heterosexuals and 52 homosexuals) with an age range between 18 and 29 years ($M = 21.16$, $SD = 2.41$). Emotional dependence was positively related to all types of psychological violence received and perpetrated, but was negatively related to self-esteem. Finally, emotional dependence was found to fully mediate the relationship between self-esteem and psychological violence received, humiliation perpetrated, psychological violence received, and control perpetrated, and partially mediated the relationship between self-esteem and psychological-social violence perpetrated. These findings suggest including emotional dependence when addressing psychological violence in couples.

Research on differences in emotional dependence according to sexual orienta-tion is scarce, although there is evidence of the presence of emotional depen-dence in same-sex couples (Flanders et al., 2016; Rollè et al., 2018). Likewise, there is some evidence indicating violence in same-sex couples, although this topic has received little attention. Our results indicate that there is no direct effect of self-esteem on violent behaviour, extending previous research to vio-lence received and psychological violence. Finally, this research incorporates the study of emotional dependence in the homosexual population, showing that this issue affects both heterosexual and homosexual couples similarly.

Resilience

Momeñe and Estévez (2019) found positive relationships between emotional dependence and permanence in violent relationships, and negative associa-tions with resilience in a sample of 237 women and 62 men, aged between 18 and 64 years (M = 29.53, SD = 10.81). These findings suggest that emo-tional dependence increases as psychological violence suffered by the partner increases, and that both emotional dependence and psychological violence increase as resilience decreases. Finally, a mediating role of resilience in the relationship between emotional dependence and psychological violence suf-fered was shown. Thus, resilience plays an important role in both emotional dependence and psychological violence suffered in the context of intimate partner relationships. Therefore, it is recommended to promote resilient be-haviour in prevention and intervention programs to avoid the establishment of relationships of dependence and psychological violence.

Emotional Dependence and Substance-Related, Addictive, and Eating Disorders

As previously mentioned, emotional dependence can be considered a non-substance-related behavioural addiction. Albeit not recognized as a psychi-atric disorder, it presents certain analogies with other behavioural addictions, such as feelings of craving and withdrawal, continuous unsuccessful attempts to break up or leave the relationship, constant ruminations, worries, and obsessions about the partner and possible abandonment, negative repercus-sions in various areas of daily life, an irresistible need and desire to be with the partner, loss of control over behaviour and constant search for contact.

Substance Use

Recently, Momeñe et al. (2021) published a study in which the sample consisted of 1,533 adolescents in school, of whom 826 were males and 707 females with ages ranging from 13 to 22 years (M = 15.76, SD = 1.25). The findings suggest a positive relationship between emotional dependence and substance use.

Similarly, substance use showed positive relationships with emotion regulation difficulties, as well as with attachment styles of parental permissiveness, self-sufficiency, and resentment against parents and childhood trauma, and negative relationships with security, family concern, parental interference, and the value of parental authority. This study is relevant because the scientific research that addresses the relationship between substance use and emotional dependence is scarce, and the present study indicates an association of both these issues with attachment styles and difficulties in regulating emotions. The mediating role of difficulties in emotion regulation and attachment styles in the relationship between substance use and emotional dependence suggests that prevention and early intervention should target these domains.

Chávez et al. (2018) analyzed the relationship between impulsivity, substance use, behavioural addictions, and emotional dependence. In addition, the authors adapted two assessment instruments for use in an adolescent population in Ecuador. The Emotional Dependence Scale in Youth and Adolescent Dating (DEN; Urbiola et al., 2014), aimed at assessing emotional dependence toward the partner, and the MULTICAGE CAD 4 (Pérez et al., 2007) screened for substance-related and non-substance-related addictive behaviours. The sample consisted of 1,533 Ecuadorian adolescents aged 14–18 years ($M = 15.76$, $SD = 1.25$). The results revealed good psychometric properties for both instruments and adequate reliability and validity values. In addition, positive and statistically significant relationships were obtained between the variables studied. This study has important implications because despite the growing research in the field of behavioural addictions, few studies assess both substance-related and non-substance-related addictions. Validation of assessment instruments that cover a wide range of addictive behaviours, including emotional dependence, in different populations is crucial to drive this field forward.

Eating Behaviour

Momeñe et al. (2020) evaluated the relationship between emotional dependence and eating disorders (ED). The sample consisted of 545 women and 167 men, with ages ranging from 18 to 30 years ($M = 21.32$, $SD = 2.94$). The findings showed that as the ED score increased, the score of emotional dependence on the partner increased. As for behavioural and psychological characteristics linked to ED, fear of maturity, inefficacy, perfectionism, asceticism, and impulsivity were the most strongly related to emotional dependence. Throughout the scientific literature, it has been pointed out that families of people with an ED often have difficulties promoting their members' independence and autonomy and tend to use overprotective parenting styles and to behave intrusively. However, to our knowledge, no studies have analyzed emotional dependence in the context of couple relationships in people with an ED. The results obtained in the present study are clinically relevant because they suggest that ED and emotional dependence are associated with each other and it is hypothesized that the presence of an ED may be a risk or vulnerability factor for the establishment of emotionally dependent relationships.

Compulsive Sexual Behaviour

Iruarrizaga et al. (2019) found significant relationships between sex addiction, difficulties in emotion regulation, early maladaptive schemas, and emotional dependence in a study composed of 1,519 adolescent students, 820 males and 699 females between 14 and 18 years of age ($M = 15.77$, $SD = 1.22$). Differences were found between men and women in sex addiction, with men reporting higher scores. The findings of the present study suggested that adolescents with sex addiction manifest greater difficulties in emotion regulation, possess more early maladaptive schemas, and are more emotionally dependent. Thus, it is recommended to address emotion regulation skills, decrease emotional dependence, and modify early maladaptive schemas to favor the establishment of healthy couple relationships.

Conclusions

Although the study of emotional dependence on a partner has received more attention in recent years, it is still a little-known topic. Emotional dependence can have negative consequences in several areas of people's lives. Despite this, it is not included in current diagnostic manuals such as DSM-5 and ICD-11. Nonetheless, its study is relevant as our research and other studies show that emotional dependence favors permanence in violent relationships, a feeling of chronic suffering, difficulties in emotion regulation, early dysfunctional schemas, negative coping styles, a tendency to constant brooding and ruminations, feelings of inferiority and low self-esteem, anxiety, and depression. The mood of people with emotional dependence fluctuates in parallel to the state of the relationship, i.e., they alternate feelings of extreme happiness and unhappiness and may even present with a picture of major depression in situations such as abandonment or the breakup of a relationship. Our research work presented earlier is relevant for determining possible etiological factors of emotional dependence. In addition, these studies allow us to extend our knowledge, better understand the problem, develop specific and effective prevention and therapeutic strategies, and prevent the establishment of emotionally dependent and/or violent relationships, while promoting the formation of healthy relationships.

References

Alonso-Arbiol, I., Shaver, P., & Yárnoz, S. (2002). Insecure attachment, gender roles, and interpersonal dependency in the Basque Country. *Personal Relationships*, *9*, 479–490.

Barroso, O. (2014). El apego adulto: La relación de los estilos de apego desarrollados en la infancia en la elección y las dinámicas de pareja [Adult attachment: The relationship of attachment styles developed in childhood on couple choice and dynamics]. *Revista Digital de Medicina Psicosomática y Psicoterapia, 4*, 1–25.

Castelló, J. (2005). *Dependencia emocional: Características y tratamiento [Emotional dependence: Characteristics and treatment]*. Madrid: Alianza Editorial.

Castelló, J. (2012). *La superación de la dependencia emocional [Overcoming emotional dependence]*. Málaga: Corona Borealis.

Castelló, J. (2019). *El miedo al rechazo en la dependencia emocional [Fear of rejection in emotional dependency]*. Madrid: Alianza Editorial.

Chávez, M.D., Estévez, A., Olave, L., Momeñe, J., Vázquez, D., & Iruarrizaga, I. (2018). Estudio de las relaciones entre adicciones comportamentales, impulsividad y consumo de sustancias en adolescentes: Validación del MULTICAGE CAD 4 y del DEN en Ecuador [Study of the relationships between behavioral addictions, impulsivity, and substance use in adolescents: MULTICAGE CAD 4 and DEN validation in Ecuador]. *Revista Española de Drogodependencias, 43*(3), 13–38.

Cubas, D., Espinoza, G., Galli, A., & Terrones, M. (2004). Intervención Cognitivo-Conductual en un grupo de pacientes mujeres con dependencia afectiva [Cognitive-behavioral intervention in a group of female patients with affective dependence]. *Revista de Psiquiatría y Salud Mental Hermilio Valdizan, 5*, 81–90.

Estévez, A., Urbiola, I., Iruarrizaga, I., Onaindia, J., & Jauregui, P. (2017). Emotional dependency in dating relationships and psychological consequences of internet and mobile abuse. *Anales de Psicología, 33*(2), 260–268. doi:10.6018/analesps.33.2.255111.

Flanders, C.E., LeBreton, M.E., Robinson, M., Bian, J., & Caravaca-Morera, J.A. (2016). Defining bisexuality: Young bisexual and pansexual people's voices. *Journal of Bisexuality, 17*(1), 39–57.

Gómez-Llano, M.N., & López-Rodríguez, J.A. (2013). Patología dual en adictos y sus parejas: La otra cara de las adicciones comportamentales. *Comunicación, III Congreso Internacional de Patología Dual Adicción y otros Desórdenes Mentales, 2013*.

Gómez, M.N., & López-Rodríguez, J.A. (2017). La dependencia emocional: La adicción comportamental en los márgenes de la patología dual [Emotional dependence: Behavioral addiction in the margins of dual pathology]. *Revista de Patología Dual, 4*(2), 2–4. doi:10.17579/RevPatDual.04.7.

Gross, J.J. (1998). The emerging field of emotion regulation: An integrative review. *Review of General Psychology, 2*, 271–299.

Henderson, E. (2009). *La resiliencia en el mundo de hoy. Cómo superar las adversidades [Resilience in today's world. How to overcome adversity]*. Barcelona: Editorial Gedisa.

Iruarrizaga, I., Estévez, A., Momeñe, J., Olave, L., Fernández-Cárdaba, L., Chávez-Vera, M.D., & Ferre-Navarrete, F. (2019). Dificultades en la regulación emocional, esquemas inadaptados tempranos, y dependencia emocional en la adicción al sexo o comportamiento sexual compulsivo en la adolescencia [Difficulties in emotion regulation, early maladaptive schemas, and emotional dependence in sexual addiction or compulsive sexual behaviour in adolescence]. *Revista Española de Drogodependencias, 44*(1), 76–103.

Laca, F.A., & Mejía, J.C. (2017). Emotional dependence, mindfulness and communication styles in conflict situations with partners. *Enseñanza e Investigación en Psicología, 22*, 66–75.

Lemos, M., Jaller, C., González, A.M., Díaz, Z.T., & De la Ossa, D. (2012). Perfil cognitivo de la dependencia emocional en estudiantes universitarios en Medellín, Colombia [Cognitive profile of emotional dependence in university students in Medellin, Colombia]. *Universitas Psychologica, 11*, 395–404.

Momeñe, J., & Estévez, A. (2018). Los estilos de crianza parentales como predictores del apego adulto, de la dependencia emocional y del abuso psicológico en las re-laciones de pareja adultas [Parenting styles as predictors of adult attachment, emotional dependence, and psychological abuse in adult relationships]. *Behavioral Psychology/Psicología Conductual, 26*(2), 359–377.

Momeñe, J., & Estévez, A. (2019). El papel de la resiliencia en la dependencia emo-cional y el abuso psicológico [The role of resilience in emotional dependence and psychological abuse]. *Revista Española de Drogodependencias, 44*(1), 28–43.

Momeñe, J., Estévez, A., Pérez-García, A.M., Jiménez, J., Chávez-Vera, M.D., Olave, L., & Iruarrizaga, I. (2021). El consumo de sustancias y su relación con la de-pendencia emocional, el apego y la regulación emocional en adolescentes [Substance abuse and its relationship to emotional dependence, attachment, and emotion regulation in adolescents]. *Anales de Psicología, 37*, 1, 12–132. doi:10.6018/analesps.404671.

Momeñe, J., Estévez, A., Pérez-García, A.M., Olave, L., & Iruarrizaga, I. (2020). La dependencia emocional hacia la pareja agresora y su relación con los trastornos de la conducta alimentaria [Emotional dependence on the aggressor partner and its relationship with eating disorders]. *Behavioral Psychology/Psicología Conductual, 28*(2) 307–325.

Momeñe, J., Jáuregui, P., & Estévez, A. (2017). El papel predictor del abuso psicológico y la regulación emocional en la dependencia emocional [The predictive role of psychological abuse and emotional regulation in emotional dependence]. *Behavioral Psychology/Psicología Conductual, 25*(1), 61–75.

Moral, M.V., & Sirvent, C. (2009). Dependencia afectiva y género: Perfil sintomático diferencial en dependientes afectivos españoles [Affective dependence and gender: Symptomatic profile in spanish affective dependents]. *Revista Interamericana de Psicología, 43*, 230–240.

Moral, M.V., García, A., Cuetos, G., & Sirvent, C. (2017). Violencia en el noviazgo, dependencia emocional y autoestima en adolescentes y jóvenes españoles [Dating violence, emotional dependence and self-esteem in Spanish adolescents and young adults]. *Revista Iberoamericana de Psicología y Salud, 8*, 96–107.

Moral, M.V., Sirvent, C., Ovejero, A., & Cuetos, G. (2018). Dependencia emocional en las relaciones de pareja como Síndrome de Artemisa: Modelo explicativo [Emotional dependence in couple relationships like the Artemis syndrome: Explanatory model]. *Terapia Psicológica, 36*(3), 156–166.

Pérez, E.P., Monje, M.R., Alonso, F.G., Girón, M.F., López, M.P., & Romero, J.C. (2007). Validación de un instrumento para la detección de trastornos de control de impulsos y adicciones: el MULTICAGE CAD-4. *Trastornos adictivos, 9*(4), 269–278.

Porrúa, C., Rodríguez-Carballeira, A., Almendros, C., Escartín, J., Martín-Peña, J., & Saldaña, O. (2010). Análisis de las estrategias de abuso psicológico en la violencia de pareja [Analysis of psychological abuse strategies in intimate partner violence]. *Información Psicológica, 99*, 53–63.

Pradas, E., & Perles, F. (2012). Resolución de conflictos de pareja en adolescentes, sexismo y dependencia emocional [Adolescent relationship conflict resolution, sexism and emotional dependence]. *Quaderns de Psicologia, 14*, 45–60.

Rollè, L., Giardina, G., Caldarera, A.M., Gerino, E., & Brustia, P. (2018). When intimate partner violence meets same sex couples: A review of same sex intimate partner violence. *Frontiers in Psychology, 21*(9), 1506.

Urbiola, I., & Estévez, A. (2015). Dependencia emocional y esquemas desadaptativos tempranos en el noviazgo de adolescentes y jóvenes [Emotional dependence and early maladaptive schemas in adolescent and young adult courtship]. *Behavioral Psychology/Psicología Conductual, 23*, 571–587.

Urbiola, I., Estévez, A., & Iraurgi, I. (2014). Dependencia emocional en el noviazgo en jóvenes y adolescentes (DEN): Desarrollo y validación de un instrumento [Emotional dependence in dating in youth and adolescents (DEN): Development and validation of an instrument.]. *Ansiedad y Estrés, 20*, 101–114.

Urbiola, I., Estévez, A., Iruarrizaga, I., & Jauregui, P. (2017). Dependencia emocional en jóvenes: Relación con la sintomatología ansiosa y depresiva, autoestima y diferencias de género [Emotional dependence in young people: Relationship with anxious and depressive symptomatology, self-esteem, and gender differences]. *Ansiedad y Estrés, 23*(1), 6–11.

Urbiola, I., Estévez, A. Iruarrizaga, I., Momeñe, J., Jáuregui, P., Bilbao, M., & Orbegozo, U. (2019). Dependencia emocional en el noviazgo: Papel mediador entre la autoestima y la violencia psicológica en jóvenes [Emotional dependence in courtship: the mediating role between self-esteem and psychological violence in young people]. *Revista Española de Drogodependencias, 44*(1), 13–27.

Urbiola, I., Estévez, A., Jauregui, J., Pérez-Hoyos, M., Londoño Arredondo, N.H., & Momeñe, J. (2019). Dependencia emocional y esquemas desadaptativos tempranos: Estudio comparativo entre España y Colombia en relaciones de noviazgo [Emotional dependency and early maladaptive schemas: Comparative study between Spain and Colombia in couple relationships]. *Ansiedad y Estrés, 25*(2), 97–104.

Yárnoz-Yaben, S. (2010). Attachment style and adjustment to divorce. *The Spanish Journal of Psychology, 13*, 210–219.

Young, J.E., Klosko, J.S., & Weishaar, M.E. (2013). *Terapia de esquemas: Guía práctica [Schema therapy: A practical guide]*. Bilbao: Desclée de Brouwer.

Chapter 22

New Therapeutic Tools Dedicated to Women with Gambling Disorder in Italy

Fulvia Prever; Francesca Picone; Maddalena Borsani; Monica Minci

The COVID-19 pandemic deeply affected our lives and our physical and mental health, and in many ways, women paid a higher prize in their personal and professional lives. The first subchapter by Fulvia Prever addresses questions such as what happened to women with gambling problems and how did we face their loneliness, isolation, depression, and fear of illness and death? Many women are torn between two contradictory needs: the desire to be independent while remaining connected with others. Their well-being is dependent on this dynamic being balanced. However, there are many situations when this balance is upset, for example through a lack of self-confidence and due to fear or an overwhelming desire to give, and relationships take a problematic or even pathological turn. In the second subchapter, Francesca Picone presents several complementary approaches to better understand the mechanisms involved in emotional dependence. The third subchapter by Maddalena Borsani introduces a study that aimed to explore how gambling is an active subject within the system and evaluate the effectiveness of "Family Life Space" as a tool to investigate gambling dynamics. Finally, in the fourth subchapter, Monica Minci discusses the use of mindfulness interventions with women gamblers.

1 WOMEN, GAMBLING, VIOLENCE, THERAPY, AND DESIRES DURING PANDEMIC TIMES IN ITALY: WHEN RESISTING WASN'T THE SOLUTION

Fulvia Prever

The COVID-19 pandemic deeply affected our lives and our physical and mental health, and in many ways, women paid a higher prize in their personal and professional lives. What happened to women with gambling problems? And how did we face their loneliness, isolation, depression, and fear of illness and death? "Holding on" wasn't always a successful strategy for them and we had to deal with their pain and domestic violence issues,

DOI: 10.4324/9781003203476-28

using new online tools to support them. We observed different reactions to gambling venue lockdowns in women with and without treatment, and we observed the importance of but also limits and barriers to our group for women with problem gambling in Milan.

Pandemic

The COVID-19 pandemic hit all five continents, and it deeply affected our lives and existence, our physical and mental health. In Italy, in many ways, women paid a higher prize in their personal and professional life as they managed child care at home and online lessons while working remotely. They provided home assistance to the elderly, exposing themselves to major sanitary risks. Moreover, women represent 66% of our National Health System's workforce and even more in private clinics and retirement homes. They were running back and forth from home to work, with anxiety of catching the virus. They were our real pandemic heroes, strong and resilient, even under pressure, but this made them vulnerable to suffering as well.

So, what happened to women with gambling problems? And how did our gambling services deal with their loneliness, isolation, depression, and fear of illness and death? After our first book *Gambling Disorders in Women* (Bowden-Jones & Prever, 2017)– finally translated to Italian in 2020 (Bowden-Jones & Prever, 2021) – and thanks to our dissemination work training professionals on a female perspective and new public funds dedicated to gambling disorder (GD), many of our addiction clinics started new *gender-oriented* treatment approaches, as you will read in the subsequent chapters. This was an additional and important resource to support women when the pandemic struck.

Women and Gambling

In Italy, we observed a significant difference among women who were already in treatment and women who weren't. Female gamblers in group or individual therapy felt the closure of all gambling venues as a relief and perceived the first lockdown as a unique moment to be completely free of gambling. They could try to find alternative activities even in times of strong restrictions. They could reconnect in a positive way with their female identity, live their family life differently, rediscover simple things such as cooking without stress, reading on the sofa, playing or talking with their kids, and it was easier for them to put into practice what they were working on in therapy sessions.

On the contrary, for women without therapeutic aid, the stressors of the COVID-19 situation, anxiety, isolation, and depression were not balanced with any support, not even gambling activities as a coping mechanism. We observed an increase in medications requests (mostly for antidepressants), overeating problems, alcohol abuse, and excessive use of Internet and sometimes online gambling. Moreover, for women with dysfunctional/violent relationship, being stuck at home during lockdown meant having no way to escape, nor the possibility to release their anxiety while gambling off line.

As clinicians we had to face all problems connected with providing therapeutic help at a distance. For a very long time, shifting our women's gambling group in Milan to an online format wasn't easy, although starting new support relationships was even more difficult. This meant that during this long pandemic period, fewer new female patients could benefit from psychological help and as soon as gambling venues were open again, women with no support could easily return to gambling on site. However, we noticed that the COVID-19 restrictions and the fear of getting sick acted as protective factors for the female population, preventing them to enter or stay too long in gambling venues. Only a minority of them shifted online, though not in a compulsive way. However, we know that this could be a future challenge in Italy, as it is already in Northern Europe, the United States, and Asia. COVID-19 has changed the perspective of relational modalities and we will have to understand how women can be better approached now, to support them in their offline *and* online gambling problems.

We all have shared a common trauma, not just a huge stress, but a long-lasting strain for all of us. Resisting, which is women's favorite coping mechanism as a way of dealing with problems without asking for help, was not the solution, but on the contrary, it could provoke a major problem.

Resisting

Laura Carniel, a skilled and sensitive physiotherapist, that knows well how soul and body are always strongly connected, wrote:

> I see bodies suffering from "accumulated pain" (patient's words), bodies subjected to immense strain, high tension, stress. Over the past year, we've experienced a collective trauma. Everyone, everybody, every nervous system. Bodies that, to resist, pay the price of acute pain treated with painkillers. Pain that slowly becomes chronic and, like annoying muzak, waits for something to change, for "this whole thing" to pass. Bodies that resist. Resistance is, in fact, a physiological mechanism, a functional characteristic, a survival strategy. But how long can you resist a force without becoming exhausted? As astrategy, it might stop working or (consciously or not) become harmful. What happens if we listen to ourselves and feel that we "can't take it anymore"? Awareness opens the vital space of self-care and ongoing adaptation that each body/nervous system activates. (Carniel, 2021)

This is a very good metaphor of what happens with female gambling as a coping strategy (a way to resist) to stress, dysfunctional and violent relationships, and love addiction: If they use it to resist in hard situations, not to leave the stage and try to survive, at a certain point gambling itself becomes their worst enemy, and shifts from a survival effort to a harmful behaviour. (Norwood, 1985).

Violence

I have described this as the cycle of violence and gambling (see Figure 22.1). Intimate violence can lead to gambling as a mechanism to cope with these experiences, then gambling itself produces self or hetero-directed violence (self-harm or impact on minors); this leads to a high risk of gambling relapses (self-harm) or future addictive behaviour for minors (hetero violence), for example. We shall break the vicious cycle down. Having a gambling problem during lockdown could create a major problem in women with gambling addiction and no therapeutical aid. We need to build awareness so that we can facilitate women to ask for help.

"Holding on" instead of "releasing and asking for help" is the same mechanism as resisting life difficulties, sorrow, and anxiety, using gambling as a coping mechanism, to resist, not to leave the scene, not to fall apart. This is the same issue as not being able to ask for help, because doing so would be to admit we are vulnerable and not perfect.

Women are not expected to ask for help and we are accustomed to doing things by ourselves. We may believe we must be strong, protective, and never weak. But even more, we think we do not deserve to be loved if we show our weakness, if we aren't the good mother, perfect wives, wonderful grandmothers. This is the universally shared fear not to be loved if we aren't perfect, this is what our female patients report during therapy, afraid to face the possibility to be refused. This is the work: To accept we are vulnerable

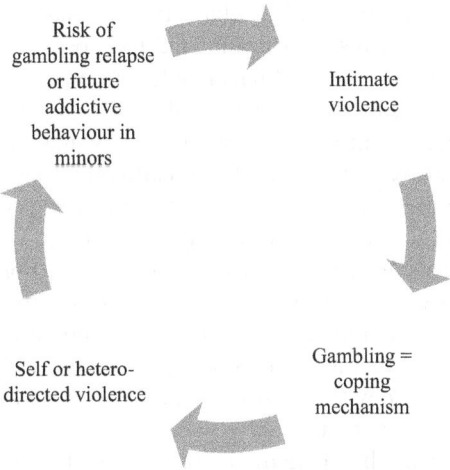

Figure 22.1 Cycle of violence and gambling.

and we may need help, being accepted as great women, loving wives, and good mothers, as women who deserve to be loved for who they are.

Resisting on all fronts – family, work, relationships – produced deep contractures and stiffness in their bodies and minds and the antidote and solutions were found in surrendering to group support, even if through online sessions, short daily communications, or deeper moments of sharing, which all avoided the creation of an abyss.

Therapy

We tried to transform wounds into strengths ... As with the Kintsughi technique (Kin = gold, tsughi = repair, reconnect) in Japan, when an object is broken it will be repaired with gold so that the vase will become even more beautiful and precious than it was before, as they bring it to new life. This exemplifies the idea that a new life, even more precious and rich, can rise from the broken pieces of the community life during the pandemic and from the intimate and painful personal events forms our image of changing. Everything is uncertain, non-programmable, unimaginable, and yet what we need in this very moment is to join together, to make networks to support women's hopes and projects that counter the pre-existing strains that lockdowns further compounded.

In the group, during the pandemic, things went differently than we expected. In other words, women behaved as most of the population did, and this was a great life lesson. During the very first moments, facing the stress of the emergency, there seemed to be a motivating drive to reach out to connect for mutual support with the spirit of "let's stick together, let's help one another because staying close will protect us from loneliness and danger."

Women did their best to shift to an online meeting modality, asking family and friends for technical support (practicing healthy behaviours of "sharing" their engagement), they experienced the benefits of expressing feelings openly in online meetings and phone calls (even with problems of having little or no privacy at all at home). We all were in the hopeful mood that people will learn something from this pandemic ... to be more generous, altruistic, to see what really matters in life.

Then the summer arrived and we were all tired of lockdown as we needed summertime and lightness. We met outside in cafes to be safer for a summer drink and happy moments together, it was great and touching to be *finally in person!!* We worked to support each of the women in our group to plan for leisure time to dedicate to themselves, as well as to explore the possibility for a short affordable holiday as a gift and reward for facing and navigating through those tough moments. We met after the summer holidays in 2020 to share the feeling of regained freedom with enthusiasm, and acknowledged the needs to see each other and talk in person.

Then, some of the women who didn't seem to have gambling problems anymore did not show up anymore, and they were no longer available to participate as life support for other group members. At first there were challenges in articulating this and we thought we may have done something wrong. We tried to understand until they finally could put into words their need to have lightness and to forget about bad things and gambling issues. We processed this temporary loss in the very small group of women who still needed our help and support.

Then autumn came and COVID-19 was still here. Stress became strain, people were getting tired and were no longer reacting positively as they began to withdraw into themselves, concentrating on their own problems instead of being open to collective mutual help. As a whole, society seemed to be in this period of "let's save ourselves individually, no time to share." Moreover, some women had full-time grandmothers' tasks, in order to allow their kids to work, or were permanently engaged as caregiver of their elderly family members. Lockdown started again, and we couldn't meet in person anymore. There was an emerging sense of abandonment, of women feeling left alone by their group pals. Some new female gamblers tried to contact us during the lockdown period, but online contact was not enough to hook them.

Online therapy wasn't so functional for the group as adherence to operating remotely began again. Privacy issues at home were one of the main problems, together with technical difficulties (for those ages 55–78), and a deep need of a real and in-person contact, but we kept the position and the group survived. As the women shared their anxiety, fears, and sorrows and their dysfunctional relationship at home, they realized the group was alive and vital again.

In our therapeutic work, violence issues (economic, psychological, physical, sexual abuse) were always a major focus because we realized how important it is to address these experiences and traumas in any woman's life history in order to support healing and recovery. Gambling was often a way to express repressed rage, a way to take a revenge in a dysfunctional relationship (operating as "I'll make you pay for it") and refund themselves for suffered harm.

Making a new connection between self-harm behaviours (cutting, etc.) and female gambling behaviour, we adopted a Dialectical Behaviour Therapy (DBT) technique (soothing box) in a new setting of female gambling issues. This experiential therapeutic process supports women in building personal positive anchors to face difficult moments and to prevent possible relapses. We found out that the mere construction process or even just the clarifying awareness of identifying what their toolbox could be was already a therapeutic process in and by itself.

The same happened with deep interviews, described as the best tools in women qualitative research (Holdsworth et al., 2012). Through deep interviews, in a sample of the Milan women's group, we looked at the connection between women's past violence experiences and their help seeking for gambling problems and we found that past violence experiences do not necessarily lead women to easily ask for help, but seeking help for this made more sense to the women. We went deeper into some women's stories that we had ever gone before, stories they had almost removed from their memories, and the interview itself became a powerful therapeutic tool (Brandt et al., 2017).

Moreover, we observed how past violence experiences can produce an incapability to live a satisfying sexual life, even in a good love relationship. Gambling often is a way to access excitement and to preserve a good love relationship where excitement is not present, therefore serving as a secondary benefit. On the other hand, *excitement* leads women to a deep guilty feeling, especially in elderly women, and we must deal with it in therapy.

It is clearly evident that to avoid relapses and finally improve women's life quality, in addition to helping them with experiencing pleasant moments and resocialization, we also must treat violence issues, trauma, guilty feelings, and overall help them to finally forgive themselves.

Desires

Let me conclude by sharing my thoughts about light as a metaphor of this moment, the light that we all need in such dark moments. Before the industrial revolution and modern life, nights were extremely dark. The discovery of light through the power of electricity, lighting up our villages and towns, produced big changes in our lives and our perspectives, while making our nights safer and more enjoyable. Before this, the night was dark, as dark as the sea, dark and mysterious, and people relied on the stars to get oriented. The dark night, dark as the sea, was ruled by stars ... and it is when stars are not visible and cannot be consulted for guidance to find the right way nor to draw auspices, that desiderium comes out.

Desiderium, meaning ardent desire or longing, comes from Latin (desidera) – lack of stars. So, we must rediscover the *strength of desiring*, starting from this darkness, from this lack of stars, because we are now living in a night without stars (Gaspari, 2022).

Women need to dream and long for a better future, so ... it's time to bring out their desires.

References

Bowden-Jones, H., & Prever, F. (Eds.). (2017). *Gambling disorders in women: An international female perspective on treatment and research*. Taylor & Francis.

Brandt, L., Tünte, M., Wöhr, A., Prever, F., & Fischer, G. (2017). Capturing experiences of violence amongst female gamblers and their connection with problem gambling. 20th conference of the European Association of Substance Abuse Research (EASAR), Nunspeet, the Netherlands, 18.-05/21/2017.

Carniel, L. (2021). When resisting is not the solution. Available at: https://www.lauracarniel.it/when-resisting-is-not-the-solution/

Gaspari, I. (2022). La versione di Fiorella. Available at: https://www.raiplay.it/video/2022/01/Ilaria-Gaspari---La-versione-di-Fiorella-24012022-b7ca7fc7-fd86-469d-b8cd-1e07fad97ed3.html

Holdsworth, L., Hing, N., & Breen, H. (2012). Exploring women's problem gambling: A review of the literature. *International Gambling Studies*, *12*(2), 199–213.

Norwood, R. (1985). *Women who love too much*. London: Arrow.

Prever, F., & Bowden-Jones, H. (Eds.). (2021). Donne e disturbo da gioco d'azzardo: Una prospettiva al femminile su trattamento e ricerca (Italian Edition). EAN-139788898726905

2 A JUNGIAN APPROACH TO UNDERSTANDING GAMBLING AND AFFECTIVE ADDICTION AMONG WOMEN

Francesca Picone

Many women are torn between two contradictory needs: the desire to be independent while remaining connected with others. Their well-being is dependent on this dynamic being balanced. However, there are many situations when this balance is upset, for example through a lack of self-confidence and due to fear or an overwhelming desire to give, and relationships take a problematic or even pathological turn. It is in these situations that gambling can become problematic. In this chapter, I will present several complementary approaches to better understand the mechanisms involved in emotional dependence. Particularly during the COVID-19 pandemic, achieving emotional balance is an opportunity to reconcile with the female archetype on a collective level, from the descent into hell to healing. Our collective journey, launched by the goddess Hestia's return, forces us to evaluate our relationships with each other and with the planet, and to see that we are all connected and dependent on each other for survival. Women gamblers pay a heavy price to sacrifice all of this.

Health professionals are well aware that gambling has had a female "hue" for many years, also in Southern Italy. Although a fact, it is well concealed since women here, like elsewhere, are unlikely to ask health services for help. They are blocked by shame and guilt, and often worried about the immoral image they would cast onto themselves, especially if they are mothers.

Sitting near a slot machine in a coffee bar, waiting for the winning Lotto numbers to be announced, holding a scratch card in one hand and a coin in the other while at the tobacco store, or sitting comfortably in a Bingo Hall are the most frequent ways in which gambling creeps into the everyday life of many Sicilian women. It is mainly housewives or pensioners while out on their daily rounds, getting the groceries, running errands, and taking children for a walk, who fit this into their routine. They start gambling later in life than men but slip toward pathology more rapidly (Prever, 2014). Driven first and foremost by wanting some innocent, harmless escapism, they are almost always just trying to distract or defend themselves from a difficult and unsatisfying love life or one that involves physical and psychological domestic violence (Echeburúa et al., 2011).

Gambling acts as an anesthetic. When it becomes pathological, it is often only the tip of an iceberg with depressive disorders, anxiety, panic attacks, and other addictions, first and foremost affective addiction, submerged in the waters below (Boughton & Falenchuk, 2007). And when these women finally ask for help, rather late in the process, it often immediately becomes clear that their primary addiction is to an unhealthy relationship they are unable to rid themselves of and which causes suffering. This is why these women do not gamble much online: even though one can easily remain anonymous in online gambling and therefore hide from being judged by others, one cannot *physically* escape those everyday obligations, one's environment or one's family and personal life story.

This is not the whole picture though: On a collective level, a culture gets handed down from one generation to the next, from mother to daughter, which attracts Sicilian women to gambling. In Sicilian culture, the female figure is strong and firmly rooted, and local folk's wisdom borders on magical thinking, and foretelling. Their dreams turn into numbers to be played in the lottery.

Generally, it is middle-aged, middle-class women, often married, who request health care services. They tend to prefer individual psychotherapy as opposed to group therapy, despite this being offered to them – and psychodynamic therapy is usually recommended because of their life story involving emotional dependence and suffering.

This kind of patient tends to be a woman who loves or has loved too much, and in therapy will let out "her fear of doing something silly," "feeling cowardly," and her guilty feelings about "being judged badly." Frequently, gambling addiction in women, in its various different forms, is rooted in frustration about the inability to be, to do, or to risk something that is worth living for. Therefore, gambling starts with an embrace by the Goddess of Fortune that first constricts then kills (Picone, 2019). By denying a wish and repressing the drive to satisfy it, a sense of guilt, unworthiness, and self-punishment emerges. The silent, apathetic acceptance of a run-of-the-mill life. A quiet accomplice, or so it seems, collides deep down with talents and inclinations that have not found an outlet. This conflict then generates gambling behaviour – an apparently mild, pleasant, and harmless activity.

In clinical work with women, gambling is an expression of deadlock, a psychic energy block, regarding her emotional-affective experience. It is a symptom of her depressed mood – a compensation, because there is often no other pleasure. It compulsively covers up trauma and all the suffering and anxiety related to it. Oftentimes, an adaptive process, self-help, laying out a rigid and precise set of rules, or bringing about a gradual transformation of the symptom via behavioural therapy is not enough when dealing with a woman's gambling addiction. Each female gambler is unique as is the suffering at the source of the gambling addiction (Prever, 2017). As health care professionals, we need to discover this while dramatically fumbling around in the dark, as we often do in our work, and dreams and the images they contain are our allies.

These women are frequently torn between two contradictory needs: wanting to be independent while remaining connected with others, and being caught up in what the other (generally a partner) needs to generate vital energy for themselves. On closer inspection, one realizes how being close to another, which is much desired, in fact conceals these women's difficulty to be alone with their fragile independence and their lack of trust and confidence. These women are unable to trust their own judgment, their evaluations, and their feelings. They doubt everything, above all their own ability to have an opinion, to choose, or to dare show initiative. So, they cling to another, as if this person had some magical power and at times was the only magical person in the world. It seems that in everything these women do they need to be authorized by someone they assign a higher power, more or less consciously. This other person, their only resource, always has to be there, near them, available, very close, too close. However, if something goes wrong and if the harmony is broken, an "addict" profile – often concealing the object of the addiction – becomes apparent in these women. Jung wrote: "One of the main characteristics of women is that they are able to do anything for the love of another human being" (Jung, 1970).

This "strong instinct to bind and loosen" is an integral part of the female, based on the principle of Eros, which woman necessarily experience during their development, beyond male patriarchal consciousness. In our patient, this part – if suppressed – is "personified" as gambling addiction. Going into these women's stories and traveling through them, while talking not so much about gambling but about self-castration, awareness of its horror, and shame, is needed so achieve "absolution" so that the patients may start living again, contemplating their pain, once the truth of the unconscious "gamble" with themselves has been unveiled.

In a physical and concrete sense, depending means "hanging from." In a psychological sense, dependence/addiction means being "taken by." In therapy, this should translate into helping women without being afraid to discover the uncontainable force that drives them ever more intensely to assert themselves. It requires helping them to express the creative impulse of maturity that dwells within them, that invites them to become independent beings endowed with a unique personality, and that defines the specific content of their personality. Being original, personal, and at the same time connected to others, loving without depending excessively on this love, and encroaching on gambling in the case of female gamblers, are forms of energy that animate the personality construction of every human being. In therapy, this is a gradual process of accepting that they are inhabited by psychic forces since birth that initially seemed contradictory: Some operate to seek a reassuring connection toward tender closeness, while others irremediably lead toward individuation. The gradual learning process includes that these two dimensions are equally necessary and do not cancel each other out but are rather complementary and give each other energy. Thus, conditions are created that enable the establishment of a balance between needing closeness and needing independence. One may move from dependence to attention, interest, and authentic feelings toward others in their relationships (Allain-Duprè, 2019). This can be the real bet – an existential bet that recognizes the other's otherness, as opposed to gambling which is a self-destructive end in itself.

And during the COVID-19 pandemic? During the pandemic, female gamblers certainly paid a high price: They were locked away at home, like all other women, and could no longer go out to bet; they were face to face with their problems and their fragilities even more than usual, despite staying in touch remotely with their therapist in this very difficult situation. Those who kept on working, perhaps from home, were often squeezed between cooking meals and looking after children and the family, the whole family. And yet, in this pandemic, in which one was "driven back" home, back to the home and hearth for Sicilian gambling women who are in such close contact with Greek culture and mythology which found its cradle in these lands, the chance to internally encounter the realm of Hestia dawned.

In Greek mythology, Hestia is the hearth at the heart of a real, physical home, a refuge where family bonds are felt and food is found. But Hestia's energy runs deeper. Hestia is the fire that animates our idea of home. This archetype is the heart that beats in our inner sanctuary; a silent core, stable and constant, that grounds us when we are calm enough to perceive its presence. Should all our terrestrial belongings vanish, this home is the heart that remains. Hestia keeps and protects this core even if the world should fall apart (Slominski, 2020).

For those female gamblers who were able to intercept Hestia inside them, this encounter represented a personal opportunity but also a collective one, shared with all other women through descending to the underworld to then heal, liberate oneself and make peace with the female archetype: an extraordinary voyage, launched by the return of the goddess Hestia who compelled these women to review and evaluate their reciprocal relationships, with themselves and with the planet, and to see that we are all connected and dependent upon one another for survival toward a new awareness of oneself and being in the world.

References

Allain-Duprè, B. (2019). *S'affranchir de ses dépendendaces affectives*. Leduc.s Éditions.

Boughton, R., & Falenchuk, O. (2007). Vulnerability and comorbidity factors of female problem gambling. *Journal of Gambling Studies, 23*, 323–334.

Echeburúa, E., González-Ortega, I., de Corral, P. et al. (2011). Clinical gender differences among adult pathological gamblers seeking treatment. *Journal of Gambling Studies, 27*, 215–227.

Jung, C.G. (1970). Woman in Europe (R. F. C. Hull, Trans.). In H. Read et al. (Eds.), *The collected works of C. G. Jung: Vol. 10*. Civilization in transition (2nd ed., pp. 113–133). Princeton University Press. (Original work published 1927).

Picone, F. (2019). *Il femminile e l'azzardo in un'ottica junghiana*. International Conference: "Il gioco d'azzardo patologico in Italia: Le Donne al centro." Palermo, 8 Marzo.

Prever, F. (2014). Il gioco al femminile. *Manuale sul gioco d'azzardo - Diagnosi, valutazione e trattamenti, a cura di Bellio e Croce*. Milano: Franco Angeli.

Prever, F. (2017). Female gambling in Italy: An international female perspective on treatment and research. In H. Bowden-Jones & F. Prever (Eds.), *Gambling disorders in women: An international female perspective on treatment and research*. London: Routledge.

Slominski, A. (2020). Social distancing, and our return to Hestia. Available at: https://www.drandreaslominski.com/post/social-distancing-and-our-return-to-hestia

3 WOMEN, RELATIONS AT STAKE: A NEW SPACE FOR FAMILY LIFE

Maddalena Borsani

Gambling women suffer because of dysfunctional family relationships. This study aimed to explore how gambling is an active subject within the system and evaluate the effectiveness of "Family Life Space" as a tool to investigate gambling dynamics. The pilot study includes women gamblers and their relatives. The sample was chosen from a group for women with problem gambling in Milan, SUN(N)COOP. Results indicate that Family Life Space facilitates communication among family members, highlighting how difficult it is for women to have support and confirming Family Life Space as a prediction and evaluation tool. Study results show where gambling is placed within family relationships. Deep interviews help understand the women's gambling experience.

Introduction

This project is experimental research in the field of clinical psychology – a qualitative study with a systemic approach and the use of the *Family Life Space* test to investigate family relational dynamics (Gozzoli & Tamanza, 1998; Mostwin, 1974). This subchapter is the result of years of scientific studies on gambling and related disorders in the fields of training, prevention, psychotherapy, and clinical activity (Borsani, 2019).

The aim of this study was to demonstrate how four female participants and their family members – chosen among the participants of the *Gioco di Donne* therapeutic group (women gambling group), which is part of the project Gambling & Women of the Milan social cooperative SUN(N)COOP – have experienced life and family dynamics, which exposed them to risk factors for developing a gambling disorder. This treatment emphasizes how gambling has tarnished, highlighted, or changed family relationships and friend networks.

Research Project

Science and gender medicine are turning their attention toward the gender factor in gambling disorder. Women are the custodians of the generative role, family stability and continuity, the care of offspring and the elderly. This "burden" can involve a strong need to escape the solicitation of too many tasks at the same time. Gambling acquires the connotation of the "best anxiolytic" on the market, expensive and effective (Prever, 2014; Prever et al., 2018). Pathological gamblers report devoting themselves to gambling as a means of escaping from stressful, unsatisfactory situations or states of depression. Caring for family issues is crucial for the onset of gambling disorder in women, as women may use gambling as a "self-medication" for mood disorders (Bowden-Jones & Prever, 2017).

During the interviews conducted for this study, the psychotherapist formulated a systemic hypothesis regarding the family and gambling disorder, including all members, to assume their overall relational functioning. Indeed, the behaviour of the woman gambler and her family member can show how every individual within the family is related with (or dependent on) all the others (Boscolo et al., 1987). Each family member enacts behaviours with a communicative intention, influencing other members, who respond with feedback, ensuring the family homeostasis.

Considering communication as an essential act (i.e., one cannot fail to communicate) makes it possible to signify the symptom of gambling disorder as a metaphorical communication of relational situations that manifest themselves in the space of family life. The therapeutic purpose is not to remove the symptom or to activate more adaptive or strategic behaviours, but to observe and modify a pattern of interaction perpetrated by the families until now.

Methodological Framework and Tool

Family Life Space, a tool validated by Mostwin (1976) and adapted in Italian by Gozzoli and Tamanza (1998), is a graphic-projective instrument administered to families. In psychotherapy, it identifies problems like triangulation, alliances, distances, alienation; measures degrees of family congruence and perceptions of the family position in the space of each member; and helps understanding the quality of family communication. This simple, effective tool was used in this clinical research project with some previously designed variations, within a mixed method framework, which included the administration of a graphic test and a systemic clinical interview.

The test was conducted with each individual participant independently from the family, graphically representing a "here and now" condition of the meaningful relationships of women gamblers and their families, and the relationships with gambling (drawn as if it was a new family member) and how it has structured and modified relational links over time. After every graphic section, the woman gambler and her relative gathered, recreating a circular-systemic setting. If the relative could not be present, the family member's presentification technique was used (Bertrando, 2002).

During an interactive session, the psychotherapist used a standard protocol of questions aimed at explaining and understanding what perceptions and thoughts the participant had while carrying out the drawing, what feelings she felt and how she felt when she performed it. The circularity, triggered by the co-built reframing with the participants, generated new possible spaces of family life: metaphorical and living images, returned at the end of every meeting.

This therapeutic act was used to explore the family system and, through hypothetical questions, to describe the family future expectations and a possible change or reshaping in the relational order, to create *a new space of family life.*

Sample

The sample was selected in agreement with Dr. Prever within the free therapeutic group "Gioco di Donne" which is part of the Gambling & Women project of SUN(N)COOP, a social cooperative based in Milan. The sample included four women gamblers, all aged between 55 and 80 years, three of whom were retired. One of them had been in a therapeutic community and was being reintegrated into the working world. One of them had a stable romantic relationship, the others came from not-problems-free divorces and separations. In two cases, the presence of the family member of reference (husband; daughter) helped to start a narrative in joint sessions, creating resonances on the reciprocal Family Life Spaces, considering how gambling had changed the family history.

In the other two cases, family members were not present (for work reasons; due to relational problems) and techniques were used, such as the *presentification of the third party* (Bertrando, 2002) and circular and hypothetical questions, to understand how the relative would develop the Family Life Space and what aspects they would report about the relationship with gambling and its effects over time on the family system.

Results

Within narrations, resonances, and restitutions in session, for privacy reasons a pseudonym has been associated with every woman gambler and her significant family member, enriching session participants with a new identity. In the first clinical case, the woman gambler was renamed Fiorenza, as she acts metaphorically – and even bodily – as a blooming flower, self-confident and endowed with a renewed hope for the future. Her husband was called Riccardo, which means strong man, as he has been a constant presence, both during the interview and in all his wife's life.

In the second case, the subject new name was Marina, following a co-built metaphor concerning the fluidity of this new life phase, which – like the dive of a dolphin into the sea – manifests a new serenity feeling. In the third case the former woman gambler has been called Lucia, which means bright, resuming her description of the change she experienced in a therapeutic community. She now recognizes in herself a new light, capable of irradiating herself and other people.

In the fourth case, the subject became Amabile, the name of an English princess, which recalls the woman gambler high-level social background, but, above all, it allows to re-signify her story and herself as the one who is worthy of love. Her daughter, instead, had the new name of Marzia, since she has always been a fighter, who now can finally experiment her independence from her parents by forming her new family.

Conclusion

During the interviews and in the analysis of relational bonds, it emerged that the presence of gambling had changed the structure of the women gamblers' families, their social and friendly relations and, in a certain way, the ones of their families, changing the meaning and giving these relations a different value.

The therapeutic choice to use the systemic-relational approach as an elective treatment in taking charge of women-gamblers and their families proved to be crucial, focusing on these four women gamblers' relational system and related problems, evident as the root of their pathology.

When a woman gambler and her relative, aided by a Family Life Space test, draw on paper their meaningful relationships narratives, this involves the whole family system, so change becomes possible. The four women gamblers would say that our "becoming-other" is recognizing one's own history and oneself as finally building new spaces of family life.

References

Barbetta, P. (2018). *La terapia familiare sistemica nel tempo della complessità. urly.it/3mggq.*

Bertrando, P. (2002). Il discorso del terzo. Tecniche di terapia sistemica individuale e di analisi del transfert. *Tecniche Conversazionali, 28*, 27–38. urly.it/3mggs

Borsani, M. (2019). *Donne, relazioni in gioco: un nuovo spazio di vita familiare.* Milano: tesi di specializzazione in psicoterapia sistemico-relazionale presso il Centro Milanese di Terapia della Famiglia.

Boscolo, L., Cecchin, G., Hoffman, L., & Penn, P. (1987). *Milan systemic family therapy: Conversations in theory and practice.* New York: Basic Books.

Bowden-Jones, H., & Prever, F. (Eds.). (2017). *Gambling disorders in women: An international female perspective on treatment and research.* London: Taylor & Francis.

Mostwin, D. (1974). Multidimensional model of working with the family. *Social Casework, 55*(4), 209–215.

Mostwin, D. (1976). Social dimension of family treatment. In D. Mostwin (Ed.), *The social dimension of family treatment.* Washington DC: NASW Press.

Prever, F., Casciani, De Luca (2018). *Specificità nella ricerca e del trattamento nel DGA femminile, in Il trattamento Psicologico e Psicoterapico del Disturbo da Gioco d'Azzardo in una prospettiva multidisciplinare, Casciani, De Luca.* Cuneo: Ed. Publiedit.

Tamanza, G., & Gozzoli, C. (1998). *Family life space. L'analisi metrica del disegno.* Milano: Franco Angeli.

4 MINDFULNESS INTERVENTIONS WITH WOMEN GAMBLERS

Monica Minci

Mindfulness-based interventions (MBIs) may be helpful to reduce craving and improve emotion dysregulation in both substance and behavioural addictions. This chapter focuses on mindfulness and women gamblers, exploring how we can consider this approach as a potential gender targeted intervention. Clinical experience has been considered in both individual and group settings, at the National Health Service, Milan's gender group and in private practice.

Mindfulness based interventions have been applied widely in both substance use disorders and behavioural addictions and they seem to have a potential utility to reduce craving and improve addiction-related symptoms like depression, anxiety, and emotion dysregulation (Sancho et al., 2018). Furthermore, women with substance use disorders (SUDs) tend to perceive that gendered groups can offer a safer and more supportive environment (Nelson-Zlupko et al., 1995).

Starting from these assumptions, the aim of this work was to explore whether mindfulness can be considered an intervention targeted at women, considering clinical experience of individual and group sessions for women gamblers in the National Health System (NHS), Milan's female gambling group, and private practice.

Gambling is often used by women to avoid pain, in the attempt not to think about everyday troubles.

> Got a call yesterday. My gran back home is in the final days of her cancer. Gambling is a distraction ... from reality. (Jenny)

Responsibilities, burdens, intense emotions can be tough for all of us. Gambling can be used as a coping strategy to avoid something too difficult to face in our lives.

> When I enter a slot hall it's like stop thinking. (Maria)
>
> Slots let me pass time far from everything and everybody ... it's my solitary island ... they bring me into a parallel world, they make me feel good. (Sonia)
>
> I feel alone and down, I struggle with anxiety. I don't need help with that, I have it under control, but I suppose I use gambling as an escape. (Eleonora)
>
> I play the slot machines. With those colors, those sounds ... it's like being in another world. It's like all the problems vanish for a while. It is like in those halls I am in a bubble. And all the mess stays outside. (Marta)

Mindfulness is a way to focus not outside, but inside, to discover or rediscover the possibility of being in contact with our internal experience. What is our internal experience? Our thoughts, emotions, and sensations. As women are keen to use gambling as a way to avoid one or all parts of their internal experience, mindfulness can be a good training to learn how to deal with it.

Accepting what's going on means that we can focus no more on *what* (the content: this belief is true or false, this emotion is good or bad, this sensation is ok or not), but on *how* (the way we react to the content). The point is not to force change in behaviour, but to practice change of our relation to internal experience, including craving. Mindfulness helps cultivating the shift from a *doing* mode to a *being* mode (Segal et al., 2002).

The doing mode is distinguished by an active mind focused on solving discrepancies between reality and desires, between how things are and how we'd like them to be; otherwise, the being mode is related to the intent of allowing whatever is present as it is, without the effort to change it in any way.

Cecilia for example realizes the utility of gambling to "manage" her unpleasant emotions and sensations, that she doesn't want to feel.

> If I'm peaceful, gambling doesn't exist. But my tinnitus is loud, I lost my friend and I'm alone. Gambling makes me not think about it.

Mindfulness can help women to learn to stay, instead of being trapped in the avoidance automatism. For example, feeling a tension in the body and trying not to immediately shift attention from something that causes discomfort makes us learn that it's feasible to be in contact with something unpleasant in the body. And this can help us manage something uncomfortable also emotionally, even for just a few seconds. Furthermore, it can make us understand that we can take care of our whole selves, without considering sometimes only the good parts, and other times only the bad ones. We are all made of vulnerabilities and resources and the challenge is to be aware of and accept them all at the same time.

A common characteristic of gambling is that it puts you in a timeless space, where time stops.

> My aim was not to bring home money, but as long as I gamble, I'm ok, I zone out. (Michela)
> When I gamble, I'm in a trance-like state, I'm on autopilot. (Manuela)
> I play slot machines. All those colours and sounds ... It's like being in another world. It's like all the troubles disappear for a while. I feel like in a bubble and all the mess stays out. (Carla)

These are some descriptions of the "Valium effect" of gambling, where everything is anesthetized. At first, it shifts attention away from problems, emotional and physical pains, and this can seem like a positive consequence in the beginning, but in the end also the rest of our life becomes numbed. Mindfulness can help us come back to the present, giving us the opportunity to stay "awake" and regain the possibility to feel alive.

During mindfulness sessions, women may experience some obstacles.

* Judgment: "It's always like that," "It's nothing," "No, I should not feel this emotion right now," and "I need to relax more" are only some examples of common ways to undermine what's going on. This reflects the constant daily judgment of what is right and wrong where women get stuck. Through mindfulness we simply listen to what's happening, whether it's pleasant, unpleasant, or neutral. The challenge is to witness, even for a few moments, the actual experience, without comparing it with something ideal.

- Avoidance: "I don't want to stay there, it's painful/boring/annoying" are classic ways to give words to the automatic reaction to unpleasant experiences: We turn our heads and attention to the other way, we get distracted or get lost in our thoughts. And then we are keen to escape physically or mentally from what we can't face.

  - A specific but less-known way to avoid is "not to feel." Some women can admit "I don't feel anything." It happens when we raise the threshold of listening. And it's interesting to explore how this tendency is spread in daily life.

Mindfulness can help women gamblers to get in contact with their body and their somatic memory. One the one hand, this may mean opening a door to some sensations and feelings that were buried and hidden within the unconscious, going beyond the mind. This is the case with Sara, who got in contact with the effects on her body of the fear related to domestic violence. This let her realize that she was not over that trauma as she thought and represented a big step in therapy.

On the other hand, mindfulness can help women to stimulate new body experiences. In fact, focusing attention on our body can improve the ability to feel our body not only when there is pain or discomfort, but also neutral sensations and pleasant ones. For example, Antonella found out that she could experience one minute without feeling her usual pains and she could also feel her body warm from inside, which was enlightening.

Even just one minute of sensation awareness of their body can help women gamblers to realize that their body is not only an automaton, of which they lose control when they gamble. They can be conscious of it, and they can actively listen to it. Observing the urge to gamble gives the possibility not to be over-taken by the impulse. When we learn how to listen, we'll find out also some-thing else apart from unpleasant feelings and we'll avoid using all our energies fighting against something that simply exists and maybe will change soon.

The challenge is simply to be there, with ourselves, whatever happens. And thoughts, emotions and sensations, at some point will change, will become something else, something will be added, something will vanish. And we will be still there. In this way, we become the "fil rouge" of our existence.

References

Nelson-Zlupko, L., Kauffman, E., & Dore, M.M. (1995). Gender differences in drug addiction and treatment: Implications for social work intervention with substance-abusing women. *Social Work*, *40*(1), 45–54.

Sancho, M., De Gracia, M., Rodriguez, R.C., Mallorquí-Bagué, N., Sánchez-González, J., Trujols, J., ... & Menchón, J.M. (2018). Mindfulness-based inter-ventions for the treatment of substance and behavioral addictions: A systematic review. *Frontiers in Psychiatry*, *9*, 95.

Segal, Z., Williams, G., & Teasdale, J. (2002). *Mindfulness-based cognitive therapy*. New York: Guilford Press.

Chapter 23

Innovative Italian Gender Approaches to Diagnosis, Treatment, and Counseling

Ornella De Luca; Amelia Fiorin and Camilla Della Pietà; Irene Ronchi, Antonella Grioni, and Tiziana Manigrasso

The first subchapter by Ornella De Luca focuses on the application of the Gambling Pathways Questionnaire (GPQ) in a group of 18 female gamblers. The outcomes are in line with existing data in the literature, specifically that female gamblers are most commonly of the behaviourally conditioned type, and the antisocial impulsive type is the least common. In the second subchapter, Amelia Fiorin and Camilla Della Pietà reflect on interventions and dedicated care for woman in Italy. Finally, in the third subchapter, Irene Ronchi, Antonella Grioni and Tiziana Manigrasso describe a bridge to help women gamblers. In 2019, their team started to look for more accessible, private, and reassuring spaces for female gamblers through the following initiatives: a dedicated self-help group, an individual listening space, and a helpline, both on the phone and in person. To promote these initiatives, the "Loosen the Knots" project was born.

1 THE COMPLEXITY OF ASSESSING AND USING THE GAMBLING PATHWAYS QUESTIONNAIRE IN A GROUP OF WOMEN WITH GAMBLING DISORDER

Ornella De Luca

This chapter focuses on the application of the Gambling Pathways Questionnaire (GPQ) in a group of 18 female gamblers. The outcomes are in line with existing data in the literature, specifically that female gamblers are most commonly of the behaviourally conditioned type, and the antisocial impulsive type is the least common. GPQ dimensions with high scores were child abuse, depression, and anxiety after the onset of gambling, and impulsivity. While antisocial traits are typically found in antisocial impulsive problem gamblers, we found them in emotionally vulnerable problem gamblers. There is a lack of acknowledgement of the complexity and differences between sexes regarding the sexual risk-taking dimension given that identical diagnostic

DOI: 10.4324/9781003203476-29

criteria are used for all sexes. Sex differences merit further investigation. Further research is needed to reflect on specific diagnostic criteria for female gamblers.

Introduction

Gambling disorder (GD), like all pathological addictions, is a very complex disorder. This complexity is due to the role of different factors and their multiple combinations, which can generate forms of suffering and severe discomfort. Gambling behaviour is sometimes part of an attempt to relieve suffering and discomfort. Every gambler, whether male or female, has its own peculiarities, as has been highlighted by some researchers who have developed etiopathogenetic models to highlight both the similarities and the differences between gamblers, and the development of the disorder (Blaszczynski & Nower, 2002; Ladd & Petry, 2002). For women gamblers, both the scientific literature and clinical experience show us that there is a need for some precautions and greater care, starting with having access to services (Grant & Kim, 2002; Grant et al., 2012).

Female Gamblers with Gambling Disorder: Peculiarities and Criticalities

In Italy, the services for taking care of patients with GD are structured territorial health services (Ser.D.) that also manage care of patients with drug addiction. For many gamblers this represents a further obstacle to access treatment because they identify with substance addiction and therefore with other users. This difficulty in accessing treatment adds to other challenging factors of various domains including:

A Socio-Cultural Factors

Gambling is commonly frowned upon, and seen as a source of harm and despised. For example, a man who gambles and squanders family assets or destroys relationships is certainly seen as a person who is not very responsible and blameworthy. For women gamblers, all this is even less acceptable, and it is more despicable. Perhaps contributing to this negative criticism is a lack of knowledge and understanding the concept of disease or disorder, particularly applied to gamblers, as it is not yet part of the common mindset. Indeed, even for professionals it is a fairly recent acquisition.

B Psychological Factors

Due to the aforementioned reasons, which can generate painful experiences, such as a sense of shame, a sense of guilt toward oneself and especially toward family members, it becomes difficult for women gamblers to ask for help from a service (Prever & Bowden-Jones, 2021). Furthermore, what has just been said is intertwined with personal frailties and personality traits that unfortunately represent fruitful ground for the development of attitudes of closure and isolation, which additionally contribute to suffering.

C Organizational (Service System) Factors

Although the lines of action of the Ministry of Health (DM n.136 16/07/2021) highlight that the regional health services or a dedicated outpatient clinic for gamblers would be desirable, in reality this has not yet been implemented. This may be due to a lack of resources but perhaps also because attention to these issues is still lacking, despite the phenomenon reaching such dimensions that it cannot be ignored. This, intertwined with socio-cultural and psychological factors described above, results in insufficient responses to the already difficult requests for help which and the specific needs of patients who require an ad hoc setting, more protection (such as a group for women only), and specific well-defined objectives (such as work on overcoming the sense of shame or on the development of certain skills such as assertiveness). In order to define treatment paths that take all this into account, an accurate assessment must be made to have a clearer and more complete view of the current and previous situation of the patient – a gambler.

Diagnosis and Assessment

For the diagnosis of GD, in both women and men, in addition to clinical observation and anamnestic assessment, we can make use of specific diagnostic tools such as the *Diagnostic and Statistical Manual of Mental Disorders*, Fifth Edition (DSM-5) and the South Oaks Gambling Screen (SOGS), which allow for the assessment of the presence or absence of the disorder and the level of severity. However, the assessment work is more complex, as well as essential, since there are numerous elements to take into account when working with women gamblers, some undoubtedly overlapping with those of men, others may be specific to women.

Consider, for example, the experiences of abuse and/or mistreatment, which are factors often present in the stories of female gamblers with GD that may negatively impact both the request for help and the development of the therapeutic relationship (Lane et al., 2016). Nevertheless, the assessment phase presents opportunities to create favorable conditions that foster the development of the therapeutic alliance necessary for the patient to develop sufficient trust in the therapist and, consequently, also develop sufficient motivation for treatment. Hence the importance of a therapeutic relationship with a female therapist for women seeking treatment for GD.

During the assessment phase, in addition to an exhaustive anamnestic assessment and clinical interviews, specific tests are used (in this case for GD) to gain a global vision of the case and to investigate issues related to GD both pre-existing and co-occurring with the disorder, such as anxiety, depression, personality disorders, etc. These problems, if not treated in parallel, with pharmacological support where indicated, would prevent us from starting a path of psychotherapy or at least make it difficult. Various standardized tests and questionnaires offer valid help to acquire further information on that specific case. However, there are limitations when they are structured on a predominantly male population, overlooking and possibly disregarding female differences due to results that may not be entirely appropriate or accurate.

In clinical experience difficulties may be encountered during the administration of tests, when certain items, at times, do not allow women gamblers to recognize themselves because they are more typical of men's experiences. For example, we can cite an item of the Gambling Pathways Questionnaire (GPQ) "I am willing to pay to have sex." On the basis of our clinical experience and the results of the questionnaires administered, we found a total lack of identification with the aforementioned behaviour on the part of women, because in Italian culture, and in the industrialized world and Western culture in general, paying for sex mainly relates to men's behaviours. In the validation work of the Italian version of the GPQ, this item was slightly mitigated to better adapt it to Italian culture.

Gambling Pathways Questionnaire and Female Gender

The Gambling Pathways Questionnaire provides clinicians with a snapshot of a client's rating (high, medium, lower) on nine etiological risk factors that lead to problem gambling: Mood Pre- and Post-Problem-Gambling Onset (anxiety, depression); Substance Misuse Pre- and Post-Problem Gambling Onset (alcohol, drugs, prescription and over-the-counter medications); Child Maltreatment (abuse, neglect, trauma); Parent or Caregiver Addiction; Narcissistic Traits; Impulsivity; Risk-Taking; Attention-Deficit/Hyperactivity Disorder (ADHD) Symptoms; and Antisocial Traits of Behaviours. It also assigns clients to one of three subgroups or types with specific implications for gambling treatment: first type (behaviourally conditioned problem gamblers), second type (emotionally vulnerable problem gamblers), third type (antisocial impulsive problem gamblers).

The above mentioned observation that paying for sex mainly relates to men's behaviours appears to be confirmed by the results of the GPQ in a sample of 18 women with GD, where the sexual risk taking dimension was completely absent. Unlike sexual risk taking, the results of the questionnaire, in general, showed different scores in the various dimensions based on the type of belonging. Most women (67%, $n = 12$) were of the behaviourally conditioned problem gambler type, 28% ($n = 5$) were assigned as emotionally vulnerable problem gamblers, and one woman as an antisocial impulsive problem gambler. This distribution of subgroups is quite similar to what is generally reported in the literature (Nower et al., 2021).

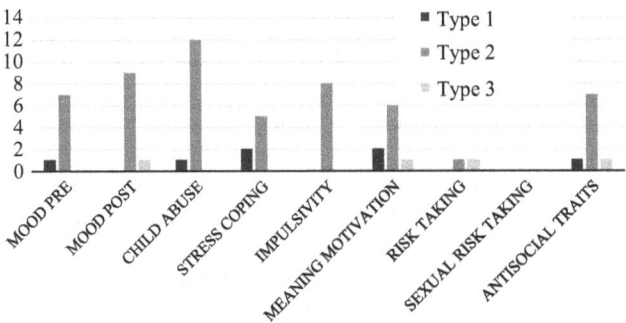

14 ■ Type 1
12
10 ■ Type 2
8
6 ■ Type 3
4
2
0

MOOD PRE   MOOD POST   CHILD ABUSE   STRESS COPING   IMPULSIVITY   MEANING MOTIVATION   RISK TAKING   SEXUAL RISK TAKING   ANTISOCIAL TRAITS

Figure 23.1 Dimension scores by type (type 1: behaviourally conditioned problem gamblers; type 2: emotionally vulnerable problem gamblers; type 3: antisocial impulsive problem gamblers).

In addition, the results of the questionnaire showed different scores in the various dimensions based on the gambling type. From the analysis of the GPQ in this sample of 18 female gamblers, the highest values across all dimensions are found in type 2 (emotionally vulnerable problem gamblers; Figure 23.1).

Within type 2, the most significant dimensions were Child Abuse (66.6%), Mood Post-Problem-Gambling Onset (50%), Impulsivity (44.4%), Mood Pre-Problem-Gambling Onset (38.8) and, unexpectedly, antisocial traits (38, 8%), while we find low values in the Risk-Taking dimension and, as already mentioned, a total absence of Sexual Risk-Taking (Figure 23.2). The high scores of the aforementioned dimensions, with the exception of antisocial traits, are typical of type 2 which is characterized by the presence of anxiety disorders, mood disorders and previous traumatic experiences in childhood, in addition to cognitive distortions. In fact, from various epidemiological investigations (Grant & Kim, 2002), it emerges that above all, women prefer those games of chance that are able to produce a high cognitive and emotional involvement that can be very reinforcing because it is capable of inducing relief and moving away from emotionally painful states.

Given that, in general, the population of gamblers assigned to type 3 is less numerous than the other two types, female gamblers are even less represented in this subgroup (Nower & Blaszczynski, 2017). In fact, in our group of female gamblers, there appears to be only one gambler of type 3. An unexpected result was that antisocial traits, typically found in type 3, were found instead in type 2 (38.8% of the total).

Clinical interviews carried out with patients allowed us to derive a hypothesis that could explain this result: most of the items relating to the "antisocial" dimension can be seen as expressions of feelings of frustration and (unexpressed) anger resulting from the passive way in which (female) gamblers have structured relationships with others and in particular with partners, while the remaining items seem to express feelings of revenge, following a history of

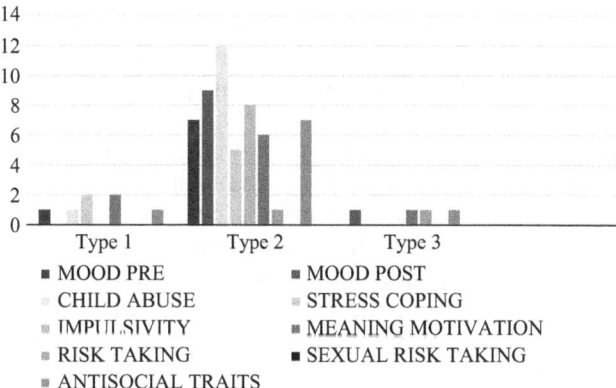

Figure 23.2 Dimension profiles by type (type 1: behaviourally conditioned problem gamblers; type 2: emotionally vulnerable problem gamblers; type 3: antisocial impulsive problem gamblers).

emotional lack, loneliness, experiences of avoidance, etc. From the collection of anamnestic data and from the patients' recent experiences depressive aspects emerge, probably as a consequence of gambling behaviour, anger for not being able to cope with problematic situations in an adequate way but also for the negative and frustrating experiences due to psychological pressure, most often experienced in the family (spouse, partner, etc.), or experiences of neglect and/ or mistreatment or abuse suffered in childhood. Because of their passivity, these patients reacted to frustration with depression or with repressed anger. Interviews at the service were for many of them a first experience of an opportunity to express themselves freely.

The analytical examination of the scores of the items in the questionnaire seems to confirm the above. The significant Mood Pre-Problem-Gambling Onset score (38.8%) could indicate the function of gambling as a mood regulator (Prever & Bowden-Jones, 2021; Rogier & Velotti, 2018), a behaviour highlighted by several studies as being the most recurrent in the female gambler population. On the other hand, the values of the Mood Post-Problem-Gambling Onset dimension (50%) may highlight a depressive and shame reaction for the consequences of gambling behaviour, which for many women seem to represent a serious failure on several levels: economic, relational, marital, social, and parental. Most of the time this sense of failure makes the need to escape even more urgent – toward lightness, lightheartedness, and for some real anesthesia, even if temporary.

Conclusion

Beyond the more strictly clinical aspects that seem to differentiate the profiles of women gamblers from men and the different meaning that gambling behaviour can have in the life system of both kinds, what is highlighted from our observation is the complex and heterogeneous nature of GD. Consequently, some critical issues arise from this complexity which must be taken into account right from the first contact with female patients:

- The complexity of the evaluation process of the clinical picture to define the level of severity and identify variables responsible for maintaining the disorder.
- There are numerous elements that feed and reinforce gambling behaviour even if the complexity lies in their interaction and combination.
- Difficulty in accessing treatment, in particular for women gamblers, due to the social stigma that weighs on them and the services that take care of people with GD, which are still closely associated with places of care for people with "drug problems."

The indication that we can draw from these considerations could be to evaluate the pre-existing situation of discomfort and to the onset of the disorder by making a classification, also with the support of ad hoc tools such as the GPQ, but above all taking into account the unique individual differences of the person who asks to be treated, in order to also elaborate specific diagnostic criteria for female gamblers, and proposing settings, when possible, that allow responding as appropriately as possible to the patient's needs.

Acknowledgements

A special thanks to Fulvia Prever for having sensitized me and stimulating my interest in female gamblers and to Onofrio Casciani for his support in work initiatives and his valuable contributions in all these years.

References

Blaszczynski, A., & Nower, L. (2002). A pathways model of problem and pathologica lgambling. *Addiction*, 97, 487–499.
Grant, J.E., Chamberlain, S.R., Scheriber, L.R., & Odlaug, B.L. (2012). Gender-related clinical and neurocognitive differences in individuals seeking treatment for pathological gambling. *Journal of Psychiatric Research*, 46(9), 1206–1211.
Grant, J.E., & Kim, S.W. (2002). Gender differences in pathological gamblers seeking medication treatment. *Comprehensive Psychiatry*, 43(1), 56–62.
Ladd, G.T., & Petry, N.M. (2002). Gender differences among pathological gamblers seeking treatment. *Experimental & Clinical Psychopharmacology*, 10(3), 302–309.
Lane, W., Sacco, P., Downton, K., Ludeman, E., Levy, L., & Tracy, J.K. (2016). Child maltreatment and problem gambling: A systematic review. *Child Abuse & Neglect*, August 2016 DOI: 10.1016/j.chiabu.2016.06.003
Nower, L., & Blaszczynski, A. (2017). Development and validation of the Gambling Pathways Questionnaire (GPQ). *Psychology of Addictive Behaviors*, 31(1), 95–109.
Nower, L., Blaszczynski, A., & Anthony, W.L. (2021, November 17). Clarifying

gambling subtypes: The revised pathways model of problem gambling. *Addiction.* doi: 10.1111/add.15745.Epub ahead of print. PMID: 34792223.

Prever, F., & Bowden-Jones, H. (2021). Donne e Disturbo da Gioco d'Azzardo. Ed. dEste, Milano.

Rogier, G., & Velotti, P. (2018, June 1). Conceptualizing gambling disorder with the process model of emotion regulation. *Journal of Behavioral Addictions*, 7(2), 239–251. doi: 10.1556/2006.7.2018.52

2 REFLECTIONS ON INTERVENTIONS AND DEDICATED CARE FOR WOMAN IN ITALY

Amelia Fiorin and Camilla Della Pietà

Previous research demonstrates that female problem gamblers are very different from their male counterparts and gambling treatment programs designed for men may be detrimental to women. Therefore, problem gambling counseling programs need to take into account the needs and issues of women gamblers with different engagement and treatment methods. The Addiction Department ULSS2 Marca Trevigiana (DDAULSS2; Italy) developed an experimental clinical approach, considering gender differences in problem gambling and changes imposed by the COVID-19 pandemic. This therapeutic path has three levels of intervention: 1) Engagement (working mainly on relationships with friends and equals that the gamblers establish as internal resources, to facilitate engagement and motivational work); 2) individual interviews during which, together with the gambler, fundamental and traumatic passages of the gambler's history are reconstructed; and 3) gender-specific group treatment for female problem gamblers to create a safe space where they feel accepted, can share their stories, gain insight about their behavior, and receive feedback.

Introduction

In services dedicated to the treatment of substance and behavioural addictions, treatment paths are structured based on research and reports that historically mainly use samples of male subjects. This is a major difficulty, on an organizational level, in these services. Crisp and colleagues highlight how treatment of gambling problems predominantly employs information and strategies based on male therapeutic needs (Crisp et al., 2000; Mark & Lesieur, 1992). However, there is a lot of research and evidence that treatments for addictions, and in particular gambling disorder, are more effective if gender differences are taken into account (Albanese et al., 2011; Grant et al., 2002; Ibáñez, Blanco, Moreryra et al., 2003; Prever & Locati, 2014; Thomas & Moore, 2003; Toneatto & Wang, 2009). Potenza et al. (2001) highlight differences in the motivations for gambling and on a diagnostic level. Women present with comorbidities more often than male gamblers, suggesting the need to equip the care system with different strategies to maximize the effectiveness of treatment. Women are often referred to as "run-away gamblers," with gambling typically triggered by emotional stressors, avoidance and significantly higher levels of psychiatric disorders (Boughton, 2003; Boughton & Falenchuk, 2007; Thomas & Moore, 2003; Trevorrow & Moore, 1998; Westphal & Johnson, 2003). As with other addictions, stories of women with problematic gambling reveal a high prevalence of childhood abuse and trauma in adulthood (Boughton, 2003; Boughton & Falenchuk, 2007; Kausch et al., 2006; Ledgerwood & Petry, 2006). Ibáñez, Blanco, de Castro et al. (2003) propose that female gamblers may respond better to treatment strategies that take into account their specific emotional needs. Based on this evidence, many services and departments focusing on addiction have developed a gendered approach, treatment protocols that take these peculiarities into account, and specific strategies to meet the needs of different population subgroups.

Before describing the intervention model used in our department in detail, it is worth briefly describing the socioeconomic and sociocultural context of the region where the intervention is implemented. The area of North Italy, Veneto, is highly industrialized, with an intact social fabric and a good standard of living where family cohesion is one of the "therapeutic" resources. The tasks of women is still bound by the traditional division of male and female roles. Changes imposed by progress and cultural transformations take place in this region though at a slow and calm pace. From 2000 onward, the gaming industry has distributed a wide range of gambling opportunities with the aim of bringing the habit of gambling also closer to the female world.

The Addiction Department ULSS2 Marca Trevigiana (DDAULSS2; Italy) developed an experimental clinical approach, considering gender differences in problem gambling and changes imposed by the COVID-19 pandemic. The two main themes of our approach are as follows:

A Engagement and First Intervention

The existing literature describes considerable difficulty gamblers face when seeking help and relying on services (Bastiani et al., 2013). In an interesting report by Boughton and Brewster (2002), 365 women who presented with problematic gambling never had access to treatment. They highlighted various obstacles that limit contact with services dedicated to problem gambling. Barriers can be practical (time, complex family schedule, distance, priority for child or parent care, financial limitations) or internal such as social stigma (including that of the service operator), fear of recognition, and exposure to criticism and guilt of family members. In relation to these aspects, the protocol at DDAULSS2 provides a first phase (3–4 session) which structured with individual interviews only between the gambler and a professional psychologist. The professional's attitude is an empathic and active listening, the management technique is to stimulate narration of events, chronology of difficulties, narration of the story of gambling, and risk factors, and to understand the possible resources and solutions that are currently available. A recent publication on linguistic analyses of self-narratives of patients with gambling disorder reinforces the choice of these techniques and the usefulness of this approach (Altavilla et al., 2020).

The autobiographical narrative and linguistic style used by gamblers are important instruments to be used in a clinical setting because they are connected to underlying emotional and cognitive processes. This "engagement intervention" ends with the achievement of two short-term objectives: The first objective is to offer, at appropriate times and in the context of brief counseling, information on coping mechanisms, stress management and management of negative emotions traced during the session, and to increase awareness and ability of reading gambling's symptom. The second objective is to engage the female gambler in a homogeneous group of gambling women – a therapy group that takes place outside the department in the evening. On the experiential level, it was found that participation of the gambler in the therapeutic group, along with connection to the service, offers an emotional experience of secure attachment.

During protocol implementation, we identified some aspects specific to the situation of female gamblers. For example, involving a friend or even a neighbour or the employer is a good resource, if they are aware of the problem. Family members, partners, or children can certainly be resources as well but they may reactivate feelings of shame and guilt and fear of abandonment. Another aspect to be carefully evaluated are debts, loans, or more generally the reconstruction of all economic parts. This is a specific phase of treatment and it is useful to agree with the patient about when to address this area, as it is often not the priority for them, while for male gamblers it is often the main reason for accessing the service. For a male gambler, it is often not only a relief to be able to share the economic burden and debt obligations with their families, but they welcome the fact that the partner takes care of the economic management. For the female gambler, this aspect is much more difficult to address and requires processing and acceptance. This process may take longer for female compared to male gamblers.

B *Creating a Homogeneous Treatment Group for Female Gamblers*

Following clinical research, behavioural interventions (CBT) are a highly effective treatment practice for the pathology of gambling in men (Ladouceur et al., 2003). However, for women these interventions present a higher degree of difficulty and less involvement. Further studies, maintaining the structure of CBT interventions, have introduced therapeutic variables that contemplate a space for narrating affective, relational and traumatic problems (Bowden-Jones & Prever, 2017; Brandt & Wöhr, 2017).

Based on existing evidence, at DDAULSS2 a group intervention for women only was implemented. The group is homogenous in terms of symptoms and gender, and there is also homogeneity in terms of elaborated themes. Therefore, the initial phase of the group is very brief, and the therapeutic work is facilitated by a process of cohesion which is encouraged by the strong similarities and identification between the members. Cohesion is a phenomenon that is assessed with punctuality, the absence of *drop-outs* and the topics covered. This homogeneous group offers women the invaluable advantage of having a support network: Sharing among peers can reduce feelings such as shame, fear, and stigma which represent barriers to crossing the threshold of services (Boughton et al., 2016). This group is also characterized by its therapeutic specificity in welcoming sharing and treating traumatic events (type I and type II following the classification of Terr, 1990), continuous episodes of neglect, and situations of loss or abandonment that easily reactivate the syndrome of addiction. The group therapy works as a collective memory that rewrites, reinterprets, and offers different meanings, repairing each single event marked as frightening, angry, distressing, fearful. Patients who have a neglectful past, interrupted by negative episodes and trauma, recognize themselves on a non-verbal level even before the conscious level, and this facilitates the emergence of "hidden" events. The therapist works to facilitate the sharing of aspects of suffering and traumatic experiences among all participants to alleviate emotional stress. The technique to facilitate this process is the construction of a single story, starting from the pieces of history of the individual members. The tool used in this process is the narrative construction of an autobiographical collective story.

References

Albanese, P., Busch, J., Evans, C., Falkowski-Ham, A., Meredith, N., Stark, S., & Zahlan, N. (2011). *Examination of the associations between problem gambling and various demographic variables among women in Ontario.* Echo.

Altavilla, D., Acciai, A., Deriu, V., Chiera, A., Adornetti, I., Ferretti, F., ... & Canali, S. (2020). Linguistic Analysis of self-narratives of patients with gambling disorder. *Addictive Disorders & Their Treatment, 19*(4), 209–217.

Bastiani, L., Gori, M., Colasante, E., Siciliano, V., Capitanucci, D., Jarre, P., & Molinaro, S. (2013). Complex factors and behaviors in the gambling population of Italy. *Journal of Gambling Studies, 29*(1), 1–13.

Boughton, R. (2003). A feminist slant on counselling the female gambler: Key issues and tasks. *Journal of Gambling Issues, 8,* 1–23.

Boughton, R., & Brewster, J.M. (2002). Voices of women who gamble in Ontario: A survey of women's gambling, barriers to treatment and treatment service needs: Ontario Problem Gambling Research Centre.

Boughton, R., & Falenchuk, O. (2007). Vulnerability and comorbidity factors of female problem gambling. *Journal of Gambling Studies, 23*(3), 323–334.

Boughton, R.R., Jindani, F., & Turner, N.E. (2016). Group treatment for women gamblers using web, teleconference and workbook: Effectiveness pilot. *International Journal of Mental Health and Addiction, 14*(6), 1074–1095.

Bowden-Jones, H., & Prever, F. (Eds.). (2017). *Gambling disorders in women: an international female perspective on treatment and research.* Taylor & Francis.

Brandt, L., & Wŏhr, A. (2017). Factors influencing treatment-seeking behavior in female pathological gamblers. A comparison of treatment centers in Austria and

Germany. In Bowden-Jones, H., & Prever, F. (Eds.). *Gambling disorders in women: An international female perspective on treatment and research.* Taylor & Francis.

Crisp, B.R., Thomas, S.A., Jackson, A.C., Thomason, N., Smith, S., Borrell, J., ... & Holt, T.A. (2000). Sex differences in the treatment needs and outcomes of problem gamblers. *Research on Social Work Practice, 10*(2), 229–242.

Grant, J.E., Kushner, M.G., & Kim, S.W. (2002). Pathological gambling and alcohol use disorder. *Alcohol Research & Health, 26*(2), 143.

Ibáñez, A., Blanco, C., de Castro, I.P., Fernandez-Piqueras, J., & Sáiz-Ruiz, J. (2003). Genetics of pathological gambling. *Journal of Gambling Studies, 19*(1), 11–22.

Ibáñez, A., Blanco, C., Moreryra, P., & Sáiz-Ruiz, J. (2003). Gender differences in pathological gambling. *The Journal of Clinical Psychiatry, 64*(3), 295–301.

Kausch, O., Rugle, L., & Rowland, D.Y. (2006). Lifetime histories of trauma among pathological gamblers. *American Journal on Addictions, 15*(1), 35–43. doi: 10.1080/1 0550490500419045

Ladouceur, R., Sylvain, C., Boutin, C., Lachance, S., Doucet, C., & Leblond, J. (2003). Group therapy for pathological gamblers: A cognitive approach. *Behaviour Research and Therapy, 41*(5), 587–596.

Ledgerwood, D.M., & Petry, N.M. (2006). Psychological experience of gambling and subtypes of pathological gamblers. *Psychiatry Research, 144*(1), 17–27.

Mark, M.E., & Lesieur, H.R. (1992). A feminist critique of problem gambling research. *British Journal of Addiction, 87*(4), 549–565.

Potenza, M.N., Steinberg, M.A., McLaughlin, S.D., Wu, R., Rounsaville, B.J., & O'Malley, S.S. (2001). Gender-related differences in the characteristics of problem gamblers using a gambling helpline. *American Journal of Psychiatry, 158*(9), 1500–1505.

Prever, F., & Locati, V. (2014). A female group: A peculiar Italian experience. Gambling as a "Way Out"? 3rd International Multidisciplinary Symposium on Excessive Gambling, Universitè de Neuchâtel, CH.

Terr, L. (1990). *Too scared to cry: How trauma affects children and ultimately us all.* Basic Books.

Thomas, A., & Moore, S. (2003). The interactive effects of avoidance coping and dysphoric mood on problem gambling for female and male gamblers. *Journal of Gambling Issues*, (8).

Toneatto, T., & Wang, J.J. (2009). Community treatment for problem gambling: Sex differences in outcome and process. *Community Mental Health Journal, 45*(6), 468–475.

Trevorrow, K., & Moore, S. (1998). The association between loneliness, social isolation and women's electronic gaming machine gambling. *Journal of Gambling Studies, 14*(3), 263–284.

Westphal, J.R., & Johnson, L.J. (2003). Gender differences in psychiatric comorbidity and treatment-seeking among gamblers in treatment. *Journal of Gambling Issues, 8*, 1–3.

3 A BRIDGE TO HELP WOMEN GAMBLERS: A FEMALE-FRIENDLY EXPERIMENTAL APPROACH

Irene Ronchi, Antonella Grioni and Tiziana Manigrasso

In Cremona, Italian women do not seek help at gambling therapy services. Many women come to our Public Clinic to support their gambling family members, but not for support or services for themselves. In 2019, our team started to look for more accessible, private, and reassuring spaces for female gamblers through the following initiatives: a dedicated self-help group, an individual listening space, and a help-line, both on the phone and in person. To promote these initiatives, the "Loosen the Knots" project was born. We involved hairdressers in delivering to their female customers our info fliers about these aid initiatives, together with a gift.

Introduction

Who really sees women gambling? Husbands? Friends? Relatives? It is unlikely.

Operators at gambling venues directly observe women gambling every day and can gather information on gambling behaviours, habits, and consequences. They claim that "women gamble just like and more than men." This phrase, which was repeated to us many times during our training and refresher courses dedicated to managers of Italian gambling venues made us reflect, drawing our attention to the problem of women's gambling.

Honestly, it is quite difficult to detect to what extent the population of gamblers is represented by women; however, it is precisely the operators who report that it could be safely estimated at 50%, although that it is not reflected in the access data of SER. D (addiction clinics) care.

Women do not seek for help at gambling therapy services. What factors might contribute to this? Reasons explored in the international literature include a strong sense of shame and guilt, the difficulties in finding time and space for self-care, the family workload and their working roles all represent important obstacles (McMillen et al., 2004).

In our experience many women come to SER. D, *The Public Service for the Treatment of Gambling*, to accompany their gambling family members but not for themselves. They are wives, girlfriends, mothers, sisters, grandmothers, friends, and we have also seen aunts and employers (Prever & Locati in Bowden-Jones & Prever, 2017). Women are accustomed to asking for help for others, although not for themselves, and this may be a contributing barrier to help seeking. In our experience, in the rare occasions that they do ask for themselves, they are always alone, they come without letting family members know their problem because they are too ashamed. A second barrier seems to be the lack of family support. Moreover, public addiction clinics in Italy are heavily stigmatized because they are connoted with a population who uses drugs and alcohol and no women friendly approaches are often found there (Prever et al., 2018).

Another reason is represented by depression, often the "real" underlying problem, from which gambling might seem to offer an escape. "When I gamble, I feel alive," is a phrase that female gamblers often tell us in clinical interviews. Gambling thus becomes an escape from a heavy and unsustainable reality, which promises to magically change their lives in an instant.

Initiatives for Women Gamblers in Cremona

Cremona is a small province, located in the Lombardy region, in northern Italy. The economy is mainly agricultural and secondly, industrial. The small size of the town has an impact on lifestyle and relationships which are still based on local habits and traditions, on the direct knowledge of people and on the bonds of trust.

After considering the above-mentioned barriers for women to access treatment, in 2019 our gambling team (a psychiatrist, a psychologist, and a social worker) started to look for more accessible, private, and reassuring spaces for female gamblers through the following initiatives:

A *A self-help group for female gamblers.* A non-therapeutic space for listening and discussion, without prejudice. The group meets every 15 days in the late afternoon.

B *An individual listening space, by phone and in person*, to voice doubts and difficulties and to receive advice. It is open to female gamblers or female family members of gamblers.

Both activities are free of charge.

The Caritas association offered an available professional volunteer educator who is an expert on female dependence, and a free, private, and protected space. This meeting place is situated far from the addiction service, considering all the recommendations relating to the setting (Piquette-Tomei et al., 2008), to guarantee a space for confidentiality, self-reflection and solidarity (Karter, 2010). The initiative arose from the partnership between the institutional service and the voluntary service.

Special leaflets have been produced to promote the initiatives, distributed on various occasions, to social and health services and to local people. The self-help group started with four female gamblers and then stopped due to the pandemic.

As already highlighted by the literature, a commonality all the participants share is a traumatic personal history, in addition to previous psychiatric diagnoses/traits (Bellio, 2009; Ibanez and others, 2001; Thomas & Moore, 2001). Another common factor is that the participants are all heavy smokers. Furthermore, for all the participants, interpersonal relationships are characterized by conflicting experiences, with difficulties related to making decisions on maintaining one's well-being, as well as experiencing behaviours of devaluation and subordination within the relational sphere.

In 2019, a conference entitled "The Other Side of the Moon" was organized as a moment of reflection on the theme and a way to start new collaborations with the speakers. In 2020, the COVID-19 pandemic led to a forced shutdown of the project and the general influx of patients to the clinic service, in parallel with the closure of gambling venues during lockdown. The pandemic has been an obstacle in helping women just as much as their fatigue and resistance to seek for help, exacerbating the already present discomfort and difficulties, accentuating dysfunctional dynamics, emotional loads, and relational fatigue. Job insecurity, managing children who are doing online learning, feelings of not being able to escape, indeed, being forced to spend more time in toxic and dangerous relationships, increased women's malaise and their burden as caregivers, which made it even more difficult for them to take care of themselves as people who already experience challenges in this domain.

Even following these initiatives, few female gamblers showed up in our care service. The main issue was: How could we better help women with gambling problems, and where could we reach them in an informal setting? We dug out an idea that had remained in the drawer for a few years, then we worked on it again in a group brainstorming: Where do all women, rich or poor, go anyway, at least occasionally? Where do they talk about their life problems with no inhibitions? The hairdresser, is that place, is it not?

The thought, which came as an insight from women and health workers, was this: "It is more common for a woman, any woman, to go to the hairdresser than to her own doctor." Hair salons are female-friendly informal places where we stop for a while to take care of ourselves and even have a chat. Hairdressers are privileged figures of contact, listening in on the female world. They are precious helpers who, through informal daily conversations, can grasp needs and difficulties, and could disseminate information on how to find help for a personal or family gambling problem.

Thanks to a regional initiative called "PIANO GAP 2019–2021," the working group found the funds to carry out the actions of the project called "SCIOGLI I NODI" ("Loosen the Knots"), involving local hairdresser organizations, which made it possible to use two psychologists who were experts in the field of addiction, and the supervision of Dr. Fulvia Prever, an international expert in the field of women's gambling.

We asked the professionals to deliver the flyer to the customers with information on the aid initiatives reserved for women, together with a gift – a nice comb with pressed on it the words "Loosen the Knots," call 335–7554210 (see Figure 23.3).

The project was carried out through the following actions:

- Contact and adhesion of the local branch of the NCA – the National Confederation of Crafts, presentation meeting for the representatives of the hairdresser category at their headquarters.
- Online meetings (due to the restrictions related to the pandemic) for planning and brainstorming between the team and supervisor to identify a gadget and formulate a slogan that would not be perceived as stigmatizing but "hook them in," such as
"brush your worries away"
"cut it out"
"did your life take a bad curl?"
"give a new twist to your life!"
- Choosing a purse comb gadget with the words "Loosen the Knots" on it and the telephone number of the service.

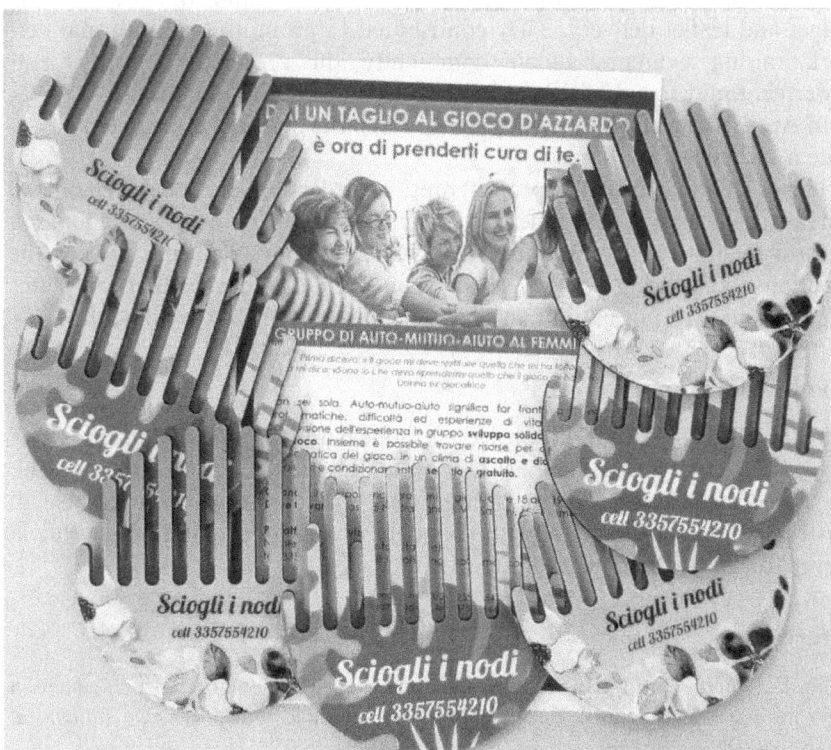

Figure 23.3 An example of a leaflet to promote initiatives for women gamblers.

- Organizing a press conference for the dissemination of the project, which was attended by four local newspapers, in addition to television interviews.
- Sharing of a project information newsletter sent to all associated hairdressers
- Short awareness-raising meeting, by appointment, directly at hair salons, with delivery of gifts and information leaflets.
- Distribution of gadgets and leaflets by hairdressers to their customers.

In March 2022, we had our first follow-up with 25% of hairdressers who joined the project, who reported:

- Info leaflets and gadgets were all distributed.
- Clients really appreciated this.
- Only a very small group of them seemed to be bothered by gadget delivery, without giving any explanation about it.

At project level, the most relevant observation was that some hairdressers took the initiative to connect their sensitive customers with specific professional roles (family doctors, leader of social organizations) during the gadget and leaflet delivery. They contributed to promoting an informal network, raising awareness in our community; this represents a further empowerment and social health promotion in our local community.

In April, we received our first phone calls to the helpline: three in ten days – quite a success!

This is a female, heartfelt project, quite a challenge in the local area but we all really believe in it very much. It is a work in progress and we are looking forward to first results. We hope that we can give a small hint toward the directions of choosing *women friendly* venues and approaches that can better reach this hidden population and have them get the help they deserve.

Acknowledgements

The "SCIOGLI I NODI" project is collegial and a work in progress. We would like to thank Dr. ssa Cristina Bassini, Nicoletta Domaneschi, Dr. Roberto Poli for their important contributions, C N A and Casa di Nostra Signora for their cooperation and network support, and Dr.ssa Fulvia Prever for her involvement as supervisor.

References

Bellio, F. (2009). Caratteristiche sociodemografiche, cliniche e differenze di genere in giocatori d'azzardo patologici in trattamento ambulatoriale, *Giornale Italiano di Psicopatologia, 15*, 39–47.

Bowden-Jones, H., & Prever, F. (2017). *Gambling disorders in women: An international female prospective on treatment and research.* Routledge.

Ibáñez, A., Blanco, C., Donahue, E., Leisieur, H.R., Pérez de Castro, I., Fernández-Piqueras, J., &Sáiz-Ruiz, J. (2001). Psychiatric comorbidity in pathological gamblers seeking treatment. *American Journal of Psychiatry, 158*, 1733–1735.

Karter, L. (2010). Therapist in women and gambling level ground therapy. Presentation at Crossroads and Roundabouts; the right way forward, 8th conference EASG, Vienna 14-17/09/2010.

McMillen, J., Marshal, D., Murphy, L., Lorenzen, S., & Waugh, B. (2004). Help-seeking by problem gamblers, friends and families: A focus on gender and cultural groups. ANU Center for Gambling Research, Camberra ACT.

Piquette-Tomei, N., Norman, E., Corbin Dwyer, S., & McCaslin, E. (2008). Group therapy for woman problem gamblers: A space of their own. *Journal of Gambling Issues, 22*.

Prever, F. (2018). Specificità della ricerca e del trattamento nel DGA femminile *in* Manuali professionali – Il trattamento psicologico e psicoterapeutico nel disturbo da gioco d'azzardo in una prospettiva multidisciplinare. O. Casciani e O. De Luca.

Prever, F., Minci, M., & Brandt, L. (2018). New cross-cultural input on female gambling disorder treatment in Italy. Presentation ICBA Koln.

Thomas, S., & Moore, S. (2001). Do women gamble for the same reasons as men. In A. Blaszczynsky (ed.), Culture and Gambling Studies Conference, Sidney, Australia, 21-24/11/2001.

Chapter 24

Gambling Therapy International and Multilingual Helpline – A Focus on Women Gamblers' Perspective

Monica Minci and Shaila Hussain

This study sheds light on women gamblers' experiences accessing a Gambling Therapy (GT) helpline. Gambling has become a significant and growing public health issue, but less than 10% of problem gamblers decide to start treatment in addiction centers. Therefore, it is important to develop alternative approaches to reach a greater number of individuals with gambling disorders. Previous literature has suggested that helplines can be a good point of reference for gamblers. This chapter will describe how the GT helpline works. Given that historically gambling studies focus on male samples and tend to generalize the outcomes to the female population, this chapter will focus on women gamblers' access to treatment. For the current study, statistical analysis was performed on sociodemographic and gambling-related information registered by GT helpline staff after each call between January 2021 and December 2021 on 3,415 service users, 647 of which were women. Another important aim of this chapter is to give voice to the subjective experience of women who access the GT helpline.

Gambling Therapy Helpline

This study aims to shed some light on the experience of women gamblers who access the Gambling Therapy (GT) helpline, a free, global online service offering practical advice and emotional support to anyone affected by problem gambling. While gambling has become a significant and a growing public health issue, less than 10% of problem gamblers decide to start treatment in addiction centers (Hodgins et al., 2011). Therefore, it is important to develop alternative approaches to reach a greater number of individuals with gambling disorders. The study described in this chapter expands the gender-blind research approach that historically focuses on male samples and tends to generalize the outcomes to female population.

GT online support consists of access through a website (https://www.gamblingtherapy.org/) and a mobile app, reaching gamblers, their families,

DOI: 10.4324/9781003203476-30

friends, and others involved. People can join the live GT helpline, a forum, and groups. The forum is accessible 24/7, groups are held every day, and the helpline is open from Mon–Sun 10 am through 3 am and Sat–Sun 10 am through 10 pm GMT. In this chapter, we are focusing on the multilingual helpline that is covered by a team of highly experienced native-speaking counselors and psychotherapists. GT is currently offering 26 hours of native-speaking Italian, whilst a multilingual software translator enables counselors to converse in over 250 languages, moving GT beyond the language barrier.

Gambling helplines may represent a crucial first point of contact for problem gamblers (Weinstock et al., 2011), especially for those who reject more traditional options (Bastiani et al., 2015). This is because helplines are less expensive than formal, in-person/in-office treatment (Gainsbury & Blaszczynski, 2011), they can serve wide geographical areas (Potenza et al., 2006; Rodda & Lubman, 2014), they are easily accessible and anonymous (Bastiani et al., 2015; Shandley & Moore, 2008), and they enable gamblers to connect with local professional treatment services. The GT helpline can also be accessed via a free app.

GT has a database of over 900 support organizations worldwide to provide specific treatment referrals. Staff provides information during consultations, like signposting to other forms of treatment on a case-by-case basis. Based on the information provided during consultations, staff refers callers to community resources such as associations that provide counseling and self-help groups.

Studying Women Gamblers' Experience with the GT Helpline

Data Collection

Quantitative and qualitative data were obtained from recorded calls to the GT Helpline received between January and December 2021, involving gamblers and affected others. Non-significant calls (from people who are not seeking information or support) were excluded.

After each online counseling session conducted by chat, the helpline staff entered some sociodemographic details into an electronic database (gender, geographical country of residence, language spoken, form of gambling, and support provided).

Characteristics of Users

In 2021, the helpline received a total of 3,415 significant calls. Of these, 2,439 (71.4%) were from men, 647 (18.9%) were from women, and 329 (9.6%) from callers who preferred not to disclose their gender.

Women users were divided into two groups: gamblers and friend and family (F&F). Women' demographic characteristics and type of gambling were summarized using percentages. Considering the country of residence,

Table 24.1 Languages most commonly spoken by women helpline callers by country

	Bulgarian	English	German	Portuguese	Romanian	Russian	Italian	Total
United Kingdom	1	178			1			180
United States of America		59						59
Canada		43						43
Ireland		17						17
Portugal				10				10
Russia						9		9
Germany		4	4					8
Italy		1					4	5

the majority of women (n = 276, 42.6%) came from the United Kingdom, 70 (10.8%) from the United States of America, and 54 (8.3%) from Canada.

The prevalence of English-speaking users was greater at 553 (85.4%) than other languages, followed by Russian (n = 17, 2.6%), Portuguese (n = 16, 2.4%), and Greek, Polish, and Spanish (n = 9, 1.3%). Italian women accessed the helpline rarely (n = 5, 0.7%), potentially related both to women struggling to ask for help and Italian women's tendency to gamble in person which may make them more likely to ask for support in person. Table 24.1 shows the languages most commonly spoken among women helpline callers by country.

Among 647 women, 190 (29.3%) were family or friends of a gambler. Focusing on women gamblers (who directly exhibit gambling behaviour), 314 (48.5%) preferred online gambling, 39 (6.0%) offline, and 44 (6.8%) both online and offline. Of the total sample, 49 (7.5%) did not disclose their gambling style. Table 24.2 shows women's gambling styles by country (most frequent ones).

Table 24.2 Women's gambling styles by country (number and percent of the most frequent ones)

Country	Gambler – Online	Gambler – Online & In-Person Location	Gambler – Physical Location	Gambler – Undisclosed Style
United Kingdom	128 (71.1%)	12 (6.7%)	13 (7.2%)	21 (11.7%)
United States of America	24 (40.7%)	10 (16.9%)	19 (32.2%)	1 (1.7%)
Canada	32 (74.4%)	5 (11.6%)	1 (2.3%)	5 (11.6%)
Ireland	13 (76.5%)	2 (11.8%)	0 (0%)	2 (11.8%)
Portugal	6 (60%)	2 (20%)	0 (0%)	2 (20%)
Russia	7 (77.8%)	2 (22.2%)	0 (0%)	0 (0%)
Italy	4 (80%)	0 (0%)	0 (0%)	1 (20%)

Qualitative Analysis

When women gamblers reach the GT helpline, they receive problem identification, emotional and practical support, and tips to start managing their
situation. Male and female gamblers may have different needs and utility
when getting in contact with helplines (Kim et al., 2016). Women seem keener
than men to realize the relationship between their gambling behaviour and
some difficult situations that they are trying to manage in their life.

Due to gender cultural differences, women represent the "glue" in the
family that keeps everyone and everything together. They take care of each
member of the family and when there is some kind of conflict, they feel the
duty of holding their family together. This is exemplified in the following
quotes from helpline callers (note that all names are pseudonyms).

Chris feels oppressed by the relational issues within her family and ends up
gambling not to feel that way:

> *Life here is hard. We are a blended family and my soon to be husband and
> daughter just don't get on. They're always arguing. And I feel stuck in the
> middle.*

Often, talking with women gamblers means talking about relationships and
emotions. For example, Linda realizes that she's using gambling to escape the
pain related to the loss of a loved one:

> *I lost my daughter and from then I've developed this habit I don't drink or
> smoke and it's like I crave gambling I think about it all the time … . When I
> can't cope I turn to gambling.*

When a disease affects someone within the family, most of the time there is a
mother, a wife, a sister, or a daughter who takes the responsibility to care for
the loved one. They are present, even if it's tough, even at the cost of their
own projects, jobs, needs, and lives.

Kate centered her life around taking care of her disabled daughter and she
ended up gambling online just to feel something exciting again:

> *My daughter had cancer. I have had to give up work to look after her. All I
> do is look after my little girl. She's very disabled. I feel like I've lost my life. I
> find this exciting but so depressing at the same time.*

Melanie started gambling in her forties about 10 years ago. She decided to
ask for help, was in recovery for about 5 years and then her husband died.
She got married again and, after discovering that her new husband was an
alcoholic, she resented it and started gambling again.

I'm watching him drink and smoke himself to death. He has emphysema as well. My late husband had a brain tumour and it took 5 years for him to die. It was cruel what happened to him but I nursed him the whole way through. I just don't want to go back there and have to become my new husband nurse … . it (gambling) is a form of escape for me.

Gambling can be a way out for a woman, after years of strict identification with the cultural role of a female, a mother who has to sacrifice almost everything to be a good woman. Danielle always focused on the needs of her family, forgetting about herself and, when exploring why she started gambling, she discloses:

I think … because we have moved house like 6 times in 10 yrs … I have 3 kids … it was always saving and felt like nothing for me.

Somehow a woman doesn't feel the right to fail, to be imperfect, to be the one who needs the support of the family. Having an addiction becomes a scarlet letter.

Maya got promoted at work and her salary increased but then she fell into gambling addiction, took all the savings, and now that she in big debt she thinks:

I'm not a good wife to my husband as well as a good mother to my 3 sons.

We know that gambling is often used to escape unpleasant feelings (Karter, 2013). Using the words of Wendy, when gambling, women are *"escaping all the frustrations and other emotions from reality."*

It is important for them to recognize that emotions can be a trigger and to find a safe place to share them. Sometimes the trigger is being on their own and/or feeling lonely and bored, like Mariana:

For sure being with my husband could help, but his work often take him away for days and this do not help. I told you about last time I played … he was at work 3 days and I was by myself (as my daughter was with the nanny all day) and this didn't help at all.

Feeling lonely is a common sensation, especially during the COVID-19 pandemic, as Fiona reports:

I'm spending an awful lot of time alone at the moment because of lockdown and it makes the feelings of "going crazy" are worse and the craving to "switch off" through gambling greater.

Other times gambling can be a way to put aside not loneliness but anxiety, like for Rose:

I am not bored and would say fed up as opposed to depressed, I have had a lot of stress so maybe it is a distraction.

And sometimes the emotion related to the urge to gamble is anger, like Amelia found out talking with us:

Okay maybe I feel anger towards my dad because he never helps me. And his step kids get everything.

In women, gambling is related to more severe psychiatric symptoms (Desai & Potenza, 2008) and can represent a way to cope with mental illness. Francine uses it to manage her OCD symptoms:

In the moment, it's the only thing that makes me feel calm and makes my thoughts quiet.

Becoming aware of the meaning and utility of gambling behaviour opens the opportunity to find a healthier way than gambling to deal with distress, like talking with a friend, using the helpline, or joining the forums and/or the groups. Support offered online lets these women find someone to talk to when they feel alone, overwhelmed, and without support.

Kylie realizes that making the decision to enter the helpline can be a new and better way to manage and take care of her pain.

Just chatting to people takes my mind off things … got lots going on in my life with illness [cancer] and now another family member has been diagnosed with tumours and I'm using it [gambling] as a getaway and I actually do find it really helpful but I need something else to take my mind away from it because I don't want it to get worse and worse.

When women arrive at the helpline, sometimes it's the first time that they have looked for help, while others have some support already but need extra help in an overwhelming moment. Therefore, joining the helpline can be helpful when NHS and treatment centers are closed (late hours and weekends). In certain cases, women tried to find support in the past but only found interventions created, led and joined by men.

As women often use gambling in a different way from men, as a specific way to cope with difficult emotions, it would be important to provide gender-specific interventions. Self-help groups are available for free all over the world but many interventions do not take gender differences into account and women end up dropping out of treatment. Like Rebecca who realizes that she needs something different:

I have tried GA in the past but as it is male orientated and I often felt uncomfortable being the only female in a group of 25–30 people. If you are able to offer or sign post me towards further routes of support I would be most grateful.

Conclusions

This is the first study that explores the characteristics of women who accessed the GT helpline in 2021. The findings show that the free, easily accessible, and widespread helpline approach can attract a large number of gamblers. As observed for other gambling helplines (Bastiani et al., 2015), an important percentage of women callers (almost one-third) were significant others who looked for help because of someone else's gambling behaviour. This confirms that women often hold a socio-cultural role that adds responsibilities and diminishes the right to take care of themselves. Therefore, women struggle to look for help, but when they do it, they show openness and interest in working on a deep level exploring both the emotional components of their urge to gamble and the relational conflicts that can trigger it.

This study provides further support that an online helpline is more likely to attract those who feel comfortable using the online medium, such as online gamblers (Lucchini & Griffiths, 2015). Looking at women's calls helped to gain a better understanding of their needs: being listened to, and accompanied in exploring their emotions and relationships, finding a place to give value to themselves, and looking for a female-friendly intervention online and locally. When women access the helpline they seem to be driven not by the urgency of the moment, but by the request to be accepted in their troubles. Therefore, the connection with the counselor becomes more important and they are keen to consider coming back on the helpline. Thanks to the internal translation system, counselors can talk to clients using the client's native language. Even if the translation isn't always perfect, this gives clients the possibility to receive live support no matter which language they speak and helps extend the range of women gamblers that can be supported all over the world. For those women who do not have access to proper local support and can't speak English fluently, GT just launched a pilot project of online psychotherapy treatment through the helpline. The new multilingual translation system represents a new way to provide tailored help for women who are isolated. Future studies should therefore explore the effect of this kind of intervention.

References

Bastiani, L., Fea, M., Potente, R., Luppi, C., Lucchini, F., & Molinaro, S. (2015). National helpline for problem gambling: A profile of its users' characteristics. *Journal of Addiction*, (2), 1–9.

Desai, R.A., & Potenza, M.N. (2008). Gender differences in the associations between past-year gambling problems and psychiatric disorders. *Social Psychiatry and Psychiatric Epidemiology*, *43*, 173–183.

Gainsbury, S., & Blaszczynski, A. (2011). Online self-guided interventions for the treatment of problem gambling. *International Gambling Studies*, *11*, 3, 289–308.

Hodgins, D.C., Stea, J.N., & Grant, J.E. (2011). Gambling disorders. *The Lancet*, *378*(9806), 1874–1884.

Karter, L. (2013). *Women and problem gambling: Therapeutic insights into understanding addiction and treatment* (1st ed.). Routledge.

Kim, H.S., Hodgins, D.C., Bellringer, M., & Abbott, M. (2016). Gender differences among helpline callers: Prospective study of gambling and psychosocial outcomes. *Journal of Gambling Studies*, *32*(2), 605–623.

Lucchini, F., & Griffiths, M.D. (2015). Preventing and treating problem gamblers: The first Italian National Helpline. *Responsible Gambling Review*, *1*(2), 20–26.

Potenza, M.N., Steinberg, M.A., Wu, R., Rounsaville, B.J., & O'Malley, S. (2006). Characteristics of older adult problem gamblers calling a gambling helpline. *Journal of Gambling Studies*, *22*(2), 241–254.

Rodda, S., & Lubman, D.I. (2014). Characteristics of gamblers using a national online counselling service for problem gambling. *Journal of Gambling Studies*, *30*(2), 277–289.

Shandley, K., & Moore, S. (2008). Evaluation of gambler's helpline: A consumer perspective. *International Gambling Studies*, *8*(3), 315–330.

Weinstock, J., Burton, S., Rash, C.J., Moran, S., Biller, W., Krudelbach, N., Phoenix, N., & Morasco, B.J. (2011). Predictors of engaging in problem gambling treatment: Data from the West Virginia problem gamblers help network. *Psychology of Addictive Behaviors: Journal of the Society of Psychologists in Addictive Behaviors*, *25*(2), 372–379.

Chapter 25

Gambling in the Life of Older Women – Benefits, Harms, and Social Perception

Bernadeta Lelonek-Kuleta

This research presents the results of the first Polish study on gambling among retired seniors. Overall, 34 women aged between 56 and 75 participated in the qualitative study, including 8 women who were problem gamblers [8 points or more on the Canadian Problem Gambling Index (CPGI)]. This chapter examines the benefits and harms of gambling for senior women and the social perception of gambling among older women in Poland. Results were analyzed in two groups of women distinguished by CPGI score, i.e., problem and non-problem gamblers. Analyzes show differences between the two groups with respect to benefits, harms, and social perceptions of gambling.

Gambling and Gambling Problems among the Adult Population in Poland

The gambling market in Poland has been strongly evolving in recent years, although certain games have been popular even before this recent growth. The most popular games of chance in Poland are lotteries, which were played by 27.4% of Poles in 2018, followed by scratch cards (16.3%), short message service lotteries (7.4%), low-volatility slot machine (3.8%), and bookmaker betting (2.1%) (Moskalewicz et al., 2019). The gambling market in Poland is regulated by the Gambling Act of November 19, 2009, and several subsequent amendments. Sports betting has been available online since 2013 (as a consequence of the Amendment of the Gambling Act of May 26, 2011), and a law concerning gambling in legal online casino only and buying lottery tickets online (both games covered by a state monopoly) has been introduced in 2018.

There is very limited nationwide data on gambling engagement. A survey by Public Opinion Research Center (CBOS) showed that 0.9% of the adult population of Poland are affected by problem gambling [8 points and more on the Canadian Problem Gambling Index (CPGI)] and 1.7% of individuals who actively gamble. Among women, the percentage of problem gamblers is 6.1%, and 15.7% among men. In terms of age, the youngest adult group (18–24 years old) has a problem gambling rate of 22.1%, while those aged 65 and older have a rate of 10.7% and are on an upward trend (Moskalewicz et al., 2019).

DOI: 10.4324/9781003203476-31

Unfortunately, there is insufficient nationwide data detailing the severity of gambling problems by gender in specific age groups.

Current Study

The first research on gambling among seniors in Poland was exploratory and qualitative in nature; therefore, no a priori research hypotheses were formulated. The aim of this study was, among other things, to understand the specifics of gambling by retired older women. Overall, 34 women aged between 56 and 75 (only one woman under the age of 60) participated in the study, including 8 women who met the criteria for problem gambling (8 points or more on the CPGI). One of the inclusion criteria for the study was retiree status. The survey was conducted using an in-depth interview method, which included the following main themes: 1) Family and social situation, 2) Actual gambling activity, 3) Gambling in the lifetime, 4) Perception of the importance of gambling, 5) Impact of gambling on a person, 6) The consequences of gambling, 7) Gambling problems, and 8) Level of awareness of gambling threats. Interviews with respondents lasted until the interviewee exhausted all topics. They were conducted in a location chosen by the interviewee (often at home), and the duration of an interview varied from 35 to 90 minutes. The material obtained in the study was processed using the thematic analysis method (Braun & Clarke, 2006) and analyzes were conducted by the research team and a clinical psychologist from outside the team, as recommended by Spiggle (1994). The results are reported according to criteria developed by Tong et al. (2007). Due to the sheer volume of qualitative data, this chapter presents results from selected topics.

Results

Benefits (Benefits from Gambling)

The benefits experienced by retired female gamblers were analyzed in relation to the severity of their problem gambling – divided into groups of problem gamblers and non-problem gamblers. Five main groups of factors perceived by women as benefits of gaming emerged during the analysis of the survey material. These were as follows: sensations, money, activity, socialization, and escape. In the group of female seniors categorized as problem gamblers, the most frequently indicated benefits were sensations, which were understood as entertainment, fun, joy, excitement, and generally positive feelings. Other common benefits mentioned by this group were the opportunity to meet other people and escape from problems. The fourth most important benefit was the hope of winning and improving one's financial situation. For non-problem gambling women, perceptions of benefit were distributed in a slightly different manner. As in the previous group, non-problem gamblers considered sensations, understood the same way as in the previous group, to be the greatest benefit of gambling. In the second place, however, this group of seniors cited hoping to win as a way to improve their and their loved ones' financial situations. They also mentioned activity, i.e., the possibility of spending time gambling, developing a habit, or avoiding boredom.

When analyzing differences between the two groups of women it became apparent that senior problem gamblers were more likely to seek social contact in gambling than the non-problem gamblers. It can be assumed that an underlying problem is loneliness, which pushes them to gamble as a means to achieve the "real" goal – relationships. This is illustrated by the following statement:

I made some new friends, and you know, when you are lonely and go to a bar, there is this urge, because you don't have anyone to really take care of you, so you go to a bar and meet various people, kind people, and you can drink a glass or two, and just like that we started to play cards.

(age 62, no. 14)

For non-problem gambling women, gambling was an addition to relationships rather than a substitute for them. These women had their circles of friends with whom they spent time on various activities, including, but not limited to, gambling. They had closer ties with these people than is expressed in just meeting at the game center and gambling together.

It is also noteworthy that older problem gamblers reported to seek escape from their problems in gambling. Gambling once again becomes a means to relieving sadness or a temporary respite from hardship. In the absence of adaptive coping mechanisms, gambling takes the role of a reliever which is a common mechanism in addiction, regardless of its object (Köpetz et al., 2013). Non-problem gambling women, on the other hand, were more likely to treat gambling as a way of spending their time, an activity that is meant to "spice up" everyday life, but not to get away from it all. The motivations of older women to gamble are described in detail in another article by the author (Lelonek-Kuleta, 2021).

Damages (Gambling-Related Harms)

Another factor that emerged from the data was the harm that gambling can generate in the lives of older women. Problem gamblers identified the following harms of gambling: disturbed family relationships (for example, worse relationship with husband), neglecting loved ones (husband, elderly mother, adult daughter), lying to loved ones, reducing other activities and narrowing the repertoire of entertainment to gambling only, loss of money, indebtedness, weakened control over gambling (awareness of risks but inability to resist), increased smoking and alcohol consumption while gambling, and severe stress while gambling, including somatic symptoms (severe digestive problems). This is illustrated by the following statements:

> *I lost a lot of things (…) my daughter is not married – the one who lives with me – and it's my fault. It is because I'm not anonymous, it's not that nobody knows about my affairs* (age 75, no. 26);
>
> *My husband even said, "not only has she got old, but also drinking and losing money" (…) and he left me, because he couldn't stand it* (age 69, no. 6);
>
> *I can see the negative impact for the family, because sometimes people get so lost in their hopes and plans (*to win*) that there is not enough space in these plans for the children; I don't even want to visit them anymore, especially my son in Southern Poland, because I have no company there (*to gamble*). I live from visit to visit (*to the casino*) just like that* (age 69, no. 13).

Among non-problem gambling women, such consequences were very rare. Small money deficits accompanied with remorse were reported in some cases, as loss of interest and ability to derive pleasure from activities other than gambling, and smoking and drinking alcohol while gambling were identified as a health detriment. Other non-problem gambling women did not indicate any potential harms from gaming. This was either due to the fact that they had never experienced difficulties related to gambling, or because they were aware of the potential dangers of gambling and perceived to have control over the activity.

It is worth noting that most of the harms experienced by female seniors due to gambling were related to family relationships, followed by financial stability, and finally health. The accumulation of negative consequences is recognized among seniors who gamble excessively, i.e., those who treated gambling as a form of escape from life's problems. These women were caught in a "vicious cycle" through using gambling as a way to escape from their problems, which in turn led to more problems.

Social Perception of Gambling among Older Women and Their Environment

We were particularly interested in the social perception of gambling among older women in Poland. The very word gambling has negative connotations in Poland. In the light of nationwide surveys, Poles identify a gambler as a disturbed person with serious financial problems who gambles on a very large scale. Interestingly, many Poles do not consider lotteries or scratch cards to be gambling (Moskalewicz et al., 2019). In the group of older female problem gamblers, almost all indicated negative perception of their activity by those around them or expressed fear of such perceptions. The only woman who made no reference to public perception of her gambling was a single person gambling alone from time to time at a casino. Regarding reactions of those around her, one problem gambler was constantly criticized by her sister, who suggested that she had a mental disorder and needed psychiatric consultation. As a result, the respondent tried to conceal her gambling from the sister. Other women declared conflicts with their husbands due to gambling. Apart from the husband, the lack of acceptance for gambling was also expressed by adult children and extended family, as well as the "wider social environment." The perception of their gambling by others is exemplified in the following account:

> *My husband said that I was an addict, (…) the children – that mum has gone crazy.*
>
> (age 61, no. 24)

Relatives would often disapprove of women's debts caused by gambling, and they also expressed concern (or fear) of their potential gambling addiction. One of the respondents persuaded herself that her relatives' anxiety about her gambling was only caused by their greed:

> *They certainly feel sorry for me losing because they could have used the money, even I could have used it in a different way. But I think they don't understand my emotions, the way I experience them, and therefore may resent them. They feel sorry because of the money.*
>
> (age 61 no. 32)

Some relatives (husband, siblings, adult children) tried different interventions, such as explaining or giving ultimatums, but these actions did not persuade the women to reduce their gambling. Such actions often resulted in weakened relationships – with an adult daughter and grandchildren, for example. In the case of some women, the disapproval of the gambling was expressed by breaking contact with them – the departure of the husband, falling out with friends, or an adult daughter and her family, or limiting contact with adult child and grandchildren due to shame caused by the mother's playing. Criticism from the environment was declared by many problem gambling women. Other women reported that they concealed their gambling from their close ones, were ashamed of this activity, and did not want to expose themselves to social criticism.

In the next step, the experiences of female non-problem gamblers were analyzed in terms of the social perception of their activity. A continuum can be observed in the attitudes of the environment in this group. Of the 26 women, about half noted more or less frequent remarks about their gambling from those around them (most often close family). A few women were gambling with their life partners and saw nothing harmful in the activity. Another woman's partner did not gamble but accepted his wife's entertainment activity and saw it as just having fun. Relatives of other women encouraged them to stop gambling but did so in a gentle manner (yet one woman made attempts to hide her gambling, ashamed of it). The families and friends of other women expressed open criticism of their gambling, resulting in different reactions. Some of them, tried to hide their gambling because of the criticism, while others did not care about the reactions of their relatives and continued gambling (one of them stated that she did it ostentatiously on purpose). One woman was criticized by her daughter-in-law, who accused the senior of teaching her children to gamble (the respondent bought scratch cards together with her grandchildren and checked the results with them). The remaining women concealed their gambling from those around them, mostly out of fear of reaction. One of them claimed that her husband would "laugh at her" knowing that she buys lottery tickets, so she hid it but sees nothing wrong in gambling herself.

It should be noted that reported negative reactions to gambling by the environment were more intense among women who gamble in a problematic manner. Problematic gambling most often was associated with a sense of shame, hiding, and negative feedback from loved ones. Those close to them often did not accept their losses and feared the development of an addiction. In contrast, positive or neutral reactions from family and friends to the senior's gambling were more often noted among women without gambling problems. Non-problematic gambling, which is less intense, was seen as a harmless pastime, although a relatively large group of close circles expressed negative attitudes towards gambling by older women in this group as well. This might be related to a generally negative social perceptions of gambling in Poland rather than harm experienced by the older women. Relatives of female gamblers in Poland may lack more objective knowledge on the real dangers of gambling and therefore their perception may be influenced by stereotypes and generalizations. This also seems to be the case for older women whose attitudes toward gambling can be diametrically opposed. On the one hand, they want to treat gambling as a simple pastime, and on the other hand, some seniors feel that they are doing something shameful that would be better kept hidden, regardless of the intensity of their gambling.

Summary

This chapter aimed to explore the perceived benefits, harms, and social perceptions of gambling among older retired women in Poland. There were notable differences in the three aspects analyzed between older women, depending on the level of severity of problems experienced due to gambling. Women who gambled in a non-problematic manner frequently mentioned pleasurable experiences related to gambling: the hope of winning to improve their own and their loved ones' financial status and the activation aspect that gambling offers. Problem gamblers, on the other hand, ranked sensation as the top benefit (as did women in the former group), followed by the opportunity to meet people while playing and to escape from problems through gambling. The perceived harms of gambling were more pronounced in the group of problem gamblers. This is an important observation given that gambling in this group of women was more often seen as a means of escaping problems. Engaging in gambling can lead to cumulative negative consequences, which should be considered in the context of gambling prevention among older women. Negative attitudes towards gambling are generally prevalent in Poland, but they were even more pronounced among problem gamblers. The consequence of such attitudes can be guilt and shame, as well as hiding gambling activity by female seniors who feel that they are doing something wrong. Shame and guilt may become a deterrent to seeking help for gambling problems (Prever & Locati, 2017). Older women in Poland are socially attributed with the role of stable mothers or grandchildren's caretakers. Any deviation from this role may lead to social ostracism, as is evident among women who gamble. In this context, it seems important to implement educational measures concerning the potential harms associated with gambling, but also responsible gambling strategies that can help older women keep gambling at the level of mere entertainment. At the same time, older people should not be excluded from this form of activity, which may have a positive role in the lives of seniors (Gaimard & Gateau, 2016; Loroz, 2004).

Study Limitations

The study was qualitative in nature, which limits the generalizability of its findings. The results of the in-depth analysis show certain directions of phenomena and possible regularities that would be worth verifying in quantitative research. Research on a representative sample would be a valuable contribution to our knowledge about the specifics of gambling among older Polish women.

This study was supported by the Ministry of Health, Fund for solving gambling problems (grant number 1/HMK/2017).

References

Braun, V., & Clarke, V. (2006). Using thematic analysis in psychology. *Qualitative Research in Psychology*, *3*(2), 77–101. DOI: 10.1191/1478088706qp063oa

Gaimard, M., & Gateau, M. (2016). Seniors and gambling: Pleasure or addiction. A French example. *Revista Universitara de Sociologie*, *2*, 25–38. https://hal-univ-bourgogne.archives-ouvertes.fr/hal-01705112

Köpetz, C.E., Lejuez, C.W., Wiers, R.W., & Kruglanski, A.W. (2013). Motivation and self-regulation in addiction: A call for convergence. *Perspectives on Psychological Science: A Journal of the Association for Psychological Science*, *8*(1), 3–24. 10.1177/1745691612457575

Loroz, P.S. (2004). Golden-age gambling: Psychological benefits and self-concept dynamics in aging consumers' consumption experiences. *Psychology & Marketing*, *21*(5), 323–349. DOI: 10.1002/mar.20008

Lelonek-Kuleta, B. (2021). Gambling motivation model for older women addicted and not addicted to gambling – a qualitative study. *Aging and Mental Health*. DOI: 10.1080/13607863.2021.1895068

Moskalewicz, J., Badora, B., Feliksiak, M., Głowacki, A., Gwiazda, Magdalena, G., Herrmann, M., Kawalec, I., & Roguska, B. (2019). *Oszacowanie rozpowszechnienia oraz identyfikacja czynników ryzyka i czynników chroniących hazardu i innych uzależnień behawioralnych – edycja 2018/2019 [Estimation of prevalence and identification of risk and protective factors for gambling and other behavioral addictions—2018/2019 edition]*. Centrum Badania Opinii Społecznej. https://www.kbpn.gov.pl/portal?id=15&res_id=9249205

Prever, F., & Locati, V. (2017). Female gambling in Italy. A specific clinical experience. In H. Bowden-Jones & F. Prever (Eds.), *Gambling disorder in women: An international female perspective on treatment and research*. London and New York: Routledge.

Spiggle, S. (1994). Analysis and interpretation of qualitative data in consumer research. *Journal of Consumer Research*, *21*, 491–503. https://www.jstor.org/stable/2489688

Tong, A., Sainsbury, P., & Craig, J. (2007). Consolidated criteria for reporting qualitative research (COREQ): A 32-item checklist for interviews and focus groups. *International Journal for Quality in Health Care*, *19*(6), 349–357. 10.1093/intqhc/mzm042

Compulsive Sexual Behaviour and Its Correlates in a Sample of Polish Treatment-Seeking Women

Ewelina Kowalewska

One of the main limitations of previous research on compulsive sexual behaviour is the fact that most study samples are comprised of men, and as a result, the current literature lacks an accurate clinical picture of women reporting issues related to these behaviours. The preliminary results of the research conducted on a sample of Polish treatment-seeking women and presented in this chapter may serve as a guideline for future research on identifying patterns of women's sexual functioning.

Introduction

Pro-women and pro-equality postulates are gaining more and more weight in Polish society. In recent years, attempts to limit or ban certain women's rights (e.g., in the field of reproductive health) have resulted in mass protests. Currently, in Poland, women's sexuality is burdened with a constant evaluation. Factors that undoubtedly contribute to this situation and prevent change are Polish conservatism and the role of the Church in maintaining the status quo. Although women engage in the same sexual activities as in other countries, in Polish society, they are often intertwined with severe embarrassment, shame, and fear of the opinion of others. These factors prevent women involved in problematic sexual activities from speaking up and problems (not only related to sexuality) remain "at home," which may contribute to the creation of barriers for help seeking.

An unstudied problem in the sexual sphere of women concerns compulsive sexual behaviour disorder (CSBD), a diagnostic entity recently included in the forthcoming 11th edition of the International Classification of Diseases (6C72, World Health Organization, 2018). The majority of previous studies were conducted on men, which results in emerging questions as to whether the criteria proposed by the World Health Organization are appropriate for women. Omitting women can also foster a greater acceptance of men reporting issues related to CSBD, which in turn, may intensify perceived shame and stigma for

DOI: 10.4324/9781003203476-32

women with CSBD. The authors of a study conducted on a sample of 719 Polish women (including 39 treatment seekers for problematic pornography use (PPU)) highlighted the role of personal beliefs about pornography and religious norms in women seeking treatment for this problem – these norms seem to be significant factors when deciding whether to enter treatment (Lewczuk et al., 2017).

Given that research on compulsive sexual behaviour (CSB) among women is in its early stages, the current chapter seeks to address this knowledge gap by exploring psychological and sexual correlates of CSB among treatment-seeking Polish women.

Method

Participants and Procedure

The data were collected through an online-based survey between July 2019 and January 2020 from a sample of Caucasian Polish women seeking treatment for CSB. The aim was to gather knowledge about CSB among women. The survey was also the first stage of recruitment for a larger project aimed at examining the neural, behavioural, and psychological aspects of CSB among this group. Upon entering, potential respondents were informed about the goal of the study and signed informed consent electronically. Inclusion criteria consisted of being female, aged 18 or older, seeking treatment for CSB, and being sexually active during the last year.

Measures

For the purpose of this chapter, we restricted analyses to participants who completed the following questionnaires: Hypersexual Behaviour Inventory (HBI; Reid et al., 2011), Sexual Addiction Screening Test-Revised (SAST-R; Polish adaptation: Gola et al., 2017), Brief Pornography Screen (BPS; Kraus et al., 2020), Hospital Anxiety and Depression Scale (HADS; Zigmond & Snaith, 1983), UPPS-P Impulsiveness Scale (Polish adaptation: Poprawa, 2014), Multidimensional Sexuality Questionnaire (MSQ; Polish version: Kowalewska et al., 2019), South Oaks Gambling Screen (SOGS; Lesieur & Blume, 1987), and Alcohol Use Disorders Identification Test (AUDIT; Saunders et al., 1993). We also asked participants to provide information about their psychoactive substance use, religiosity, and (if possible) information about sexual activity such as dyadic sexual activity and solitary practices.

The analysis included 103 women aged 19–66 [$M = 30.92$; $SD = 8.06$]. With regard to sexual orientation, a majority of women ($n = 91$; 88.3%) declared themselves as exclusively or predominantly heterosexual on the Polish adaptation of the Kinsey Scale (Wierzba et al., 2015). Of the total sample, 59 women (57.3%) were married or in an informal relationship and 43 women (41.7%) declared themselves as religious or believers.

Statistical Analyses

A series of Pearson chi-square tests and non-parametric Mann-Whitney U tests were used to examine possible differences between treatment-seeking women who met the HBI cut-off score of 53 and those who did not. All analyzes were performed using SPSS-23 (IBM SPSS Statistics for Windows, Version 23.0).

Ethics

This study was carried out in accordance with the basic principles of Declaration of Helsinki. The Research Ethics Committee of SWPS University in Warsaw approved the study. All participants were informed about the scope, as well as the anonymous, voluntary, and non-monetary nature of this study.

Results

Severity of CSB Symptoms

This study was conducted before the emergence of official CSBD diagnostic criteria. Therefore, severity of CSB was measured using the HBI questionnaire (Reid et al., 2011), which is based on the criteria of Hypersexual Disorder available at that time (Kafka, 2010). Using the HBI the sample was divided into two groups – treatment-seeking women who met the clinical cut-off value of 53 (+TS; $n = 61$) and treatment-seeking women who scored lower than 53 (−TS; $n = 42$) (see Table 26.1). Analysis revealed a significant difference between groups in total HBI score [$Z = 8.60$, p < 0.001, $r = 0.63$] and each subscale [*Control: Z = 22.65*, p < 0.001, $r = 0.91$; *Coping: Z = 6.74*, p < 0.001, $r = 0.52$; *Consequences: Z = 8.14*, p < 0.001, $r = 0.63$]. Results obtained in SAST-R were also significantly higher in the +TS group [$M = 11.56$, $SD = 3.68$] compared to −TS [$M = 6.88$, $SD = 3.58$; $Z = 5.32$, p < 0.001, $r = 0.45$]. The mean score in both groups exceeded the SAST-R's cut-off value of 6 (Carnes et al., 2010). In terms of severity of PPU assessed by the BPS (Kraus et al., 2020), the +TS group obtained a significantly higher mean score [$M = 4.23$, $SD = 3.40$] that exceed the cut-off value of 4 as proposed by Kraus and colleagues (2020) compared to the −TS group [$M = 2.38$, $SD = 2.50$; $Z = 2.72$, p < 0.01, $r = 0.20$].

Sexual Activity

A significant intergroup difference was revealed in terms of the number of sexual partners during the last year, with the +TS group having more partners [$M = 5.61$, $SD = 7.70$] than the −TS group [$M = 3.65$, $SD = 8.56$; $Z = 2.87$, p < 0.01, $r = 0.21$]. Moreover, women from the +TS group devoted more time (in minutes) to pornography during the last 7 days [$M = 123.84$, $SD = 124.61$) than

Table 26.1 Sexual activity and psychological assessment of Polish treatment-seeking
women (N = 103) divided into groups by the HBI cut-off score of 53

Study characteristics	Above (+TS) (n = 61) % / M (SD)	Below (−TS) (n = 42) % / M (SD)	x² / Z
Hypersexual Behaviour Inventory	**66.36 (10.42)**	**38.88 (9.39)**	p < 0.001
Control	28.43 (5.84)	15.21 (4.35)	p < 0.001
Coping	25.62 (5.30)	16.62 (5.06)	p < 0.001
Consequences	12.31 (3.13)	7.05 (2.23)	p < 0.001
Sexual Addiction Screening Test-Revised	11.56 (3.68)	6.88 (3.58)	p < 0.001
Brief Pornography Screen	4.23 (3.40)	2.38 (2.50)	p < 0.01
Onset of first sexual intercourse	17.59 (2.88)	17.88 (4.02)	ns
Number of sexual partners during the last year	N = 56 5.61 (7.70)	N = 34 3.65 (8.56)	p < 0.01
Number of dyadic sexual intercourse during the last 7 days	N = 37 3.59 (4.17)	N = 27 2.89 (3.47)	ns
Onset of first pornography exposure	N = 59 12.63 (4.44)	N = 39 12.69 (4.39)	ns
Time spent on pornography during the last 7 days (in minutes)	N = 37 123.84 (124.61)	N = 24 85.96 (125.21)	p < 0.05
Number of masturbations during the last 7 days	N = 54 5.13 (4.49)	N = 35 2.83 (2.11)	p < 0.05
Subjective feeling of experiencing a loss of control over sexual behaviour (yes/no)	**91.8%**	**50%**	p < 0.001
Pornography	34.4%	9%	ns
Masturbation	42.6%	21.4%	p < 0.05
Paid sexual services	3.3%	-	ns
Casual sexual contacts	37.7%	9.5%	p < 0.001
Fantasizing	59%	16.7%	p < 0.001
Web chats, webcams	9.8%	4.8%	ns
Other	8.2%	16.7%	ns
Religious practices (minutes a week)[A]	N = 21 181.29 (270.74)	N = 22 133.64 (109.27)	ns
Does your sexual activity conflict with your religious or moral beliefs?			
Yes	39.4%	16.7%	p < 0.01
No	24.6%	54.8%	
Hard to say	8.2%	14.3%	
Does not matter to me	27.8%	14.2%	
Hospital Anxiety and Depression Scale			
Anxiety	13.39 (4.58)	10.07 (4.70)	p < 0.001
Depression	8.64 (4.32)	6.00 (4.19)	p < 0.01

(Continued)

Table 26.1 (Continued)

Study characteristics	Above (+TS) (n = 61) % / M (SD)	Below (−TS) (n = 42) % / M (SD)	x^2 / Z
UPPS-P Negative Urgency	38.16 (5.00)	31.86 (5.18)	$p < 0.001$
UPPS-P Lack of Premeditation	26.10 (4.86)	24.31 (4.25)	$p < 0.05$
UPPS-P Lack of Perseverance	24.11 (5.85)	22.12 (5.55)	ns
UPPS-P Sensation Seeking	34.84 (7.11)	32.10 (7.77)	ns
UPPS-P Positive Urgency	38.93 (7.81)	34.02 (7.07)	$p < 0.01$
Multidimensional Sexuality Questionnaire	**128.48 (19.15)**	**109.95 (19.75)**	$p < 0.001$
Sexual esteem	14.42 (5.20)	13.57 (4.31)	ns
Sexual preoccupation	11.70 (2.90)	7.93 (3.19)	$p < 0.001$
Internal sexual control	10.59 (3.55)	13.76 (2.91)	$p < 0.001$
Sexual consciousness	13.02 (3.68)	13.02 (2.90)	ns
Sexual motivation	15.21 (4.31)	12.38 (5.28)	$p < 0.01$
Sexual anxiety	9.93 (4.61)	6.57 (4.40)	$p < 0.001$
Sexual assertiveness	12.07 (5.54)	12.62 (4.70)	ns
Sexual depression	9.10 (5.14)	6.34 (4.68)	$p < 0.01$
External sexual control	10.67 (5.03)	5.29 (4.70)	$p < 0.001$
Sexual monitoring	5.87 (5.24)	2.07 (2.74)	$p < 0.001$
Fear of sexual relationships	6.82 (4.16)	6.36 (4.31)	ns
Sexual satisfaction	9.07 (5.76)	10.26 (5.82)	ns
South Oaks Gambling Screen	1.07 (2.54)	0.69 (1.66)	ns
Alcohol Use Disorders Identification Test	N = 50	N = 36	ns
Low risk (0–7 points)	11.52 (7.32)	9.14 (4.75)	$p < 0.05$
Risky or hazardous level (8–15 points)	31.1%	35.7%	
High risk or harmful level (16–19 points)	27.9%	42.9%	
Very high risk (20 points or more)	6.6%	7.1%	
Not drinking	16.4% 18%	- 14.3%	
Psychoactive substances use during last 2 months			
Stimulants (e.g., amphetamine, cocaine)	19.7%	14.3%	ns
Hallucinogens (e.g., LSD)	8.2%	4.8%	ns
Nicotine	41%	33.3%	ns
Marijuana	47.5%	42.9%	ns
Other (e.g., MDMA, GBL, air duster, dextromethorphan, antidepressants, tramadol, codeine, benzodiazepines, sedative-hypnotics)	3.3%	-	ns

*** $p < 0.001$, ** $p < 0.01$, * $p < 0.05$

Note
A Only participants who declared themselves as religious or believers were asked about average weekly time spent on religious practices, such as religious gatherings, meditations, prayers, and reading of religious books.

women from the −TS group [M = 85.96, SD = 125.21; Z = 2.05, p < 0.05, r = 0.26]. Number of masturbations during the last 7 days was also higher in the +TS group [M = 5.13, SD = 4.49] compared to the −TS group [M = 2.83, SD = 2.11; Z = 2.25, p < 0.05, r = 0.21]. No significant differences were noted for the onset of first sexual intercourse, onset of first pornography exposure, and number of dyadic sexual intercourse during the last 7 days.

A majority of women from the +TS group (91.8%) and half of the women from the −TS group (50%) reported experiencing a subjective feeling of a losing control over sexual behaviour. Specifically, problematic sexual behaviours that diversified the groups were masturbation [x^2 = 4.98, p < 0.05, Phi = 0.22], casual sexual contacts [x^2 = 10.21, p < 0.001, Phi = 0.32], and fantasizing [x^2 = 18.34, p < 0.001, Phi = 0.42].

The 12 individual propensities related to sexual relationships were assessed using the MSQ (Kowalewska et al., 2019). The total score ranges from 0 to 240 points and the scores on subscales range from 0 to 20 with higher scores indicating the greater intensity of the relevant sexual tendency. The +TS group obtained significantly higher MSQ total score [M = 128.48, SD = 19.15] than the −TS group [M = 109.95, SD = 19.75; Z = 4.26, p < 0.001, r = 0.38]. Furthermore, women from the +TS group scored significantly higher on subscales related to the following tendencies: becoming obsessed with thoughts about sexual aspects of life [*Sexual Preoccupation*; Z = 5.33, p < 0.001, r = 0.45], desire to be involved in a sexual relationship [*Sexual Motivation*; Z = 2.70, p < 0.01, r = 0.20], feeling anxious about sexual aspects of life [*Sexual Anxiety*; Z = 3.45, p < 0.001, r = 0.29], feeling depressed about sexual aspects of life [*Sexual Depression*; Z = 2.68, p < 0.01, r = 0.20], belief that sexuality is determined by influences beyond personal control [*External Sexual Control*; Z = 4.93, p < 0.001, r = 0.38], and awareness of the public impression that one's sexuality affects others [*Sexual Monitoring*; Z = 4.22, p < 0.001, r = 0.38]. On the other hand, women from the −TS group obtained significantly higher scores on a subscale concerning the belief that sexual aspects of one's life are determined by one's own personal control [*Internal Sexual Control*; Z = 4.28, p < 0.001, r = 0.38]. No significant differences were found in terms of the tendencies to positively evaluate one's ability to relate sexually with others [*Sexual Esteem*], reflect on the nature of one's sexuality [*Sexual Consciousness*], be assertive about sexual aspects of life [*Sexual Assertiveness*], fear of engaging in sexual relationships [*Fear of Sexual Relationships*], and sexual satisfaction [*Sexual Satisfaction*].

Anxiety, Depression, and Impulsivity

The severity of anxiety and depressive symptoms were assessed by HADS (Zigmond & Snaith, 1983). According to the authors, a total subscale score of >8 points out of a possible 21 denotes notable symptoms of anxiety or depression (depending on the analyzed subscale). However, recommended cut-off scores are 8–10 points for doubtful cases and ≥11 for definite cases. In this study, the +TS group (as compared to the −TS group) scored significantly higher both, on the *Anxiety* [$Z = 3.40$, $p < 0.001$, $r = 0.29$] and *Depression* subscale [$Z = 3.00$, $p < 0.001$, $r = 0.29$]. Moreover, women from the +TS group obtained a score on the *Anxiety* subscale that may indicate definite cases.

Regarding the level of impulsivity (assessed by the UPPS-P; Poprawa, 2014), women from the +TS group (compared to the −TS group) obtained significantly higher results on three subscales, related to the tendency to act rashly under extreme negative [*Negative Urgency*; $Z = 5.31$, $p < 0.001$, $r = 0.45$] and positive [*Positive Urgency*; $Z = 3.04$, $p < 0.01$, $r = 0.29$] emotions and the tendency to act without thinking [*Lack of Premeditation*; $Z = 1.98$, $p < 0.05$, $r = 0.10$]. No intergroup differences were noted in terms of the inability to remain focused on tasks [*Lack of Perseverance*] and the tendency to seek out novel and thrilling experiences [*Sensation Seeking*].

Other Addictions and Religiosity

Eleven women from the +TS group (18%) and 5 women from the −TS group (14.3%) declared that they had been drinking in the past but not currently. The analyzes did not show a significant difference between the groups in terms of the total AUDIT score (Saunders et al., 1993) – the +TS group obtained a mean score of 11.54 [$SD = 7.32$] and the −TS group a score of 9.14 [$SD = 4.75$]. It is worth noting that 50.9% of the +TS group and 50% of the −TS group achieved a result that ranks them at least in the risky or hazardous level of drinking alcohol.

The analysis did not reveal significant differences between groups in terms of results obtained on the SOGS (Lesieur & Blume, 1987) – no group exceeded the cut-off value of 5. In addition, the percentage distribution of women taking psychoactive substances in the last 2 months did not differ by group.

Interestingly, 39.4% women from the +TS group (compared to 16.7% from the −TS group) declared that their sexual activity conflicts with their religious or moral beliefs ($x^2 = 17.50$, $p < 0.01$, *Cramer's V* $= 0.41$). Moreover, an association between personal religious or moral beliefs and subjective feeling of losing control over sexual behaviour was found [$x^2 = 11.23$, $p < 0.05$, *Cramer's V* $= 0.33$]. The analysis of the average weekly time (in minutes) devoted to religious practices was restricted to women who declared themselves as religious or believers (41.7%). The +TS and −TS groups did not differ in time spent on practices such as religious gatherings, meditations, prayers, and/or reading of religious books.

Discussion

The aim of this small sample study was to explore psychological and sexual correlates of CSB among treatment-seeking Polish women ($n = 103$). The

HBI (Reid et al., 2011) cut-off score was used to divide the sample into two groups: treatment seekers with high severity of CSB symptoms (+TS, $n = 61$) and treatment seekers with low CSB symptoms severity (−TS, $n = 42$). +TS women scored higher in all psychometric instruments measuring CSB compared to −TS women. Only women from the +TS group exceeded the cut-off scores of HBI and PPU, whereas results obtained from the SAST-R were above the cut-off score in both groups. Considering these ambiguities, it would be important to validate these questionnaires on large samples of women to assess its usefulness in measuring the severity of CSB in this group. Another point that deserves more attention is the fact that a significant number of women from this study who did not meet cut-off score (−TS group) were looking for help and volunteered to participate in this study.

The groups differed in terms of three sexual behaviours that, according to the subjective feelings of the women included in this study, were getting out of control – excessive masturbation, engaging in casual sexual contacts, and recurrent fantasizing. Furthermore, women from the +TS group had more sexual partners during the last year, spent more time on pornography consumption in the last 7 days, and had masturbated more often during the last 7 days. Previous research has identified excessive pornography use coupled with masturbation as the dominant pattern of functioning among men with CSB (Kowalewska et al., 2020). The percentage distributions presented in this chapter clearly show that women engage in other problematic behaviours as well, which is partially in line with a study of Klein & colleagues (2014), who found that pornography use, masturbation, and number of sexual partners were associated with hypersexual behaviour in women.

Another aspect measured in this study concerned individual tendencies associated with sexual relationships assessed by the MSQ (Kowalewska et al., 2019). Results showed that women from the +TS group exhibit higher sexual preoccupation, sexual motivation, sexual anxiety, sexual depression, external sexual control, and sexual monitoring, while women from the −TS group scored significantly higher on the subscale measuring internal sexual control. The results of this study indicate similarities and differences between men and women with CSB in terms of multidimensional aspects of sexuality. A prior study conducted on 72 Polish men seeking treatment for CSBD and 208 men from the general population (Kowalewska et al., 2019) revealed significant intergroup differences in 9 of the 12 MSQ subscales. Similar to this study, CSBD men (compared to men without CSBD) presented higher sexual anxiety, sexual depression, and external sexual control; however, men exhibited greater fear of sexual relationships as well. Similar to the present study, internal sexual control has been found to be higher in men without CSBD. In addition, men with CSBD (compared with those without CSBD) had lower tendencies related to sexual esteem, sexual consciousness, sexual assertiveness, and sexual satisfaction. These differences were not found in the female groups of the present study. Interestingly, +TS women exhibited a stronger desire to be involved in a sexual relationship than −TS women, while in men, those with CSBD showed more fear of sexual relationships (compared to men without CSBD).

In our study, CSB symptoms severity was associated with anxiety and depression, and three dimensions of impulsivity – the tendency to act rashly under extreme negative and positive emotions, as well as the tendency to act without thinking. In terms of drinking behaviour, mean scores obtained in AUDIT (Saunders et al., 1993) did not indicate levels of drinking that would meet diagnostic criteria for alcohol use disorder in either group. Symptoms of CSB were not related to the scores in the questionnaire; however, half of the women within each group were consuming alcohol at least at a risky or hazardous level. Additionally, the groups did not differ in terms of the frequency of psychoactive substance use in the last 2 months or problematic gambling behaviour (Lesieur & Blume, 1987).

CSB symptoms severity was not related to the mean time spending on religious practices. However, a significantly higher proportion of women from the +TS group (compared to the −TS group) reported that their sexual activity conflicts with their religious or moral beliefs. This association between personal religiosity or moral-based beliefs and the subjective feeling of losing control over sexual behaviour is partially in line with previous work indicating such a relationship between religiosity/morality and self-perceptions of CSB (Grubbs et al., 2020). The present results should be further investigated, especially since a prior study on Polish women showed that the number of religious practices is the strongest predictor of treatment seeking for PPU in this group (Lewczuk et al., 2017).

Limitations

Results of the present study are preliminary; thus, caution should be exercised when attempting to generalize these findings. The main limitation is the small sample size, online-based recruitment, and the risk of selection bias due to the self-selected treatment-seeking sample. Future studies on larger samples of women are needed to verify these results. Given that the severity of CSB symptoms was measured using an instrument based on criteria for Hypersexual Disorder (Kafka, 2010), the number of women from the present sample who meet official criteria of CSBD proposed by World Health Organization (2018) remains unknown. Another limitation is that the groups differed in the number of answers to questions about sexual activity (e.g., number of dyadic sexual intercourse during the last 7 days), which makes results difficult to interpret.

Conclusions

Women seeking treatment for CSB who exhibit high symptom severity may differ from those with a low CSB symptom severity in the level of anxiety, depression, impulsivity, and psychological tendencies associated with sexual relationships, such as sexual preoccupation, internal sexual control, sexual motivation, sexual anxiety, sexual depression, external sexual control, and sexual monitoring. The abovementioned aspects warrant replication and further investigation in future studies on CSBD in women.

References

Carnes, P., Green, B., & Carnes, S. (2010). The same yet different: Refocusing the sexual addiction screening test (SAST) to reflect orientation and gender. *Sexual Addiction & Compulsivity*, *17*(1), 7–30.

Gola, M., Skorko, M., Kowalewska, E., Kołodziej, A., Sikora, M., Wodyk, M., Wodyk, Z., & Dobrowolski, P. (2017). Polish adaptation of sexual addiction screening test - revised (SAST-PL-M). *Polish Psychiatry*, *51*(1), 95–115. 10.12740/PP/OnlineFirst/61414

Grubbs, J.B., Hoagland, K.C., Lee, B.N., Grant, J.T., Davison, P., Reid, R.C., & Kraus, S.W. (2020). Sexual addiction 25 years on: A systematic and methodological review of empirical literature and an agenda for future research. *Clinical Psychology Review*, *82*(82), 101925. 10.1016/j.cpr.2020.101925

Kafka, M.P. (2010). Hypersexual disorder: A proposed diagnosis for DSM-V. *Archives of Sexual Behavior*, *39*(2), 377–400. 10.1007/s10508-009-9574-7

Klein, V., Rettenberger, M., & Briken, P. (2014). Self-reported indicators of hypersexuality and its correlates in a female online sample. *Journal of Sexual Medicine*, *11*, 1974–1981. 10.1111/jsm.12602

Kowalewska, E., Gola, M., Kraus, S.W., & Lew-Starowicz, M. (2020). Spotlight on compulsive sexual behavior disorder: A systematic review of research on women. *Neuropsychiatric Disease and Treatment*, *16*, 2025–2043. 10.2147/NDT.S221540

Kowalewska, E., Kraus, S.W., Lew-Starowicz, M., Gustavsson, K., & Gola, M. (2019). Which dimensions of human sexuality are related to compulsive sexual behavior disorder (CSBD)? Study using a multidimensional sexuality questionnaire on a sample of Polish males. *The Journal of Sexual Medicine*, *16*, 1264–1273. 10.1016/j.jsxm.2019.05.00

Kraus, S.W., Gola, M., Grubbs, J.B., Kowalewska, E., Hoff, R.A., Lew-Starowicz, M., Martino, S., Shirk, S.D., & Potenza, M.N. (2020). Validation of a brief pornography screen across multiple samples. *Journal of Behavioral Addictions*, *9*(2), 259–271. 10.1556/2006.2020.00038

Lesieur, H.R., & Blume, S.B. (1987). The South oaks gambling screen (SOGS): A new instrument for the identification of pathological gamblers. *American Journal of Psychiatry*, *144*, 1184–1188. 10.1176/ajp.144.9.1184

Lewczuk, K., Szmyd, J., Skorko, M., & Gola, M. (2017). Treatment seeking for problematic pornography use among women. *Journal of Behavioral Addictions*, *6*, 445–456. 10.1556/2006.6.2017.063

Poprawa, R. (2014). Znaczenie impulsywności dla stopnia zaangażowania młodych mężczyzn w picie alkoholu. *Alcoholism and Drug Addiction*, *27*, 31–54. 10.1016/S0867-4361(14)70003-3

Reid, R.C., Garos, S., & Carpenter, B.N. (2011). Reliability, validity, and psychometric development of the hypersexual behavior inventory in an outpatient sample of men. *Sexual Addiction & Compulsivity*, *18*, 30–51. 10.1080/10720162.2011.555709

Saunders, J.B., Aasland, O.G., Babor, T.F., De la Fuente, J.R., & Grant, M. (1993). Development of the alcohol use disorders identification test (AUDIT): WHO collaborative project on early detection of persons with harmful alcohol consumption-II. *Addiction*, *88*, 791–804. 10.1111/j.1360-0443.1993.tb02093.x

Wierzba, M., Riegel, M., Pucz, A., Leśniewska, Z., Dragan, W.Ł., Gola, M., Jednoróg, K., & Marchewka, A. (2015). Erotic subset for the Nencki Affective Picture System (NAPS ERO): Cross-sexual comparison study. *Frontiers in Psychology*, *6*, 1336. 10.3389/fpsyg.2015.01336

World Health Organization. (2018). ICD-11 for mortality and morbidity statistics. Retrieved on November 01, 2021, from: https://icd.who.int/browse11/l-m/en

Zigmond, A.S., & Snaith, R.P. (1983). The hospital anxiety and depression scale. *Acta Psychiatrica Scandinavica*, *67*(6), 361–370. 10.1111/j.1600-0447.1983.tb09716.x

Chapter 27

The Gendering of Gambling in Sweden

Jessika Spångberg and Klara Goedecke

In 2018, a follow-up study of a 2015 study on the prevalence of gambling in Sweden indicated that women were in the majority among problem gamblers. This suggests a change in the gendering of gambling in Sweden. However, no such change is recognized in help-seeking data. This raises questions: are women in the majority among problem gamblers? If so, what is the significance of this? In this chapter, we discuss gender and gambling in Sweden, giving an overview of recent developments. We argue for a deepened engagement with gender, the gendering of gambling, and a greater methodological diversity within gambling research.

Introduction

In the spring of 2019, several major news outlets, including Swedish Svenska Dagbladet (April 1, 2019) and UK-based BBC (April 4, 2019), reported that Swedish women were now in the majority among problem gamblers. Seemingly, this corresponds to the feminization of gambling hypothesis introduced by the Australian Productivity Commission in late nineties and further explored by Volberg (McCarthy et al., 2019; Svensson, 2013). This hypothesis suggests that more women than before gamble, develop problems, and seek help for gambling problems. This development is surprising in the light of both older and more recent Swedish research, which indicates that men still gamble more than women and that men constitute the majority among problem gamblers.

According to the European Gaming & Betting Association, in 2019, Sweden had the highest share (58.8%) globally of gambling activity taking place online. According to international reviews, the majority of online problem gamblers are men (Mora-Salguerio et al., 2021). Yet, some researchers suggest that online gambling increasingly exposes, appeals to, or targets women (McCarthy et al., 2019). In online casino gambling, one of the most problematic gambling forms in Sweden, there seems to be no or minor differences between the sexes regarding gambling involvement, which implies that women are equally involved and affected as men. However, it is possible

DOI: 10.4324/9781003203476-33

that a gender change might have taken place in the most severe spectrum of problem gambling. The gendered implications of online gambling, including online casino gambling in Sweden, remain to be studied.

Altogether, this raises questions about the gendering of gambling in Sweden. Are women in the majority among problem gamblers? If so, what is the significance of this, and does it correspond to changes in gender relations, gambling practices, or the gendering of gambling? How do the health systems and treatment services respond? In this chapter, we discuss gender and gambling in contemporary Swedish research, with a special focus on the alleged changes in the gender balance of Swedish gamblers. We also include a brief discussion on potential effects of the COVID-19 pandemic on gambling behaviour in Sweden.

Perspectives on Gender in Gambling Research

The field of gambling research is dominated by medical and psychological perspectives (McGowan, 2004) and quantitative methods. Gambling research is thus comparable to the empiricist, positivist research fields discussed by Sandra Harding (1986, p. 34). Gambling research has a history of gender blindness, with men's gambling used as point of departure and a lack of gender-specific discussions of results (Mark & Lesieur, 1992). Lately, gender has become more integrated in gambling research even if it is not yet axiomatic in quantitative gambling studies. Often, separate analysis of women and men's gambling is missing, which raises risks of omitting gender differences (Volberg et al., 2016).

Even if gender is integrated into analyses, a limited understanding of this construct prevails. It is "a property of individuals," not related to "social structures and conceptual systems," that is, it is seen as a variable (Harding, 1986, p. 34). This resembles the integration of gender perspectives in other fields, such as science education, as discussed by Hussénius et al. (2013, p. 302), who differentiate between three approaches: most commonly, research addressing gender uses gender or sex as analytical categories. Gender research uses a gender theoretical framework that may involve analysis of power, and feminist research highlights different power relations with an intention to change them. These categories are often combined or blurred in practice. Given as follows, we use them to distinguish approaches to gender in Swedish gambling research. As very little research exists in the latter two categories, we discuss them together.

A Feminization of Gambling in Sweden? – Contradictory Findings in Population Studies

The first category of approaches to gender in research, research addressing gender, discusses gender or sex, but does not use gender theory or discuss gender in terms of power (Hussénius et al., 2013, p. 302). This approach is valuable as it covers large-scale changes in the Swedish gambling landscape and can be useful in examining an eventual feminization of gambling. Most quantitative Swedish research can be classified as part of this category.

In 2015, only 18% of the problem gamblers in Sweden were women according to the Public Health Agency of Sweden (PHAS). As mentioned above, the Swelogs[1] 2018 study indicated a threefold increase of women problem gamblers; in 2018, they constituted 64% of severe problem gamblers (Problem Gambling Severity Index, PGSI 8+). Regarding moderate risk gambling (PGSI 3+), there were no differences in men and women in any age groups besides 18–24 year olds (0% women, 3.2% men).

If there is indeed a preponderance of women at the most severe end of the problem gambling spectrum, a dramatic gendered shift in problem gambling has occurred in Sweden. However, the data were not derived from a prevalence survey, but from a follow-up study to the 2015 prevalence study. In 2015, 9,400 of 21,000 persons aged 16–84 years responded to the survey. The follow-up study in 2018 contacted the 9,400 from the 2015 study and added 4,000 new individuals aged 16–18. The response rate was 38%. The actual number of women and men (non-weighted) in the PGSI 8+ bracket was very low, indicating that the results are not necessarily generalizable to the population of severe problem gamblers in Sweden and leave room for interpretation.

Meanwhile, in 2018, PHAS published data from the National Public Health Survey, which has a random sample of 40,000 individuals aged 16–84 years. This survey showed a remaining large gender gap, with 1% of the women scoring as risk gamblers compared to 6% of the men (using an abbreviated version of the PGSI). A yearly national representative school survey from the Swedish Council for Information on Alcohol and Drugs (CAN) shows the same uneven gender distribution among students in 2018 and 2019 as well as in earlier years.

Men – Still the Majority of Help-Seeking Gamblers

According to data on gambling operators' customers from the Swedish Gaming Board, in 2019 and 2020, over 70% of active players were men. The register of self-exclusion from online gambling (68,000 individuals in total, in 2020) has a similar gender distribution. Regarding help seeking, data from the National Helpline for Gamblers show that in 2021, much like in earlier years, men constituted 80% of the callers. However, help-seeking relatives to problem gamblers consist of 80% women, an interesting finding that warrants more attention. In addition, both clinical studies and data from the National Board of Health and Welfare Register show a preponderance of men among people receiving in- or outpatient care for gambling problems in Sweden: of 779 patients in 2020, 79% (n=617) were men.

Thus, apart from the Swelogs follow-up study in 2018, there are few indications of feminization of gambling in Sweden. In general, men still gamble more frequently than women do, and men and women gamble in different gambling domains. However, women who gamble as frequently as men in gambling forms such as Electronic Gambling Machines (EGMs) seem to be just as likely to develop problems as men, or are even more vulnerable (Svensson, 2013, Volberg et al., 2016). This is supported by a recent web panel survey addressing online gamblers (past year online gambling on 10 or more occasions) with a sample of 1,004 respondents (78% men) which found that the prevalence of problem gambling (PGSI > 7) was higher in women (24%) compared to men (10%, p<0.001) (Håkansson & Widinghoff, 2020).

Gambling and COVID-19 in Sweden

The effects of the COVID-19 pandemic on Swedish gambling are still unclear. In April/May 2020, professional sports and physical state-owned casinos were closed; the latter continue to be closed as of June 2021. Despite decreased availability of some gambling forms, the revenue from gambling in 2020 was similar to the revenue in 2019 according to the Swedish Gambling Board, probably attributable to a shift from land-based gambling to online gambling. A follow-up study of the National Public Health Survey 2018 from the autumn of 2020 did not indicate any major changes in problem gambling prevalence. Regarding increased gambling problems, there was no statistical difference between men and women (men 1.0% and women 0.7%). However, increased problems with gambling were detected among the unemployed, people who already had gambling problems, and persons who had experienced canceled leisure activities. Before the pandemic, 25% of the low-risk gamblers (PGSI 1+) in the sample were women compared to 20% during COVID-19. For moderate risk (PGSI 3+), the ratio was 23% before and 39% during the pandemic. The gender ratio in help seeking did not change during the first year of the pandemic.

Thus far, the research discussed is based on quantitative methods, and while gender or sex are present as analytical categories, they remain variables. Simply put, this is what Mark and Lesieur (1992) called for – research that is not gender-blind but uses gendered categories and points to differences or similarities between them. Large-scale quantitative studies are vital to understand and address changes in the gendering of gambling but approaching gender or sex as variables has limitations.

A Need for Gender and Feminist Research on Gambling in Sweden

Whether or not a feminization of gambling is taking place in Sweden, and if/how the pandemic might affect the gendered patterns in gambling behaviour, is unclear. Thus far, it has not been seen or addressed in clinical work. Regardless, the gendered patterns briefly outlined above indicate that gambling in Sweden is highly gendered in ways that need to be explored more fully. To understand the significance of such findings, how they matter, and why they occur, other tools are needed.

Gender and feminist research "emanates from a gender theoretical framework that may involve power analysis" (Hussénius et al., 2013, p. 302) and critically scrutinizes empirical material and previous research with the aim of changing existing power imbalances. These approaches understand gender as multifaceted and as a social category, but they are unusual within gambling research, both internationally and in Sweden. Our overview suggests that these studies encompass several methodologies and have the potential to problematize the gendering of gambling. More developed and contextualized understandings of gender in quantitative research are possible (Spierings, 2012).

For instance, Jessika Spångberg's [Svensson's] research (Svensson, 2013) applies a gender perspective on quantitative data while examining gendered gambling spaces and patterns. Svensson argues for the need to go beyond gender as a category, using it in combination with age, class, and gambling arena (domestic/public) to study gendered gambling patterns in Sweden and suggests that gambling is a form of "doing gender," which may both reproduce and destabilize traditional gender patterns (2013). Frida Fröberg (2015) examined gambling problems among young men and women. In addition to identifying differences, Fröberg discusses them in relation to gendered expectations of young men and women. While gambling can be viewed as a "normative" behaviour, a part of a developmentally accepted pattern of risk-taking behaviours among young men, for young women, gambling is viewed as a deviant behaviour connected to severe social and psychological problems.

In his ethnography of Swedish EGM gamblers, Philip Lalander (2004) notes that gambling spaces, often pubs or restaurants, were masculinized both socially and symbolically, as were some male gamblers' approaches to their gambling – they sought to exercise power over the machines. Lalander problematizes the common designation of women as "escape gamblers," noting that male gamblers also escaped into the world of the game where they, unlike in their ordinary lives, could access resources and power, however illusory. Similar to Svensson (2013), Lalander introduces intersectional perspectives in his discussion of gender and gambling and sees gambling as an arena where gender is "done." Ethnographic methods are unusual within Swedish gambling research but hold much potential for in-depth understandings of the gendering of gambling (Cassidy, 2014).

Perspectives that include power analysis can also be found in gender and gambling advertising research. International studies have pointed to stereotypical gendered portrayals (Jouhki, 2017) but Swedish research points to a centring of women and problematization of stereotypical masculinity. Kroon (2021) discusses a feminized address in three Svenska Spel (the state-owned, formerly oligopolistic gambling company) commercials and Håkansson and Widinghoff (2019) point to a focus on female gamblers in televised commercials for online casinos. Contrastingly, Goedecke (2021) discusses men and masculine positions in sports betting commercials and shows that gender constructions are explicitly addressed, played with, reproduced, and subverted (cf. Jouhki, 2017). Goedecke argues that "responsible" gambling is connected to constructions of Swedish, gender-equal men, pointing to a shift in the gender politics of sports betting advertising.

This research combines features from the second and third categories – gender and feminist research. While it cannot answer questions about a numeral feminization of gambling, it demonstrates that gambling is entangled with ideas about gender, nationality, age, and class. A possible feminization of gambling aside, there are signs that the cultural construction of gambling, at least with regard to some gambling forms, is becoming less masculinized (McCarthy et al., 2019). It also acknowledges that gender is relational – it is not only about women, but about how different categories are produced together, situated in a specific context and point in time. Gender and feminist perspectives have the potential to further develop and expand Swedish gambling research.

Conclusion

It is unclear whether a feminization of gambling has taken place in Sweden. Definitive answers will have to wait for the upcoming prevalence study, conducted in autumn 2021 by PHAS. If it confirms that the number of women with (severe) gambling problems has increased as suggested in Swelogs 2018, further research and evaluation are acutely needed, not least in the field of gender and treatment and the significance of online gambling technologies. As the National Board of Health and Welfare noted in an Aftonbladet article (April 16, 2021), women with substance use disorders get less treatment and treatment of poorer quality. If that is also the case in the treatment for problem gambling remains to be studied.

The gambling field in Sweden is dominated by quantitative methods and, at best, uses gender as a variable. The male dominance in many gambling practices risks obscuring women and women's gambling, which demonstrates the need for more sophisticated methodologies as well as more developed views of gender, that go beyond the individual and highlight gendered on structural and symbolic levels in quantitative research. We also suggest that more qualitative work is needed, covering more forms of gambling and women, men, and other gendered categories, as well as other categorizations and power relations. Methodologically diverse research is necessary to understand the gendering of gambling in Sweden on structural, individual, symbolical, and discursive levels.

Update

In the spring of 2022, after writing the above and just before the publishing of this book, the Swelogs 2021 numbers arrived. They show that almost 80% of people with problem gambling (PGSI 8+) were men. In addition, men were heavily overrepresented in all PGSI categories. The results suggest that the results of Swelogs 2018 regarding women with severe problem gambling might have been affected by methodological bias.

Note

1 The Swedish longitudinal gambling study (Swelogs) is a long-term prospective population study on gambling comprising four waves of data collection among Swedish citizens aged 16–84 years at baseline, conducted by the Public Health Agency (PHAS) in Sweden. Swelogs also includes qualitative in-depth studies, the 2015 prevalence study, the 2018 follow-up study as well as the forthcoming 2021 prevalence study. PHAS also conducted the COVID-19 study in 2020, based on a sample from the National Public Health Survey.

References

Cassidy, R. (2014). "A place for men to come and do their thing": Constructing masculinities in betting shops in London. *The British Journal of Sociology*, 65(1), 170–191. DOI: 10.1111/1468-4446.12044

Fröberg, F. (2015). Problem gambling among young women and men in Sweden [Doctoral dissertation, Karolinska Institutet]. https://openarchive.ki.se/xmlui/bitstream/handle/10616/44557/Thesis_Frida_Fr%C3%B6berg.pdf

Goedecke, K. (2021). "Be soft": Irony, postfeminism, and masculine positions in Swedish sport betting commercials. *Men & Masculinities*. DOI: 10.1177/1097184 X211012739

Harding, S.G. (1986). *The science question in feminism*. Ithaca: Cornell Univ. Press.

Hussénius, A., Andersson, K., Gullberg, A., & Scantlebury K. (2013). Ignoring half the sky: A feminist critique of science education's knowledge society. In N. Mansour and R. Wegerif (Eds.), *Science education for diversity: Theory and practice, cultural studies of science education* (8, pp. 301–315), Springer.

Håkansson, A., & Widinghoff, C. (2019). Television gambling advertisements: Extent and content of gambling advertisements with a focus on potential high-risk commercial messages. *Addictive Behaviors Reports*, 9, 100182. DOI: 10.1016/j.abrep.2019.100182

Håkansson, A., & Widinghoff, C. (2020). Over-indebtedness and problem gambling in a general population sample of online gamblers. *Front Psychiatry*, 11(7). DOI: 10.3389/fpsyt.2020.00007

Jouhki, J. (2017). The hyperreal gambler. On the visual construction of men in online poker ads. *Journal of Extreme Anthropology*, 1(3), 83–101. DOI: 10.5617/jea.5441

Kroon, Å. (2021). "Moderate" gendering in Swedish gambling advertisements. *Feminist Media Studies*, online first. DOI: 10.1080/14680777.2021.1916771.

Lalander, P. (2004). *Den statliga spelapparaten. Mellan dröm och verklighet.* Stockholm: Sorad

Mark, Marie E., & Lesieur, Henri R. (1992). A feminist critique of problem gambling research. *British Journal of Addiction, 87*(4), 549–565. DOI: 10.1111/j.1360-0443.1992. tb01957.x

McCarthy, S., Thomas, S.L., Bellringer, M.E., & Cassidy R. (2019). Women and gambling-related harm: A narrative literature review and implications for research, policy, and practice. *Harm Reduction Journal, 16*(18). DOI: 10.1186/s12954-019-0284-8

McGowan, V. (2004). How do we know what we know? Epistemic tensions in social and cultural research on gambling 1980–2000. *Journal of Gambling Issues, 11*. DOI: 10.4309/jgi.2004.11.11

Mora-Salgueiro, J., García-Estela, A., Hogg, B., Angarita-Osorio, N., Amann, B.L., Carlbring, P., Jiménez-Murcia, S., Pérez-Sola, V., & Colom, F. (2021). The prevalence and clinical and sociodemographic factors of problem online gambling: A systematic review. *Journal of Gambling Studies*. Online first. DOI: 10.1007/s10899-021-09999-w

Spierings, N. (2012). The inclusion of quantitative techniques and diversity in the mainstream of feminist research. *European Journal of Women's Studies, 19*(3), 331–347. DOI: 10.1177/1350506812443621

Svensson, J. (2013). Gambling and gender: A public health perspective [Doctoral dissertation, Mid Sweden University]. http://urn.kb.se/resolve?urn=urn:nbn:se:miun:diva-19046

Volberg, R.A., Romild, U., & Svensson, J. (2016). A gender perspective on gambling clusters in Sweden using longitudinal data. *Nordic Studies on Alcohol and Drugs, 33*(1), 43–59. DOI: 10.1515/nsad-2016-0004

Chapter 28

Problem Use of the Internet and Social Media among Young Women in the Russian Federation

Eugenia V. Fadeeva

In Russia, like in other countries, there is a high prevalence of Internet and social media use, as well as related manifestations of addictive behaviour: impaired control, increasing priority over other life interests, continuation despite negative consequences, and impairment of important areas of functioning. Several researchers from Russia point out that prevalence of Internet addiction is higher among women, compared to men, and that the most frequent type of Internet activity among women is the use of social media, which in some cases meets the criteria of problem use. Among personal features of girls and young women with problem Internet and social media use are high social anxiety, fear of negative assessments, and difficulties in accepting their own emotions and emotions of others.

General Introduction

Digital mobile devices and social media have become an essential part of daily life of people all over the world. Even though the development of the Internet and Internet-based technologies is undoubtedly a positive phenomenon, and benefits including those in the field of public health are very significant, there is a growing concern among specialists in the field of psychiatry, addictology, and psychology related to Internet problem use and increasing prevalence of Internet addiction. A significant obstacle for specialists in the field of diagnosis, prevention, and treatment of addictive behaviour is insufficient systematization of certain addictive phenomena and diagnostic criteria for problem use of the Internet or social media. Currently, assessments of the Internet-dependent behaviour phenomenon are usually carried out using psychometric scales, particularly the Chen Internet Addiction Scale (CIAS), without a clinical diagnosis. However, on January 1, 2022, the 11th edition of the International Classification of Diseases (ICD-11) will be introduced, with a new medical condition "gaming disorder" included under a specific diagnostic code. This was a result of World Health Organization expert meetings, analysis of available

DOI: 10.4324/9781003203476-34

evidence in the scientific literature and case series, as well as clinical experience provided by international experts in psychiatry, clinical psychology, internal medicine, family practice, epidemiology, neurobiology, and public health (Rumpf et al., 2018).

Problem Use of the Internet

According to the global project "We are social" (Digital, 2021), nowadays 124 million people in Russia (85% of the country's population) are using the Internet. The average time that users aged 16–64 spend on the Internet, using any device, is almost 8 hours per day, including 3 hours 29 minutes using mobile devices (smartphones). On average, users spend 2 hours 28 minutes communicating on social networks, 55 minutes reading texts, over 3 hours watching video content, 47 minutes listening to music, and 33 minutes playing computer games (Digital, 2021).

According to international and Russian researchers, Internet addiction is a behavioural disorder associated with increasing time and loss of control over the time spent on the Internet, adverse consequences in professional and social life, and physical or mental problems associated with excessive use of the Internet. Internet addiction is observed mainly among the young part of the population, older adolescents, and young adults (Gerasimova & Kholmogorova, 2020; Grechaniy et al., 2020; Solodnikov & Zajczeva, 2021), and its prevalence in Russia is estimated between 4.3% and 22.6% (Merkur`eva & Maly`gin, 2020). In order to assess prevalence of Internet-dependent behaviour symptoms, a study among 1,119 school students 15–18 years of age was conducted by Trusova et al. (2020) using the CIAS scale. Pronounced risk of developing Internet addiction was identified among 10.4%, moderate risk among 58.4%, and minimum/no risk among 31.2%. Girls appear to be more vulnerable to developing Internet addiction than boys, due to emotional distress, alexithymia, fear of negative evaluation, and social anxiety. Internet-dependent behaviour is characterized by certain psychopathological phenomena: obsessive-compulsive disorder, depression, anxiety, and symptoms of distress, as well as social activity decrease or impaired social adaptation (Antonienko, 2014; Skvorcova & Lushkina, 2021; Solodnikov & Zajczeva, 2021). Another study of school students aged 15–17 years [8.208 boys (45%) and 10.014 girls (55%)] showed that the prevalence of alcohol use as well as frequent alcohol use are significantly higher among adolescents who are using the Internet for 3 hours a day or more, compared to with adolescents who do not use the Internet excessively (Skvorczova & Lushkina, 2020).

The aim of a study conducted by Trusova et al. (2020) was to assess prevalence of Internet-dependent behaviour and to investigate gender-related features of Internet addiction and individual psychological factors that are significant for its development. Significant gender differences were observed for manifestations of Internet-dependent behaviour, as well as for specific individual psychological risk factors for Internet addiction in teenagers aged 15–19. Overall, girls showed more pronounced key manifestations of Internet-addicted behaviour, including compulsive symptoms, withdrawal symptoms, and tolerance (see Table 28.1). In the group with high risk of

Table 28.1 Individual psychological characteristics among teenagers aged 15–19

Indicator	Girls (N = 565) Me [Q1; Q3]	Boys (N = 554) Me [Q1; Q3]	U-test value, p
Chen Internet Addiction Scale (CIAS)			
Compulsive symptoms	10.0 [8.0; 12.0]	9.0 [7.0; 11.0]	130,998.0 p < 0.001***
Withdrawal symptoms	10.2 [8.0; 13.0]	9.0 [7.0; 12.0]	134,798.0 p < 0.001***
Tolerance	8.0 [7.0; 10.0]	8.0 [6.0; 9.0]	126,997.0 p < 0.001***
Key symptoms of Internet addiction	29.0 [24.0; 34.0]	26.0 [21.0; 31.0]	126,174.5 p < 0.001***
Total scores	50.0 [42.0; 58.0]	46.0 [36.0; 54.0]	134,123.5 p < 0.001***
Positive and Negative Affect Schedule (PANAS)			
General negative affectivity	23.0 [17.0; 30.0]	21.0 [15.0; 26.2]	133,673.5 p < 0.001***
Brief Fear of Negative Evaluation Scale-Revised (BFNES-R)			
Total scores	31.0 [23.0; 40.0]	21.0 [15.0; 26.2]	127,296.0 p < 0.001***
Liebowitz Social Anxiety Scale (LSAS)			
Total score for "Fear"	22.0 [13.0; 34.0]	27.0 [19.0; 35.0]	130,821.0 p < 0.001***
Total score for "Avoidance"	23.0 [14.0; 34.0]	22.0 [11.0; 30.0]	138,608.0 p < 0.001***
Fear of interpersonal contact situations	12.0 [7.0; 18.0]	10.0 [4.0; 16.0]	130,410.0 p < 0.001***
Fear of verbal communication and interaction situations	8.0 [5.0; 13.0]	8.0 [3.0; 11.0]	133,853.5 p < 0.001***
Fear of doing something in public place	2.0 [0.0; 4.0]	1.0 [0.0; 3.0]	137,668.0 p < 0.001***
Avoiding interpersonal contact situations	8.0 [4.0; 11.0]	11.0 [5.0; 17.0]	136,191.0 p < 0.001***
Avoiding situations of verbal communication and interaction	8.0 [4.0; 11.0]	7.0 [3.0; 11.0]	144,859.0 p < 0.031*
Avoiding taking action in public places	3.0 [1.0; 5.0]	2.0 [0.0; 4.0]	142,401.0 p < 0.008**
Total scores	45.0 [29.0; 67.0]	41.5 [22.0; 58.0]	132,940.0 p < 0.001***

Me = median, [Q1; Q3] = 1–3 quartile.

Note

This table was first published by Trusova et al. (2020). We would like to thank Anna Trusova for permitting us to re-print the table in this chapter.

Internet addiction development, only withdrawal symptoms were more pronounced among girls, i.e., when it was impossible to use the Internet or a device with Internet access, they were more prone to mood changes, irritability, anxiety, and depressive manifestations than boys.

The study has shown that pronounced differences were shown virtually for all parameters of Internet addiction: girls had higher overall CIAS scores, higher severity of compulsive and key symptoms, and higher tolerance and withdrawal symptoms ($p < 0.001$). According to the results of the Brief Fear of Negative Evaluation Scale-Revised (BFNES-R) scale, girls had more pronounced manifestations of fear of negative evaluation. This personal psychological characteristic is the basis of social anxiety. Significant differences were also obtained on the Positive and Negative Affect Schedule (PANAS); girls had more pronounced manifestations of negative affectivity than boys. In addition, girls had higher values for a vast majority of indicators of social anxiety, which manifests itself in situations of social interaction, measured by Liebowitz Social Anxiety Scale (LSAS). Gender-specific perception of parenting style was revealed in groups of boys with moderate and high risk of Internet addiction, but only in relation to the figure of the father. This study may serve as a basis for developing targeted and gender-specific programs for prevention of Internet addiction and early intervention among adolescents (Trusova et al., 2020).

At the same time, foreign and Russian scientists note that the severity of addictive behaviour depends on the type of activity on the Internet (communication in social networks, viewing educational and entertainment content, etc.), and online gaming has a relatively greater "addictiveness" (Antonienko, 2014; Gerasimova & Kholmogorova, 2020; Korchagina et al., 2016). According to a survey by Antonienko (2014) among 214 adolescents [110 boys (51.5%), 104 girls (48.5%)] aged 14–17 years, among adolescents who prefer online games, the overall score on the CIAS scale was significantly higher ($p \leq 0.05$) than among adolescents who prefer online communication. Adolescents with Internet-addicted behaviour who prefer computer games are showing increased tolerance, have difficulty controlling time spent on the Internet, and have a higher prevalence of eating disorders and insufficient sleep (less than 4 hours a day; Antonienko, 2014).

Research of computer gaming prevalence among more than 18,000 adolescents (15–17 years old) from 17 rural regions of Russia [8.208 (45%) boys and 10,014 (55%) girls] provided insight into gender differences in online gaming as a specific Internet activity. The prevalence of computer games use is lower among girls: only 38.3% of girls were playing computer games, while among boys this value reached 76.8% ($p < 0.001$). Among girls, 11.9% played for more than 3 hours during a day, and 5% played 5 hours or more (Skvorczova & Lushkina, 2020). Similar results were obtained by a group of researchers from St. Petersburg and Moscow who studied forms and content of online activity, gender differences, as well as signs of mental and substance-related disorders in individuals with Internet addiction. According to this study, the most frequent form of Internet activity for women was "using social networks" (91.8%, p = 0.047). While the group who predominantly used social networks showed anxiety level, depression, prodromal psychotic symptoms, and general psychopathological profiles statistically comparable to other groups, there was a greater severity of compulsive Internet addiction symptoms and withdrawal symptoms (according to CIAS; Grechaniy et al., 2020).

Problem Use of Social Media

Despite the fact that Internet addiction is a multidimensional problem, an increasing number of studies and monitoring projects show that involvement in social networks communication plays an important role in shaping Internet addiction behaviour. The Health Behaviour in School-aged Children (HBSC), one of the largest international youth monitoring projects, highlighted a number of problems related to online communication, which included intensive use of electronic communications, preference to online communication with friends compared to interpersonal, and problem use of social networks among school students. A number of problem aspects of electronic communications use that was typical for girls from Russia were revealed: 31% of 11-year-old girls intensively used electronic communications (HBSC average 28%). In addition, according to the 2020 Health Behaviour in School-aged Children study, girls from Russia more often preferred online communication to interpersonal ones: 13% among 11-year-olds, 17% among 13-year-olds, and 22% among 15-year-olds compared to HBSC averages of 8%, 14%, and 16%, respectively.

A number of surveys conducted in Russia were devoted to problem use of social media. Sirota et al. (2018) adapted and tested the Problematic Facebook Use Scale (PFUS) for adolescents and young adults in a Russian-speaking sample. The study involved 900 participants, including 670 women (74.4%) and 230 men (25.6%), with an average age of 28.6 ± 7.5 years. All participants were active users of social networks. The findings indicate that age (r = −0.327; p = 0.001) and education (r = −0.204; p = 0.001) contribute to reduction of over-engagement and intrusive thinking about social media. A higher level of education is also associated with lower values on the compulsive use scale (r = −0.150; p = 0.04) and older age was associated with lower values on the negative consequences scale (r = −0.180; p = 0.01). In addition, lower scores on the scales "cognitive absorption," "regulation of emotions," and "compulsive use" were typical for participants with higher level of education and older age. However, the study has not revealed gender-related associations with social media problem use scales (Sirota et al., 2018).

However, a study by Gerasimova and Kholmogorova (2018) came to the opposite conclusion. To assess convergent validity, a sample of 1,100 students aged 14–21 years (mean age = 16.31; SD = 1.76) was studied, among them 1,036 girls. A psychopathological symptoms severity questionnaire, Symptomchecklist-90-Revised (SCL-90-R), was used to measure inter-correlation validity and assess risks of problem Internet use for mental health. For three scales of the questionnaire – preference for online communication ($p \leq 0.01$), cognitive absorption ($p \leq 0.05$), and compulsive use ($p \leq 0.01$) – results for girls and young women were significantly higher than for boys and young men. The authors concluded that girls are more inclined to use online communications and have higher compulsiveness and cognitive involvement; however, they appear to be less likely to use the Internet as a strategy for mood regulation.

Problem Use of the Internet and Social Media during the COVID-19 Pandemic

In a study of coping strategies, psychological well-being, and problem Internet use among girls and young women (aged 13–22) located in Russia during the COVID-19 pandemic (Gerasimova & Kholmogorova, 2020), respondents with problem Internet use were more likely to report an increase in stress, anxiety, and obsessive-compulsive symptoms. Moreover, the study revealed that the problem of Internet use was closely related to family conflicts and a subjective desire for social distancing (Gerasimova & Kholmogorova, 2020). Results of a pilot study of the use of social media and Internet gaming disorders among 192 students from Yaroslavl (142 young women and 50 young men) during the COVID-19 pandemic demonstrated an increase in duration and frequency of social media use and gaming sessions. The authors used the modified PFUS and Internet Gaming Disorder Scale – Short-Form. During the pandemic, the majority of respondents began to use social media (65.1%) and play video games (33.2%) more often, and the duration of sessions increased significantly. Such changes may indicate the development of addictive behaviour. Around one-third of participants subjectively assessed their use of social media during the COVID-19 pandemic as problematic (Lanovaya et al., 2021).

Conclusions

Currently, in Russia and elsewhere, there is no clear distinction between the concepts of "problem use of social media" and "problem use of the Internet." However, several validated psychometric tools are available to objectively assess the prevalence of excessive Internet and/or social media use. In view of the relatively high prevalence of problem use of social media among girls and young women, risk factors associated with such behaviour and related psychological and clinical phenomena require further research. There are significant gender differences in activities that adolescents and young adults take up on the Internet – the use of social media is more common among girls, while online gaming is more common among boys. At the same time, girls demonstrate more pronounced key manifestations of Internet-dependent behaviour: compulsive symptoms, withdrawal symptoms, and tolerance, as well as mood changes, irritability, depression, and anxiety. These problems may have profound impacts on the health of young women and require further detailed research using reliable methods to explore the effectiveness of specific prevention interventions.

References

Antonienko, A.A. (2014). Internet addiction of adolescents to computer games and online communication: Clinical and psychological characteristics and prevention [Internet-zavisimost` podrostkov ot komp`yuterny`kh igr i onlajn-obshheniya: kliniko-psikhologicheskie osobennosti i profilaktika], Moscow, 105. (In Russ., abstr. in Engl.).

Gerasimova, A.A., & Kholmogorova, A.B. (2018). The generalized problematic internet use scale 3 modified version: Approbation and validation on the Russian sample. *Konsul'tativnaya psikhologiya i psikhoterapiya [Counseling Psychology and Psychotherapy]*, *26*(3), 56–79. DOI 10.17759/cpp.2018260304. (In Russ., abstr. in Engl.).

Gerasimova, A.A., & Kholmogorova, A.B. (2020). Coping strategies, psychological well-being and problematic internet use during a pandemic. *Psychological Science and Education [Psikhologicheskaya nauka i obrazovanie]*, *25*(6), 31–40. DOI 10.17759/pse.2020250603. (In Russ., abstr. in Engl.)

Grechaniy, S.V., et al. (2020). Internet addiction in young adults: Types of online activities, gender differences, comorbid mental and substance use disorders. *4*(187), 78–102. (In Russ., abstr. in Engl.).

Korchagina, G.A., Fadeeva, E.V., Golubinskaya, O.I., & Vy`shinskij, K.V. (2016). The main trends in the study of computer and gaming addiction, excessive use of the internet in the Russian Federation. *Journal of Addiction Problems [Voprosy` narkologii]*, *7–8*, 17–23. (In Russ., abstr. in Engl.).

Lanovaya, A.M., Shakun, E.U., Fadeeva, E.V., Volkov, A.V., Minakov, M.A., & Amelina, S.V. (2021). Social networks use and computer internet gaming among students of Yaroslavl region during the COVID-19 pandemic. *Journal of Addiction Problems [Voprosy` narkologii]*, *4*(199), 5–30. (In Russ., abstr. in Engl.).

Merkur`eva, Y.A., & Maly`gin, V.L. (2020). Features of socio-psychological adaptation and psychopathological phenomena accompanying internet addiction in adolescents. *Journal of Addiction Problems [Voprosy` narkologii]*, *4*(187), 63–77. (In Russ., abstr. in Engl.).

Rumpf, H.J., et al. (2018). Including gaming disorder in the ICD-11: The need to do so from a clinical and public health perspective. *Journal of Behavioral Addictions*, *7*(3), 1–6. DOI 10.1556/2006.7.2018.59

Sirota, N.A., Moskovchenko D.V., Yaltonsky V.M., & Yaltonskaya A.V. (2018). Development of the Russian version of the questionnaire for the problematic use of social networks. *Konsul'tativnaya psik- hologiya i psikhoterapiya [Counseling Psychology and Psychotherapy]*, *26*, 3, 33–55. DOI 10.17759/cpp.2018260303. (In Russ., abstr. in Engl.).

Skvorczova, E.S., & Lushkina, N.P. (2020). Computer games among Russian rural schoolchildren (prevalence, consequences, problems). *Issues of Mental Health of Children and Adolescents [Voprosy` psikhicheskogo zdorov`ya detei i podrostkov]*, *20*, 1, 24–33. (In Russ., abstr. in Engl.).

Skvorcova, E.S., & Lushkina, N.P. (2021). Daily long-term internet use and alcohol consumption among rural adolescents. *The Russian Journal of Preventive Medicine and Public Health [Profilakticheskaya meditsina]*, *24*(1), 53–59. DOI 10.17116/profmed2021

Solodnikov, V.V., & Zajczeva, A.S. (2021). The use of social networks and the socialization of Russian adolescents. *Sociological Science and Social Practice [Socziologicheskaya nauka i soczial`naya praktika]*, *9*, 1, 23–42. DOI 10.19181/snsp.2021.9.1.7870. (In Russ., abstr. in Engl.).

Trusova, A.V., et al. (2020). Internet addiction predictors: Analysis of psychological factors. *V.M. Bekhterev Review of Psychiatry and Medical Psychology*, (1), 72–82. (In Russ.) Retrieved from 10.31363/2313-7053-2020-1-72-82 (In Russ., abstr. in Engl.).

Trusova, A.V., et al. (2020). Gender differences in individual psychological characteristics in adolescents with different levels of manifestations of internet-addicted behavior. *Journal of Addiction Problems [Voprosy` narkologii]*, *4*(187), 45–62. (In Russ., abstr. in Engl.).

We Are Social (2021). Digital 2021 – Global Overview Report. Available at https://wearesocial.com/digital-2021

Chapter 29

The Impact of Internet and Gaming Addiction on Women and Gender Minorities in Sweden and Europe

Emma Claesdotter-Knutsson and Niroshani Broman

Equality between men and women has also affected women in non-expected ways. Today, the prevalence of female substance abuse is slowly approaching the male level. A similar trend has been seen in gambling with increased numbers of women gambling and developing problems but also seeking help for problems related to gambling. There is reason to believe the same is applicable for gaming. Several studies have revealed that differences in gaming patterns are greater between sexual minority women and heterosexual women than between sexual minority men and heterosexual men. This is an emerging field of study with more research needed.

Introduction

In 2021, Sweden was one of the most "equal" countries in the European Union. The country has held this position since 2005. The European Institute for Gender Equality oversees the monitoring and they measure gender equality based on constructs such as work, income, knowledge, time, power, and health. Is this equality also reflected in gaming behaviours?

In Sweden, equality between men and women is a basic constitutional norm and a political goal. Men and women shall have the same rights to form their own lives. Since 2010, Sweden has a gender-neutral military service, the salary gap between comparable professions is among the lowest in the world, all taxes and social services are individually based, and Sweden is also leading in efforts to put an end to male violence against women.

But this has also affected women in non-expected ways. Today, the prevalence of female substance abuse is slowly approaching the male level. Women took over traditionally male domains before men had a chance to do the reverse. As a result, women experience more negative stress and are overwhelmed with a place in society that is often still subordinated. On the other hand, men still have a risky lifestyle and but now in combination with a loss of previous privileges. This changing trend has also affected life

DOI: 10.4324/9781003203476-35

expectancy. Women still live longer than men, but men have more power and resources and better self-reported health.

The internet has become a constant in our lives. We gained a lot from the internet like communication and information but at the same time, potential problems emerged. Internet addiction (IA) defined as "psychological dependence on the internet," although not yet accepted in either DSM-5 or ICD-11, has been found to be related to comorbidities such as anxiety and depression (Broman et al., 2021). Gender is a central factor in understanding behavioural addiction including IA. Traditionally men were reported to have higher IA than women but more recent studies that have differentiated IA in social and gaming domains have shown different gender patterns: men are more engaged in gaming whereas women tend to be more engaged in the social aspects of the internet using it as a tool for social interaction.

Women tend to use social media to counteract feelings of emptiness and they state not being satisfied with "real life," increasing the risk of addiction. Gaming is a traditional male activity but during the past decades female gaming has increased and today women represent up to half of the gaming population. Despite these observations, almost all research on gaming is conducted with male gamers (Broman & Håkansson, 2018). There is a knowledge gap regarding female perspectives on both the positive and negative aspects of gaming.

Female Experiences of Gaming

Male predominance is a well-known feature of problematic gaming, with a reported male-to-female ratio of 3:1 (Wang et al., 2019). The exact reason for the male predominance in problematic gaming is unknown. However, one plausible explanation for gender differences are motivations for gaming. Women tend to seek challenges or immersing themselves in other worlds while the main reason for gaming given by men is to destroy things.

In 2003, Volberg (2003) described a "feminization" of gambling in the US. The author was the first to name this phenomenon which is now seen worldwide: an increased number of women gambling and developing problems but also seeking help for problems related to gambling. There is reason to believe the same is applicable for gaming. For example, our research group looked at self-reported gaming during the second wave of the COVID-19 pandemic and our results suggest that female participants were just as likely as the male to increase their time gaming during the pandemic (Claesdotter-Knutsson et al., 2021). However, in general, women tend to play less video games than men. This could be due to experiences of harassment online and/ or because the characters in these games are mostly males making many women choose a male character when playing (Lopez-Fernandez et al., 2021).

Most professional gamers are male. There is a problematic conceptualization of the "female gamer" who is marginalized and looked upon as not "true" or "hard-core." This results in a low female gamer identification, women are often discriminated against by male players, and female characters are often sexualized or objectified. Most female characters are dependent on the male hero character. Women are less encouraged to participate in playing video games as video games are largely designed and developed for a male audience, focusing on male players and including sexualized content in language or actions (Lopez-Fernandez et al., 2021). Many women state that when playing a female character, they are faced with harassment and bullying online. To avoid this, they prefer to play a male character (Lopez-Fernandez et al., 2021). There is also evidence that male players take on a female character when wanting additional support or pity in the game and gender swapping within games is very common (Hussain & Griffiths, 2008). Therefore, gender swapping is a strategy used by both genders in order to receive advantages (Hussain & Griffiths, 2008).

Gaming among Sexual and Gender Minorities

The health disparities between the LGBT and the general population are well documented. Yet, sexual minorities are typically reached to a lesser extent by clinical interventions and in research (Russel & Fish, 2016).

Transgender youth report more gambling as well as problematic gambling (Rider et al., 2019). Transgender women report the same rate of gambling as cismen but a higher prevalence of problem gambling (Rider et al., 2019). Among sexual and gender minorities, certain features could be present that play a role for the development of addictive behaviours, such as social isolation and increased risk of other psychiatric problems.

There is a well-known association between stigma in the form of discrimination, violence, or less satisfying economic and social features and a higher risk for mental health and substance use problems among lesbian, gay, bisexual, and gender minority populations (Bränström & Pachankis, 2018; Bränström et al., 2020). Several studies have revealed a pattern where differences are greater between sexual minority women and heterosexual women than between sexual minority men and heterosexual men. In a Swedish report on same-sex marriages, women in same-sex marriages had the same level of alcohol problems as male groups (social board on health and welfare, 2016). In some studies, women with a bisexual orientation were more likely to report alcohol problems and illicit drug use than women with a homosexual and heterosexual orientation (Coulter et al., 2018). It seems that the minority stress theory (Meyer, 2003) stating that disparities in health could be a result of minority stress is well applicable in this group. Online activities have been described in qualitative research as a part of social isolation among young LGBT individuals when experiencing stigma from the surrounding society (Steinke et al., 2017).

Video games tend to be heteronormative in their layout and some even display negative attitudes toward non-heterosexual identities (Krobová et al.,

2015). For example, in a 2014 report by the Swedish Federation for Lesbian, Gay, Bisexual, Transgender, Queer and Intersex Rights on gaming from an LGBT perspective, sexism and homophobia in online chat forums are described. One could speculate that this would not appeal to sexual and transgender minorities. Nevertheless, a pilot study showed that both gaming and gambling in this group are extensive (Broman & Håkansson, 2018). Sexual minorities give the anonymity of the online world as reason for extensive online activity. The online world is a place to explore sexual and gender identity, independent of their lived sexual orientation or gender identity, not having to worry about passing as a man or woman (Devlin & Holohan, 2016). This dualism might add to the complexity of sexual identification and gaming behaviour – the online world can be homophobic and transphobic but also the place to be if one wants to express one's wanted identity. This might be problematic since more time spent on gaming could be associated with a greater risk for developing behavioural addictions.

Our research group has looked at problematic gambling, gaming, and internet use in the European context to see if these behaviours are affected by sexual orientation (Broman et al., 2021 in press). We only found an independent association between belonging to a sexual minority and these behavioural addictions among women defining themselves as having another sexual orientation status than lesbian, gay, bisexual, and homosexual. In addition, while not statistically significant, we observed an overrepresentation of screening positive for problematic gambling, gaming, and internet use *and* belonging to a sexual minority looking. These findings seem to be explained by social factors such as experienced psychological distress and loneliness. The difference between European countries in living conditions and economic and social factors such as acceptance in the society for minorities might also affect the willingness to seek help for mental conditions and behavioural addiction. Sexual and gender minorities might encounter stigma due to mental health problems and their sexual or gender identity. The result of our study, indicating a higher prevalence of problematic gambling and gaming behaviour among sexual minority women, raises the question whether sexual minority women engage in these activities as a way of coping with psychological distress, stigma, and isolation.

Other studies among sexual minorities in Sweden have revealed a link between stigma and psychiatric problems (Bränström, 2017). Specifically, women stating a sexual minority status were more likely to report problematic gambling and gaming after controlling for age and nationality. For units treating behavioural addiction, this underlines the importance of including perspectives of women with a sexual minority status. They may experience comfort and a sense of belonging in the online world (Lucassen et al., 2018) while living in fear of not being accepted in offline world. Increased knowledge about living conditions for sexual and gender minorities might be of importance for treatment outcomes if these conditions are different from the general population.

Women in the general population are underrepresented in substance use and behavioural addiction. One explanation could be that most research is done in clinical samples. We know that women have a high threshold for admitting they have an addiction, have problems finding time to devote to therapy, and coming out as having an addiction problem might lead to fear of losing custody of their children or of not being understood. Few clinics are devoted to women which makes it more difficult for them to be acknowledged for their specific needs. This might be a problem since women with problematic gaming who define themselves as a sexual minority stated considerable psychological distress and hence would need professional help. Our research on LGBT people on the other hand has shown that this group is more willing to seek help for their behavioural addiction than heterosexual women.

Is it possible that women belonging to sexual minorities utilize their problematic internet use to seek general assistance and support? Perhaps, this leads the health care system to overlook their minority status, making it "safe" for them to seek help without being afraid of being stigmatized for their sexual minority status. Research on differences in internet and gaming addiction regarding gender differences but also differences related to gender minorities is scarce. We have seen in other addictions the importance of addressing gender differences in order to tailor both therapy but also prevention.

A Clinical Perspective on Gaming among Patients with Gender Incongruence

I have worked at an adult transgender clinic since 2014. Due to the enormous rise in young people defining themselves as transgender, we were bound to open a clinic for youth under 18 years of age. There have been speculations regarding this sudden and steady rise in under-aged people. Could the rise be due to environmental factors such as hormones in the water, more and easier access to health care, more knowledge regarding gender identity in society in general due to information on internet, less stigmata resulting in adolescents of today making gender identity a natural part of their identity development, or something else? It is worth noting that being transgender is still very unusual, but more and more adolescents define themselves as gender neutral. In my clinic, the majority of my patients state that acting out their "true" gender identity online was one of the first tentative steps in exploring their wanted gender. They might be bullied at school or have problem passing as their wanted gender but online they can be free to be whoever they want and in whatever gender they want. For most of them, it is not possible to participate in sports due to the early division in boys' and girls' teams and they might not feel comfortable in sharing changing rooms with others. Transgender youth that are engaged in music often encounter problems when reaching adolescent due to their voice cracking. But then the online world is a free zone, attractive for its anonymity. They can play their favorite game but in their wanted gender to see how it feels, as a good way to explore their wanted name and gender identity. Many of them report sexism and homophobia in online communities supporting the above statement that online games are heteronormative and that transgender youth experience a duality regarding gaming. I also find that the young transgender community drinks less alcohol and uses less drugs than non-transgender youth. They report much more social isolation and much more online gaming activity where it seems like they have most of their social network. Young transgender individuals see gaming as their lifeline. Perhaps, one could use this interest in gaming and online activities to break social isolation and negative thought patterns.

Acknowledgment

We would like to thank Prof. Anders Håkansson and his team for data and support.

References

Broman, N., & Hakansson, A. (2018). Problematic gaming and internet use but not gambling may be overrepresented in sexual minorities–a pilot population web survey study. *Frontiers in Psychology, 9*, 2184.

Broman, N., Prever, F., di Giacomo, E., Jiménez-Murcia, S., Szczegielniak, A., Hansson, H., & Håkansson, A. (2021). Gambling, gaming and internet behavior in a sexual minority perspective. A cross-sectional study in seven European countries. *Frontiers in Psychology*, in press.

Bränström, R. (2017). Minority stress factors as mediators of sexual orientation disparities in mental health treatment: A longitudinal population-based study. *Journal of Epidemiology and Community Health, 71*(5), 446–452. 10.1136/jech-2016-207943

Bränström, R., & Pachankis, J.E. (2018). Sexual orientation disparities in the co-occurrence of substance use and psychological distress: A national population-based study (2008-2015). *Social Psychiatry and Psychiatric Epidemiology, 53*(4), 403–412. 10.1007/s00127-018-1491-4

Bränström, R., van der Star, A., & Pachankis, J.E. (2020). Untethered lives: Barriers to societal integration as predictors of the sexual orientation disparity in suicidality. *Social Psychiatry and Psychiatric Epidemiology, 55*(1), 89–99. 10.1007/s00127-019-01742-6

Claesdotter-Knutsson, E., André, F., & Håkansson, A. (2021). Gaming during the COVID-19 pandemic: A cross-sectional study focusing on young people and possible changes in gaming behavior. *JMIR Serious Games*.

Coulter, R., Jun, H.J., Calzo, J.P., Truong, N.L., Mair, C., Markovic, N., Charlton, B.M., Silvestre, A.J., Stall, R., & Corliss, H.L. (2018). Sexual-orientation differences in alcohol use trajectories and disorders in emerging adulthood: Results from a longitudinal cohort study in the United States. *Addiction (Abingdon, England)*, 10.1111/add.14251. Advance online publication. 10.1111/add.14251

Devlin, C., & Holohan, A. (2016). Cultures of experimentation: Role-playing games and sexual identity. In *Communication and information technologies annual*. Emerald Group Publishing Limited.

Hussein, Z., and Griffiths, M. (2008). Gender swapping and socializing in cyberspace: An exploratory study. *Cyberpsychology & Behavior*, 11, 47–52. doi: 10.1089/cpb.2007.0020

Krobová, T., Moravec, O., & Švelch, J. (2015). Dressing commander shepard in pink: Queer playing in a heteronormative game culture. *Cyberpsychology: Journal of Psychosocial Research on Cyberspace*, 9(3), Article 3.

Lopez-Fernandez, O., Williams, A.J., Griffiths, M.D., & Kuss, D.J. (2021). Female gaming, gaming addiction, and the role of women within gaming culture: A narrative. *Psychopathology Among Youth in the 21st Century: Examining Influences from Culture, Society and Technology.*

Lucassen, M., Samra, R., Iacovides, I., Fleming, T., Shepherd, M., Stasiak, K., & Wallace, L. (2018). How LGBT+ young people use the internet in relation to their mental health and envisage the use of e-therapy: Exploratory study. *JMIR Serious Games*, 6(4), e11249.

Meyer, I.H. (2003). Prejudice, social stress, and mental health in lesbian, gay, and bisexual populations: Conceptual issues and research evidence. *Psychological bulletin*, 129(5), 674.

Rider, G.N., McMorris, B.J., Gower, A.L., Coleman, E., & Eisenberg, M.E. (2019). Gambling behaviors and problem gambling: A population-based comparison of transgender/gender diverse and cisgender adolescents. *Journal of Gambling Studies*, 35(1), 79–92.

Russell, S.T., & Fish, N.J. (2016). Mental health in lesbian, gay, bisexual and transgender (LGBT) youth. *Annual Review of Clinical Psychology*, 12, 465–487.

Steinke, J., Root-Bowman, M., Estabrook, S., Levine, D.S., & Kantor, L.M. (2017). Meeting the needs of sexual and gender minority youth: Formative research on potential digital health interventions. *The Journal of Adolescent Health: Official Publication of the Society for Adolescent Medicine*, 60(5), 541–548. 10.1016/j.jadohealth.2016.11.023

Volberg, R.A. (2003). Has there been a "feminization" of gambling and problem gambling in the United States? *Journal of Gambling Issues*, (8).

Wang, Z., Hu, Y., Zheng, H., Yuan, K., Du, X., & Dong, G. (2019). Females are more vulnerable to Internet gaming disorder than males: Evidence from cortical thickness abnormalities. *Psychiatry Research: Neuroimaging*, 283, 145–153.

Part VI

Oceania

Chapter 30

All That Glitters Is Not Gold

Women's Experiences of Using Gambling Venues to Escape Intimate Partner Violence

Lydia Mainey, Nerilee Hing, Cathy O'Mullan,
Helen Breen, and Elaine Nuske

One in four Australian women have experienced intimate partner violence (IPV). Personal, systemic, and societal barriers prevent many women from leaving abusive relationships and some look to other outlets for safety and emotional support. Gambling venues can provide a safe, friendly environment that some victims of IPV find attractive. Playing electronic gaming machines also provides an emotional and physical escape but poses a significant risk of further harm and addiction and can result in more abuse. This chapter explores the context and complexities in which women victims of male partner violence use gambling venues as safe spaces.

Introduction

Intimate partner violence (IPV) refers to violence between current or previous partners. One-quarter of Australian women have been subjected to IPV; it is a major public health issue (Australian Institute of Health and Welfare, 2019). Leaving an abusive relationship is notoriously difficult due to a range of personal, systemic, and societal barriers such as community attitudes towards domestic violence victims, inadequate police and justice responses, lack of safe and affordable housing, and inflexible work arrangements and childcare for single mothers (Diemer et al., 2017; Halket et al., 2014). Given these difficulties, some women cope with escalating physical violence, emotional conflict, coercive control, and social isolation by distancing themselves from their spouse and using other outlets for emotional support and physical safety (Zink et al., 2006). Gambling venues, which are often comfortable social outlets with daycare centers, extended trading hours, and security staff, present an environment that women coping with IPV can find attractive (Hing et al., 2017). Within these venues, electronic gaming machines (EGMs or pokies) offer women an immersive emotional escape from their problems but pose a significant risk of further harm and addiction (Thomas & Moore, 2003). This chapter highlights how male partner violence can contribute to problem gambling when women victims use gambling as a coping mechanism or gambling venues as "safe spaces."

DOI: 10.4324/9781003203476-37

Methods

We interviewed 24 Australian women whose IPV victimization was linked to their own harmful gambling. Participants were recruited from services that provide counseling for people experiencing financial hardship, problem gambling, and family violence. Analysis occurred using the Grounded Theory extension, Situational Analysis (Clarke, 2018). The full methods and findings are detailed in Hing et al. (2020). Here, we present two case studies that shed light on the context and complexities of IPV victims using gambling venues as safe spaces. All names in the case studies are pseudonyms.

Findings

Julie's Story

Julie is a professional in her 60s and has been married to Richard since she was in her early 20s. Julie believes that marriage is forever, its purpose is to have children, and it forms the fundamental support structure for children. Richard lost his white-collar job early in the relationship and took up farming. Financial hardship ensued and Julie has borne the burden of working to support the family as well as running the household and raising their two daughters.

Richard soon became depressed, an alcoholic, and resistant to medical or psychological help. Most afternoons Julie would come home to a drunk husband, and the children locked in their rooms. Fights would escalate over his drinking and Richard began stealing from Julie to buy alcohol. He became emotionally abusive and threatened to hit her on a few occasions. He put her down, gaslighted her, and criticized her mothering and housekeeping skills:

As for the violence business, it was shocking, it was horrid ... He sometimes did stupid things, like hitting a wall and breaking it, or breaking something else ... Calling me an idiot ... he tried to make me doubt myself, and that wasn't very hard to do, because I did not have a very high opinion of myself ... So, when he criticised me or made any kind of a comment about my mothering, or housewife skills, it really hurt, and I would curl up like a fish worm.

Julie blames herself for Richard's unhappiness and violence and feels that Richard may have been happier if she had complained less about their situation. She felt unsupported by family or friends who suggested she was making life hard for everyone and should just leave the relationship. She did not tell them the full extent of her relationship problems and his abuse.

Julie found excuses to stay back at work to avoid the conflict at home. One day Julie decided to call into her local club on the way home.

From going from total loneliness ... There were all these people, and free snacks, and lights, and noise and music; and I thought, "Oh, this is nice."

Julie's feelings of loneliness and low self-worth temporarily disappeared as she interacted with the friendly hospitality staff.

At the time, it wasn't gambling, it was just an excuse to spend time in this lovely environment, which was so welcoming, and unlike anything else I had to go to … Girls would come over to wipe your table, and they'd say, "How's your day going?" … Otherwise nobody would have talked to you all day … Just loved it.

The club offered little more than gambling and drinking, and as Julie no longer drank alcohol, she started playing the pokies. She enjoyed the ambience of the gaming room, the simple interaction with the cashiers and other patrons, and the thrill of exploring new games. The repetitive and hypnotic effect of the EGMs would allow Julie to disassociate every afternoon after work. Julie developed a gambling addiction that continued for many years.

I started using the pokies … but it rapidly got, I felt, out of control. You know, "Just one more. Just one more. It's just about to pay out." That sort of stuff. I started with $5 notes, and then it was $20 notes, and I couldn't see how I was going to control that. So, I was frightened by the gambling. So, in the end, I cut it off, and I haven't been back. And I still have trouble. I want to, and I won't, and that's where we are now.

She has never told anyone about her gambling addiction. She still cohabits with Richard, who continues to drink. She has found limited success with counseling services or medication for her ongoing depression but is managing to successfully resist her ongoing urges to gamble.

Brenda's Story

Brenda had gambled only a few times in her life before she started a new relationship when aged in her early 40s. Her new partner, Roy, quickly started using violence against her, hospitalizing her several times in the first 18 months. After they moved to a new town, Brenda had no family or friends nearby. Roy forbade Brenda from answering the phone, insisted she pays for most expenses and treated her with contempt when he felt like it. Brenda told how he had held her down on the floor and urinated on her. Roy was "a big drinker" and went to the pub frequently. His violence became "a fairly regular event" especially when he was affected by alcohol.

He would come home … and he had that glassy eyed look. I just knew if I closed the drawer the wrong way, or if I didn't answer a question correctly, I was going to cop a backhander … you couldn't pacify that. There was no reasoning with him when he had that glassy-eyed look.

Brenda sometimes went to the pub with Roy, but she did not like to drink much and instead started playing the pokies and keno. She found that if she won and gave him money, he would not become violent even if he had been drinking.

> *That's actually how it started. He was at the bar having a drink ... So, I'll go and play the pokies. It was great. You'd have a win and it's wonderful, and then he'd be happy. It started that if I had a win, I'd give him money ... Effectively, try and buy his affection ... For me, it became, "alright, I've had a win, it will be fine."*

Brenda continued gambling in the hope of winning so that she could please Roy and avoid his abuse. At the same time, she became increasingly anxious about the relationship. She discussed her low self-esteem, concerns that Roy would leave her for someone else, and feeling that she constantly needed to win his approval: "everything became focused on the relationship and how can I make this better, and I can change him, and things will be okay if I make him happy." She played the pokies to relieve her anxiety and numb her worries, but soon found that her gambling was becoming a habit.

> *It was like a relief to watch the things spin around ... the old brain freeze ... the anxiety just quietly dissipates and – oh I got two little Indian fellas and I've won something – and that was refreshing from everything else that was going on. It was relief and a distraction ... I could escape. I didn't have to think ... Then it became habitual. You start chasing the money.*

As Roy's violence "got worse" and "psychotic," Brenda sought physical safety in gambling venues whenever she saw "that look in his eyes" or whenever he went out drinking. She recounted a typical episode.

> *He walked in the door and he started an argument ... emotional abuse ... he said I was horrible and stupid and useless ... he'd leave me there feeling like absolute crap ... I was then thinking oh my God, what is he going to be like when he gets home? ... He's probably going to come home drunk ... So, I would run away ... and play the pokie machines ... I wouldn't leave until the club was closed and maybe he was home and hopefully asleep. Then, I would creep in and go to bed in the spare room ... because I didn't know what I was in for ... Basically, I would stay away to avoid confrontation.*

Roy also used violence when Brenda lost at gambling. She recounted: "he said 'did you lose it all?'. He just gave me a hell of a hiding with this walking stick ... He broke it into three pieces over my back and the back of my legs."

Brenda lost about $90,000 from the sale of her house on the pokies in 18 months. With no money and nowhere else to live, it was difficult for her to leave, even though the police had warned her that "you've got to leave him before he kills you." After he tried to drown her after pushing her into the backyard swimming pool, she finally escaped to a refuge, and eventually moved to a different town close to her parents. With support from family and friends, as well as counseling, Brenda managed to regain control over her gambling but still struggles with gambling urges and the legacy of her victimization. She reflected:

> *It's been quite a few years for me, and it's taken a long time to get a handle on it ... every now and then I get that urge where I just want to go and sit and get lost with a pokie machine. But I pull myself up ... To this day, it's still has scars. It's an ongoing battle and it's not something that leaves tomorrow. It does not go away overnight.*

Discussion

Julie's and Brenda's stories highlight the role that expressions of gender inequality play in male violence against women, including stereotypical gender expectations and a sense of entitlement in some men to exercise power and control over their female partners (Our Watch et al., 2015). Their stories also show how the harmful use of alcohol can greatly exacerbate this violence and reveal the added complexity when victims and/or perpetrators experience mental health issues such as low self-esteem, anxiety, and stress.

The case studies particularly highlight the attraction of EGMs for women looking to gain emotional respite from an abusive partner and from relationship and domestic pressures. EGMs have well-known immersive qualities that facilitate absorption and dissociation, and many players describe escaping into a trance-like "zone" during play where they can temporarily forget life's problems (Livingstone, 2005). Continuing to play may become the primary goal, with money losing its usual value except as a means to sustain play and time out from a difficult reality (Schüll, 2012). Due to these immersive qualities, EGM gambling can become a means of avoidance-based coping, and individuals are at heightened risk for problem gambling if they frequently play EGMs to self-regulate negative emotions (Scannell et al., 2000). Women are particularly drawn to EGMs to gain an emotional escape from stress, anxiety, boredom, loneliness, and difficult life circumstances (Hing et al., 2017). Gambling venues can also reduce the social isolation often experienced by women experiencing IPV. Julie's story especially highlighted the social connection that venues can provide for women, particularly interactions with venue staff. These frequent but often superficial connections help reduce social isolation, while allowing women to maintain their privacy and keep their domestic problems hidden.

The case studies also highlight the attraction of gambling venues for women seeking a safe physical space to avoid their partner's abuse. EGM venues are highly accessible throughout suburban Australia, and they are often the only venues open late at night where women might feel welcome, reasonably safe, and socially accepted (Hing et al., 2017; Rintoul et al., 2013; Thomas et al., 2011). However, while venues might provide physical safety, a woman's gambling and subsequent losses can result in further violence from a male partner. In the two case studies, abuse from their partner preceded the women's development of a gambling problem, demonstrating how IPV can catalyze and exacerbate harmful gambling. Women can then become caught in a reinforcing cycle of gambling and abuse, where the abuse prompts further gambling by the woman, with her partner then responding with more violence. Further, as shown in Brenda's case, gambling might be seen as a way to avoid violence by generating wins that buy a temporary reprieve. This desperation to win can further fuel gambling and loss chasing by a victim of IPV. An Australian examination of crime and gambling harm reported that women were advised by some specialist help services to use gambling venues to escape IPV (Campbell, 2017). Julie's and Brenda's stories show the real dangers of this approach. Not only is there a risk of gambling addiction, financial harm, and violent backlash, women who use emotional-focused coping behaviours, like gambling, are more likely to stay in the IPV situation (Zink et al., 2006).

Conclusion

Women who use gambling to cope with IPV or use gambling venues as safe physical spaces to escape from violence have been neglected in the broader literature on problem gambling and on violence against women. Julie's and Brenda's stories demonstrate how women can become trapped in violent relationships and turn to gambling to cope with their situation. Best-practice guidelines such as those available here (https://www.anrows.org.au/wp-content/uploads/2020/12/ANROWS-Hing_Gambling-and-DFV-Practice-Guide.pdf) should be available to specialist services, including counseling and domestic violence services, to reduce the additional risk of harm to women.

References

Australian Institute of Health and Welfare. (2019). *Family, domestic and sexual violence in Australia: Continuing the national story 2019*. Cat. no. FDV 3. Canberra: AIHW. https://www.aihw.gov.au/getmedia/b0037b2d-a651-4abf-9f7b-00a85e3de528/aihw-fdv3-FDSV-in-Australia-2019.pdf.aspx?inline=true
Campbell, E. (2017). Compulsion, convergence or crime? Criminal justice system contact as a form of gambling harm. https://apo.org.au/node/116126
Clarke, A.E. (2018). *Situational analysis: Grounded theory after the interpretive turn* (2nd ed.). Los Angeles: SAGE. https://us.sagepub.com/en-us/nam/situational-analysis/book238990

Diemer, K., Humphreys, C., & Crinall, K. (2017). Safe at home? Housing decisions for women leaving family violence. *Australian Journal of Social Issues*, *52*(1), 32–47. 10.1002/ajs4.5

Halket, M.M., Gormley, K., Mello, N., Rosenthal, L., & Mirkin, M.P. (2014). Stay with or leave the abuser? The effects of domestic violence victim's decision on attributions made by young adults. *Journal of Family Violence*, *29*(1), 35–49. doi:10. 1007/s10896-013-9555-4

Hing, N., Nuske, E., & Breen, H. (2017). A review of research into problem gambling amongst Australian women. In H. Bowden-Jones, & F. Prever (eds.). *Gambling disorder in women: An international female perspective on treatment and research* (Ch 18, pp. 235–246). London: Routledge. https://www.routledge.com/Gambling-Disorders-in-Women-An-International-Female-Perspective-on-Treatment/Bowden-Jones-Prever/p/book/9781138188327

Hing, N., O'Mullan, C., Nuske, E., Breen, H., Mainey, L., Taylor, A., ... & Rawat, V. (2020). *The relationship between gambling and intimate partner violence against women: Research report*. Sydney: ANROWS. https://20ian81kynqg38bl3l3eh8bf-wpengine. netdna-ssl.com/wp-content/uploads/2020/09/RP.17.01-RR-Hing-GamblingDFV.pdf

Livingstone, C. (2005). Desire and the consumption of danger: Electronic gaming machines and the commodification of interiority. *Addiction Research & Theory*, *13*(6), 523–534.

Our Watch, ANROWS, & VicHealth. (2015). *Change the story: A shared framework for the primary prevention of violence against women and their children in Australia*. Melbourne: Australia. https://media-cdn.ourwatch.org.au/wp-content/uploads/sites/ 2/2019/05/21025429/Change-the-story-framework-prevent-violence-women-children-AA-new.pdf

Rintoul, A.C., Livingstone, C., Mellor, A.P., & Jolley, D. (2013). Modelling vulnerability to gambling related harm: How disadvantage predicts gambling losses. *Addiction Research & Theory*, *21*(4), 329–338. 10.3109/16066359.2012.727507

Scannell, E.D., Quirk, M.M., Smith, K., Maddern, R., & Dickerson, M. (2000). Females' coping styles and control over poker machine gambling. *Journal of Gambling Studies*, *16*(4), 417–432. 10.1023/a:1009484207439

Schüll, N.D. (2012). *Addiction by design: Machine gambling in Las Vegas*. Princeton: Princeton University Press. https://press.princeton.edu/books/paperback/9780691160887/ addiction-by-design

Thomas, A.C., Bates, G., Moore, S., Kyrios, M., Meredyth, D., & Jessop, G. (2011). Gambling and the multidimensionality of accessibility: More than just proximity to venues. *International Journal of Mental Health and Addiction*, *9*(1), 88–101. 10.1007/ s11469-009-9256-7

Thomas, A., & Moore, S. (2003). The interactive effects of avoidance coping and dysphoric mood on problem gambling for female and male gamblers. *Journal of Gambling Issues*, *8*. 10.4309/jgi.2003.8.16

Zink, T., Jacobson, C.J., Pabst, S., Regan, S., & Fisher, B.S. (2006). A lifetime of intimate partner violence: Coping strategies of older women. *Journal of Interpersonal Violence*, *21*(5), 634–651. 10.1177/0886260506286878

Chapter 31

Women's Participation in "Card Circles" in Remote Australian Aboriginal Communities

Megan Whitty and Charlotte Boyer

Gambling practices of women in minority groups are often characterized as being multifaceted and informal in nature, which contributes to them not being widely researched or understood. This chapter illustrates possible reasons why women living in remote Aboriginal communities in Australia may engage in card-based gambling and the implications of such activities. Narrative interpretation and data analysis bring together qualitative evidence to show the context and cultural complexities in which Aboriginal women play cards. Focussing on card circles primarily as a social activity, we also explore how gambling-related harms can present in this population setting.

Introduction

In Australia, gambling is widely recognized as a public health issue that can have serious adverse effects on individuals, families, and communities, including those arising from a gambling disorder. However, gambling is also a popular recreational activity that can have important social, recreational, and communal functions that should not be overlooked. Due to the unique social and regulatory characteristics of Aboriginal communities, gambling is a common public spectacle. Aboriginal people are reportedly at greater risk of experiencing gambling-related harm (McMillen & Donnelly, 2008), even more so for those living in remote, compared to non-remote, areas (Fogarty, 2013; Stevens & Young, 2009). Research into the nature, extent and impact of gambling in remote Aboriginal communities is relatively limited but one prominent example is unregulated community card games (Fogarty, 2013; Stevens, 2017). Card gambling may be perceived as "endemic," dysfunctional, and contributing to many community harms, but for Mob[1] it is often seen as an innocuous way to socialize, pass the time, combat boredom, and make money.

Early research suggests that women, whether they be Tiwi people (Goodale, 1987), Wik (Martin, 1993), Gunwinggu (Altman, 1987), or Kimberly[2]

DOI: 10.4324/9781003203476-38

(Hunter & Spargo, 1988), were the main participants in card games. Card gambling using small stakes in long slow games is still seen primarily as women's gambling. This chapter explores gender identity, motivations, and social interactions being played out in remote Aboriginal community card circles.

Methods

This case study is based on qualitative data collected as part of the Northern Territory Gambling Project.[3] A total of 114 interviews with community members and services providers were conducted in 3 remote Australian Aboriginal communities[4] from 2017 to 2019. Full study details and research findings are reported elsewhere (Paterson et al., 2020). Restorying is a form of narrative data analysis that employs a three-dimensional space approach (Connelly & Clandinin, 2000). This technique uses three aspects (interaction, continuity, and situation) to create a "narrative text that promotes an account of participants' lived experiences" (Ollerenshaw & Creswell, 2002). The following vignette, describing women playing cards in a remote Aboriginal community, represents a number of individual stories that have been condensed into one narrative. All names are pseudonyms and italics indicate verbatim quotes.

Findings

It is three o'clock on a Tuesday afternoon and six women are sitting under a large tree. The shade provides some relief from the scorching desert sun. The women are engaged in a complicated game of klinka[5] while a throng of small children play and skip around in the dust beside the card circle. The women – aged between 19 and 55 – are all from one extended family group. The conversation centers on community gossip (new romances, which relatives are visiting, who is fighting with whom).

All the women have come to the card circle today for different reasons. Kylie, the youngest present, sits with a sleeping baby in her lap. She is a first-time mum. Her own mother died when she was young. She comes to play as much to ask for advice and gain support from the older aunties, as to try and double the pay check from her partner's part-time job. Kylie's older cousin Milika sits next to her. An attractive woman in her mid-30s, Milika is explaining to the compassionate ears and downcast eyes of the group ...

He's threatening me again, making me go look for money for grog.[6] Saying "you don't make any money today, I will kill you." He wants me to play cards to win money and if I don't take money home this time, he'll punch me.

Rosanna looks across at her brothers' daughter who is speaking. She has seen the bruises on her face and arms before. Last week Rosanna had taken her to the Safe House again, after being woken by the frantic but familiar tapping on her window. Milika nursed a black eye and Rosanna a hot cup of tea, as they waited together in the early morning for Night Patrol to come.

Mavis waited impatiently for the conversation to change, looking forward to more local gossip, she thinks to herself – ... that's why family play cards, to communicate and be happy. That's what some do. I do that to communicate too, to be happy. The big cycle there when you're losing money, it goes around to family, because if you're a gambler, that's you in the middle, then there's a circle around it. That could be yourself and your family around you. Because we've all got brothers and sisters, nieces and nephews, sons and daughters, and uncles and aunties.

Ria, perched on the milk create, also likes these "friendly games." When the money being gambled is communal in a sense, and if you lose – it's okay because someone in the family will win and the money therefore is not really "lost." She will always have enough for her kids to get a coke and hot chips for dinner from the store next door.

Sylvie is the most serious gambler playing today; she never misses the opportunity to throw her money into a card game and is always the last to stop playing. Her mood is intense, her frustration at slow games obvious. The others know she would play until three or four o'clock in the morning if she could. They leave it with her, it is her business, and no one wants to disrespect the elder matriarch. There is nothing much going on in the community this time of year anyway, and card playing is a way to pass the time, win some extra money, and sometimes teach the kids about counting.

Hours pass this way, people come and go but the game never skips a beat. The shade from the tree has disappeared into the darkness of the night. The women continue to play cards, bathed in the bright light of the community's only store. The new store floodlights are not facing the road in front, they are trained on the block beside the small carpark, where the women sit and a number of other card circles have sprung up.

There is serious anticipation as the crowd watching the game next to the women grows in size and intensity. They also play Klinka but stakes in the neighboring game are much higher. Even though it is unlikely that the tension will turn into genuine conflict, the women (with the exception of Sylvie who is chasing last games losses) agree it is a good hand to end on. They slowly stand, brush the fine red dust off their long, brightly colored skirts and walk the short distance to their homes. They will meet tomorrow for another game and another day of conversation around the card circle.

Discussion

Gambling is visible in many Aboriginal communities, particularly in remote parts of Australia, where vast distances, limited infrastructure, and persistent poverty mean access to alternative forms of entertainment is relatively restricted (Breen et al., 2010; Fogarty, 2013). For some women in such settings, card circles provide a safe space (most often not afforded in over-crowded housing) for lengthy conversations about day-to-day life: gossip, joys, worries, and discussions regarding local politics and community issues (Fogarty, 2013). For others, who are addicted or rely on winnings to subsidize the household income or fund their (or an intimate partner's) alcohol or cannabis use, the consequences of card games are more worrying.

When analyzing the motivations and social regulation of gambling, it is important to consider that gender plays a significant role. Research into community level gambling in other rural and remote settings, such as in South Africa, has also focused on women as a vulnerable group because of their significant levels of participation in informal or illegal gambling activities (de Vries, 2017). Be it unregulated card games, such as in remote Aboriginal communities in Australia, or increased commercial gambling activities resulting from a more globalized market, significant harms can arise for women who have a gambling disorder. For example, a Canadian study focusing on Aboriginal women's experiences of social trauma and gambling disorder highlights how the former creates a desire to escape life problems which contributes to the development and maintenance of the latter (Hagen et al., 2013).

Back to our example, the most prominent form of gambling-related harm in Australian Aboriginal communities where gambling is commonplace is the negative impact it has on children. Indeed, our research indicated that the concern expressed most consistently across fieldwork sites was the neglect of children as a result of the amount of time, money, and attention afforded to card games (Paterson et al., 2020). A key finding of our evaluation was that community members and service providers alike, recognized the multifaceted harms gambling can have on children. Such harms – including issues of nutrition, education, and safety – need to be acknowledged and addressed.

Conclusion

Our story briefly explores possible reasons why Australian Aboriginal women participate in card-based gambling (see Figure 31.1): to engage with networks, for enjoyment, to reduce boredom, to escape stress, and – of course – to win money. Card circles can be a site of complex social, economic, and political processes in remote Aboriginal communities. It is important to understand the benefits and the harms of such a culturally imbued practice.

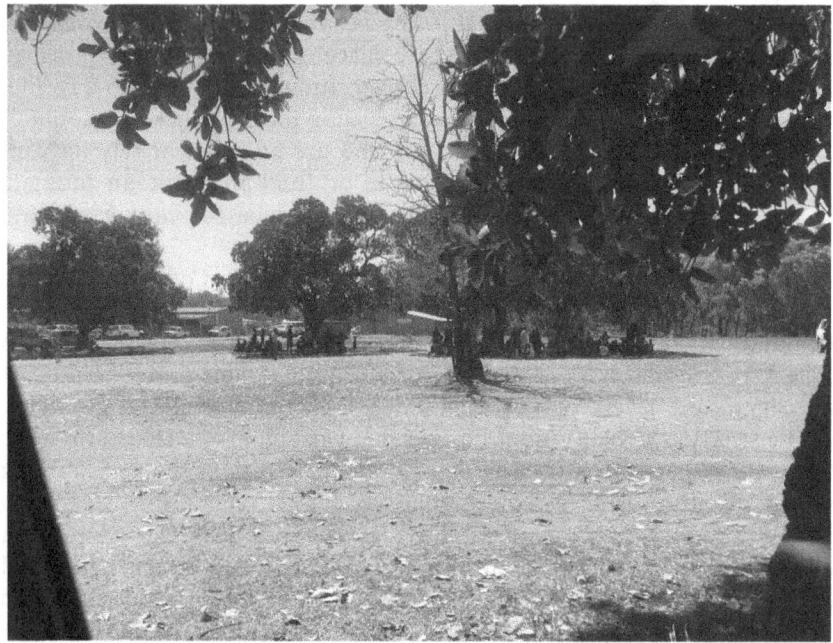

Figure 31.1 Bush Casino. Central desert community, 2019.

Notes

1   "Mob" is a colloquial term identifying a group of Aboriginal people associated with a particular place or country. Mob can be used in reference to one's family group, clan group, or wider Aboriginal community group. www.deadlystory.com
2   Tiwi, Wik, Gunwinggu, and Kimberly are all names of Aboriginal language families or groups.
3   Funded by the Northern Territory Department of Business, Australian Government.
4   Pmara Jutunta and Willowra in Central Australia, and Wurrumiyanga, Tiwi Islands. Ethics approval was granted from the Central Australian Human Research Ethics Committee and the Australian National University Human Research Ethics Committee.
5   *Klinka* is a popular card game played with four people who use picture and number cards to gain sets, similar to poker.
6   Common Australian slang for beer or alcohol.

References

Altman, Jon C. (1987). *Hunter-gatherers today: An Aboriginal economy in north Australia.* Australian Institute of Aboriginal Studies Canberra.
Breen, H., Hing, N., & Gordon, A. (2010). *Exploring indigenous gambling: Understanding indigenous gambling behaviour, consequences, risk factors and potential interventions.* (pp. 1–242). Lismore: Southern Cross University.

Connelly, F. Michael, & Clandinin, D. Jean. (2000). Narrative understandings of teacher knowledge. *Journal of Curriculum and Supervision, 15*, 315–331.

de Vries, L. (2017). Gambling amongst South African women: An exploration of the impact of gambling over the past twenty years. In *Gambling disorders in women*. Routledge.

Fogarty, M.A. (2013). *From card games to poker machines: Gambling in remote Aboriginal communities in the Northern Territory*. Charles Darwin University.

Goodale, J.C. (1987). Gambling is hard work: Card playing in Tiwi society. *Oceania, 58*, 6–21.

Hagen, B., Kalishuk, R.G., Currie, C., Solowoniuk, J., & Nixon, G. (2013). A big hole with the wind blowing through it: Aboriginal women's experiences of trauma and problem gambling. *International Gambling Studies, 13*, 356–370.

Hunter, E.M., & Spargo, R.M. (1988). 'What's the big deal?: Aboriginal gambling in the Kimberley region'. *Medical Journal of Australia, 149*, 668–672.

Martin, D.F. (1993). Autonomy and relatedness: An ethnography of Wik people of Aurukun, western Cape York Peninsula.

McMillen, J., & Donnelly, K. (2008). Gambling in Australian Indigenous communities: The state of play. *Australian Journal of Social Issues (Australian Council of Social Service), 43*, 397–426.

Ollerenshaw, J.A., & Creswell, J.W. (2002). Narrative research: A comparison of two restorying data analysis approaches. *Qualitative Inquiry, 8*, 329–347.

Paterson, M., Boyer, C., Stevens, M., & Whitty, M. (2020). *NT gambling project: Development and pilot of a health promotion initiative addressing gambling harm in Indigenous communities in the Northern Territory*. Final Report. Canberra, Australia: The Australian National University.

Stevens, M. (2017). 2015 Northern Territory Gambling Prevalence and Wellbeing Survey Report (Menzies School of Health Research & the Northern Territory Government: Darwin).

Stevens, M., & Young, M. (2009). Betting on the evidence: Reported gambling problems amongst the Indigenous population of the Northern Territory. *Australia and New Zealand Journal of Public Health, 33*, 556–565.

Index